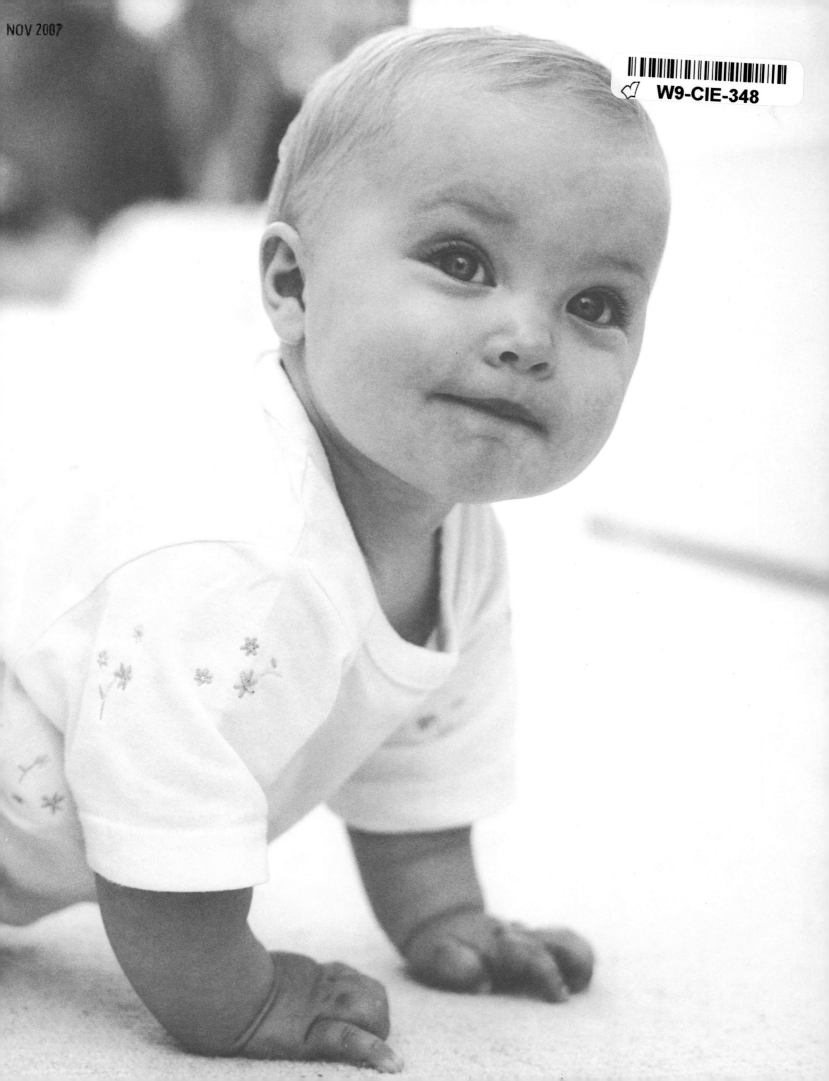

BABY & CHILDCARE
the pure and natural way

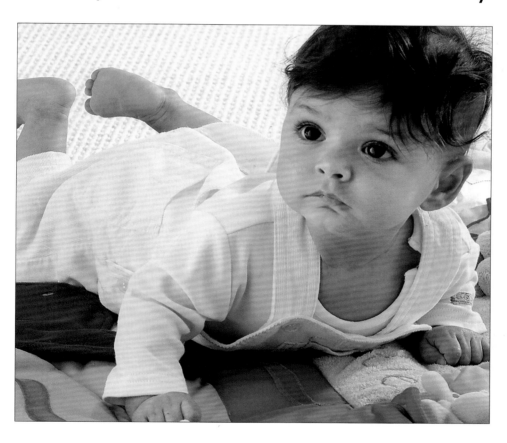

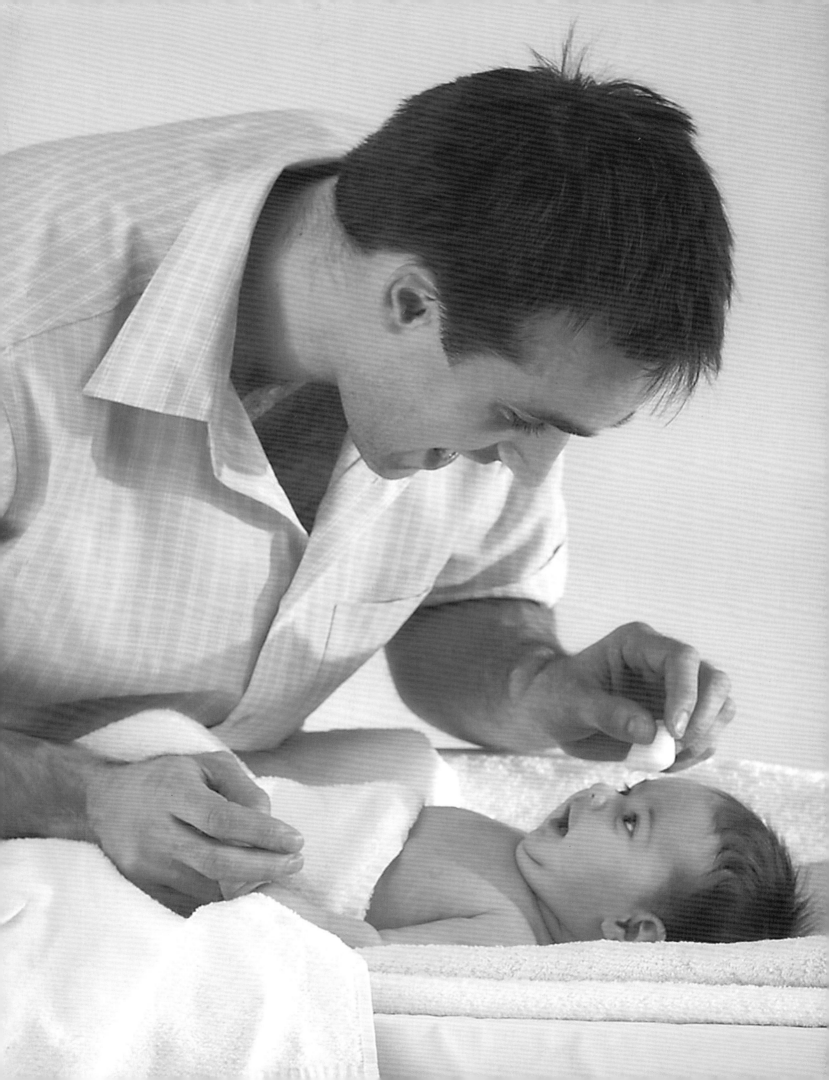

BABY & CHILDCARE
the pure and natural way

raising your baby and child the way nature intended, from
birth right through to the age of 5

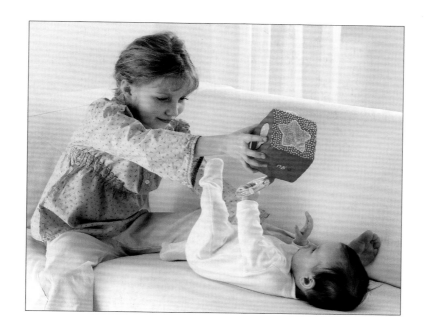

Kim Davies

LORENZ BOOKS

contents

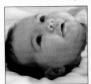

Introduction

There is nothing more natural than having a baby, and many parents would tell you that there is no life-experience more rewarding. The sense of achievement that many women feel when they look back on childbirth is unlike any other – even if the birth turned out very differently than they expected, and forty years after the event, most fathers can remember every detail of the moment they saw their child being born.

The birth of your child, however, is just the beginning of the journey of being a parent. Raising a son or daughter is a lifelong project, one that involves, over the course of the years, thousands of separate judgments and decisions that will affect the way your child grows up, and the kind of person he or she becomes. Those decisions, when repeated across the population, also have far-reaching effects on the world at large. For example, there is an ecological price to be paid if everyone, or nearly everyone, exclusively uses disposable nappies (diapers).

This book is intended to help parents to make choices that are soundly natural, responsibly ecological and roundly sensible. Childcare, like any other social activity,

Breastfeeding is the most natural way to feed your new baby, and there is plenty of support out there to help you get the hang of it, and continue.

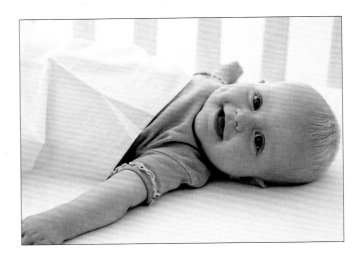

Parents have to make thousands of decisions when they bring up their children. But ultimately the most important thing is that they feel loved and special.

is subject to fashion – but this book is not a trendy guide to green parenthood, and has no ideological axe of its own to grind. The aim of the book is primarily to give parents the means to bring up their children in a way that does as little harm to the environment and the community as possible, but more importantly in a way that is also good for the child.

Natural remedies can help you treat some of the common ailments that all children often experience.

Your physical closeness, loving touch and communication are three of the most precious gifts you can give your child.

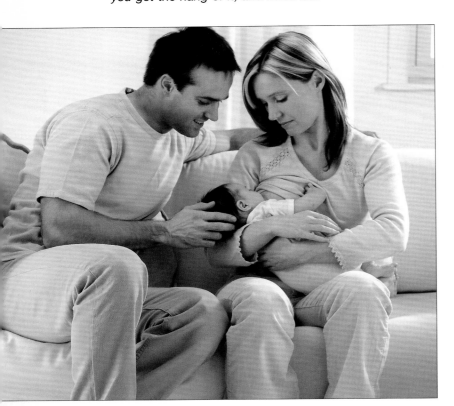

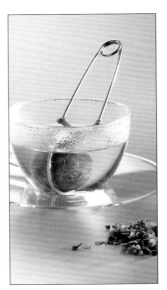

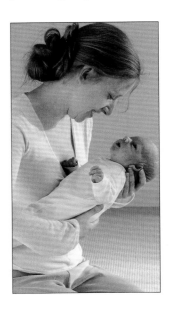

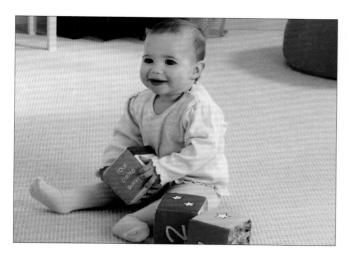

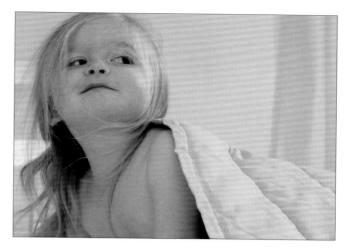

Children have a natural curiosity about the world, and need the chance to explore it through sight, smell, touch, hearing and taste.

Every child has a unique personality that needs to be nurtured and appreciated. The fun of parenthood is in discovering who your child really is.

In practice, natural childcare is an amalgam of old practices (such as cooking real meals rather than using jars of processed babyfood) and of the best new thinking in paediatrics (such as the revelation that cold, fresh air is the best treatment for croup). There is nothing regressive about using time-honoured methods, nor is it a denial of modern technology. The claim, for example, that breastmilk is the best food for your baby is undeniable; but formula milk and other options are there if you cannot manage it at any point. And the business of using 'real' nappies is much easier in today's society than it was a generation ago: there are washing services, there are shaped nappies with poppers that are almost as easy to put on as disposables. All these nappy options are better for the world and, crucially in this instance, better for your

baby's skin than the bleached, indestructible, chemical-rich disposables that were once seen as a mother's best friend, and the only option readily available.

Any mother or father who aims to take a natural approach to childcare will find much guidance in these pages – but this is not a manual, and the advice contained in the book should not be seen as a blueprint. From the moment of birth, every child is an individual with a unique personality and set of circumstances, and every parent has an instinctive way of caring for their child. The most natural thing a mother or father can do is to rely on their growing knowledge of their own child's way of being, to learn from experience as much as possible, and above all to trust to instinct. Follow these principles, and you won't often go far wrong.

You can protect your child from exposure to many household chemicals by using essential oils and items such as oil and vinegar instead of ordinary cleaners.

Healthy eating starts young. Feeding your child good, healthy food now will stand him or her in good stead for many years to come.

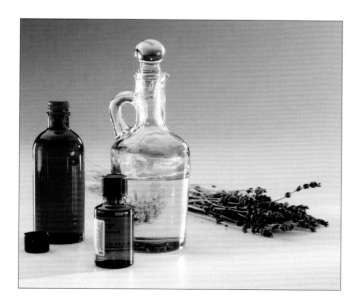

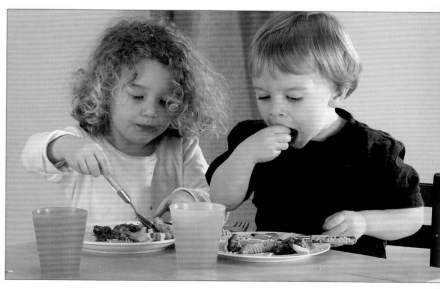

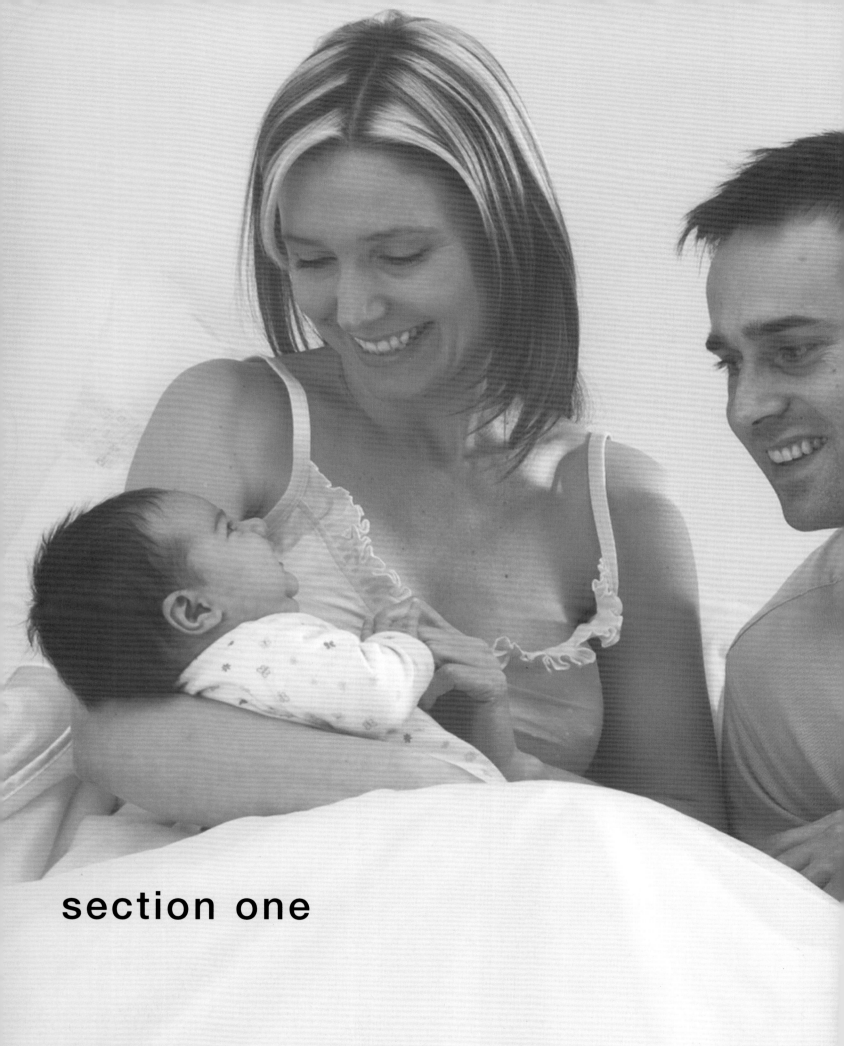

section one

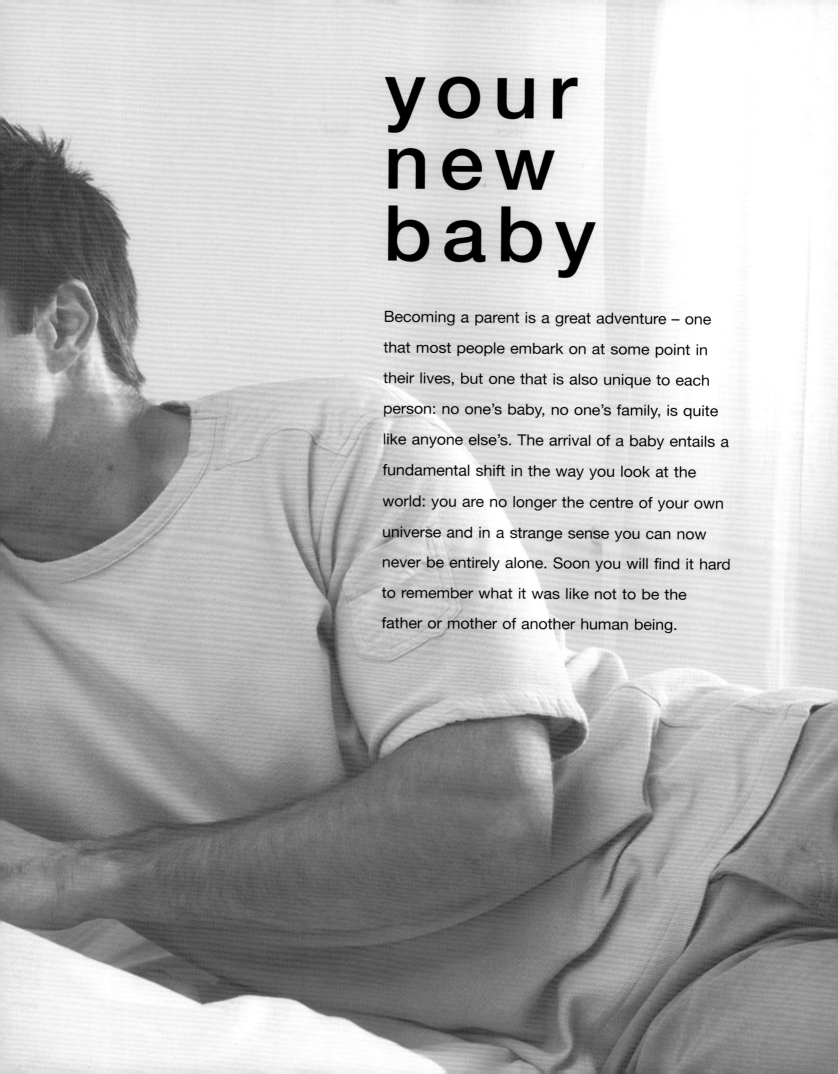

your new baby

Becoming a parent is a great adventure – one that most people embark on at some point in their lives, but one that is also unique to each person: no one's baby, no one's family, is quite like anyone else's. The arrival of a baby entails a fundamental shift in the way you look at the world: you are no longer the centre of your own universe and in a strange sense you can now never be entirely alone. Soon you will find it hard to remember what it was like not to be the father or mother of another human being.

The first days and weeks

" No two babies, not even twins, are the same, and yours will have likes and dislikes right from the start. "

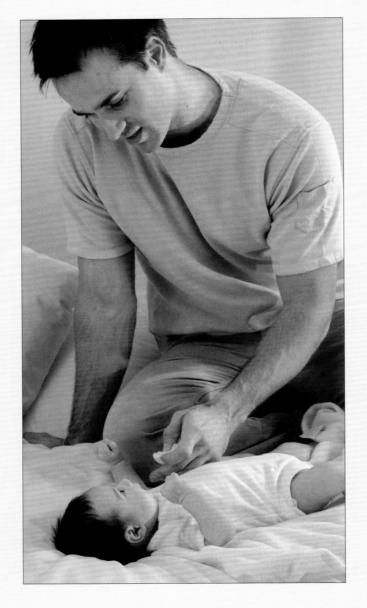

The weeks after a child is born are a time of great transformation for your family. If this is your first baby, you and your partner have stepped over the threshold of parenthood. Here at last is the baby you have been looking forward to for so long. Your life – wonderfully and irreversibly – will never be the same again.

It will help you to enjoy and appreciate this special time if you can give it the importance it deserves. Spend as much time as you can together as a family, limit your visitors to those who will help and support you, and try to let go of other anxieties and concerns – work, money, family problems and so on. Above all, rest and recuperate as much as you can.

There will inevitably be moments – or even long interludes – when you feel you have taken on an almost impossible task. It is entirely normal and extremely common to struggle with fatigue and disorientation at first. You may have feelings of confusion or even despair when, say, your baby is crying and you don't know why. All new parents

The most important thing that a new father can do is to spend time with his baby and partner. Most hospitals will leave the family alone to facilitate bonding.

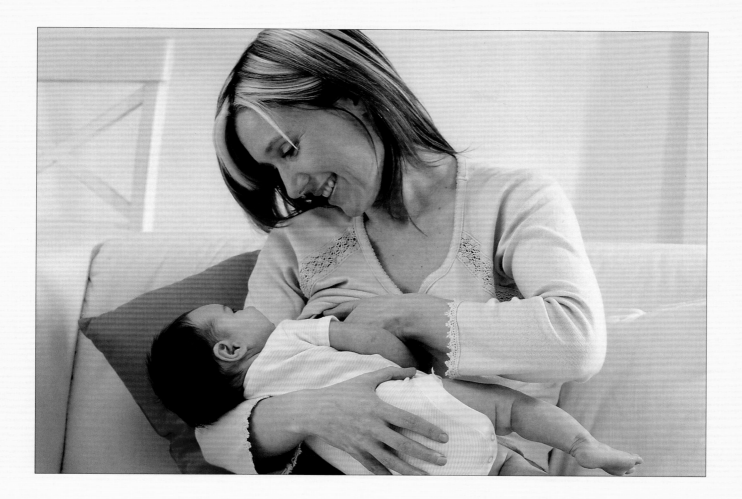

know this experience, and there will come a time when you can look back on the sleepless nights with a rueful smile.

It helps to remember that your child is a unique individual. No two babies, not even twins, are the same, and yours will have likes and dislikes right from the start. You will need to experiment to discover exactly how your baby likes to be held, and whether stroking or patting, for example, soothes him or her more easily. This is much easier if you take a flexible approach, rather than trying to follow a set routine from the outset. Spending these first weeks observing, listening to and cuddling the baby will help you to get to know your child and to understand his or her needs in a way that will store up benefits for the months and years to come.

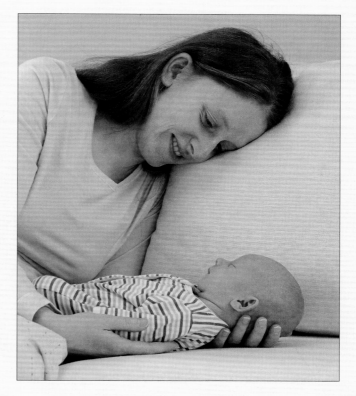

Top: Spend plenty of time getting to know your new baby. An alert baby will be just as curious about you and will gaze upon your face.

Some mothers fall in love with their babies at the first instant, but many women find that they take longer to form a really close attachment.

Bonding with your baby

A lot is said about the importance of bonding straight after the birth, and it is wonderful if the new family can be given the quiet and privacy they need to enjoy these first moments together. Your baby has been propelled from the dark, familiar cocoon of the mother's womb into a bright and noisy world, and is being bombarded with new sensations. In your arms is the most comforting and reassuring place to be.

The hour or so after delivery is also the ideal time to start breastfeeding. It not only encourages bonding but also stimulates digestion and ensures that the baby gets the protective benefits of the first milk (colostrum) straight away. Babies practise the sucking movement while in the womb, and if placed on the mother's stomach may find their own way to the nipple using their sense of smell.

At this time bright lights should be dimmed to create as relaxing and unobtrusive an environment as possible. Any weighing or non-urgent checks should wait, so that mother and baby can get to know each other. The room should be warm so that the baby can be placed naked on the mother's bare skin. If the father is there, he shouldn't feel that he has to immediately rush off to telephone relatives with the news. It is far more important that he stays to share the first few minutes of his baby's life. Everything else can wait.

All babies need loving touch. Research shows that premature babies who are stroked gain more weight, are more responsive and spend fewer days in hospital.

WHEN BONDING IS DELAYED

In the past, mothers and babies in hospital were separated soon after the birth to allow the mother to rest. Fathers' visiting rights were strictly limited. Bonding is now seen as so important that midwives and hospital staff do everything they can to facilitate a new family's need for time alone together. But the safety and health of the baby and mother come first, and if the delivery has been tricky or there are concerns about either, they may have to be separated for a while.

Even if the mother is physically close to her newborn, she may not feel the rush of love that she may have expected. She may be too exhausted from the labour and delivery to be able to feel anything other than relief that it is over; she may be in pain or shock or feeling woozy from the effect of drugs, or she may feel initial disappointment if the child is, say, a boy rather than a girl or has a physical defect such as a hare lip or a birthmark. If she had strong ideas about the type of birth she wanted and it turned out differently, she may be distracted by disappointment and less able to appreciate the beautiful baby in front of her.

Similarly, the father may have found the birth a much more distressing experience than he imagined, especially if there were complications. He may be too worried about his partner to feel much for his child. He may be disturbed

Many new mothers find that they cannot sleep the night after the birth, because they don't want to miss a minute of the child's first hours of life.

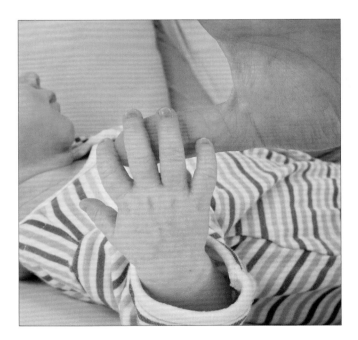

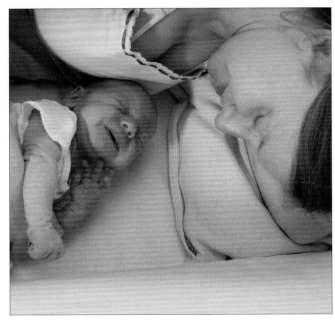

to find that the blood-streaked, blotchy newborn that he sees before him does not match the image of the angelic-looking baby he expected. And the realization that he is now responsible for this tiny being may feel overwhelming rather than exciting.

Some parents feel guilty if they do not feel instant love for their baby, and being separated from the child early on can be devastating. But it is a mistake to think that any delay in the bonding process will have a permanent effect on your relationship.

Bonding often starts slowly and grows over time. There is nothing special that you need to do to help this process along. It will unfold naturally as you get to know your baby, as you learn about his or her likes and dislikes, and – especially – as you tend to the baby's needs: changing, cleaning, bathing, comforting, rocking and feeding. Your baby will not remember those first hours of life, but over the months and years that follow will gradually become aware of being encompassed by your love and care.

SPECIAL CARE

Some babies need to be looked after in a special care unit. It can be very hard to see your baby in an incubator or covered in tubes. But even if you cannot yet bring the baby home, there is a lot you can do. Spend as much time as possible by your baby's side, talking softly so that he or she gets to know your voice. Hold the baby's hand and stroke him or her through the holes in the side of the incubator. Cuddle the baby as much you are able: skin-to-skin contact helps to regulate a baby's heartbeat, body temperature and breathing, and it is very calming.

Breastfeeding helps you to bond. It gives you the satisfaction of knowing that you are giving your baby the best possible nourishment and is also the one thing that you can do for your child that nobody else can. If the baby can't be taken out of the incubator, then you can express milk to be given through a tube. The hospital should help you to do this by lending you an efficient breast pump and giving you privacy to use it. It can be hard to establish a good milk supply by expressing alone, so ask for support from a breastfeeding counsellor.

Occasionally a baby needs to be taken to a different hospital for special care while the mother is too ill to travel. This is very distressing, and it will help if the father can become the main carer for a while. If you are a mother in this situation, it is important to remember that you will be able to start the bonding process later on. In the meantime, keep a photograph of your baby with you. Some hospitals use webcams so that parents can see their babies even when they cannot be with them.

Holding a young baby can feel daunting at first. It takes several weeks before new parents feel confident about handling their baby.

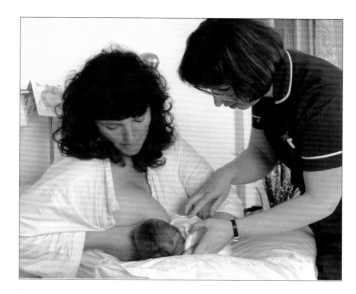

Nursing your baby soon after birth gets breastfeeding off to the best possible start. The antibodies in colostrum will help to protect your newborn from infection, and babies who are nursed early on may be less likely to develop sucking problems later.

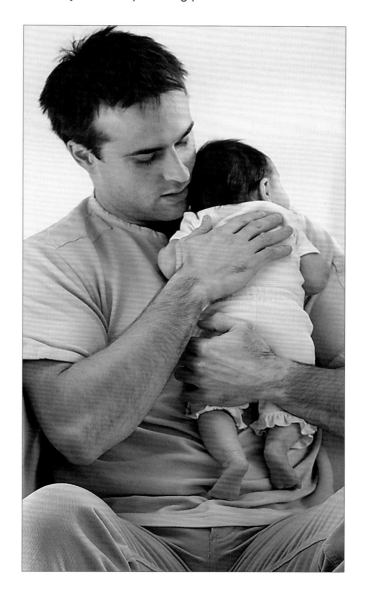

Your newborn baby

Not all newborn babies are cherubic visions of beauty. Their heads may be an odd shape after the birth (especially if the delivery was by ventouse or forceps) and their noses may look squashed. Their eyes may be puffy; their skin (especially if they were overdue) may be wrinkly and flaky, look greasy or be covered in downy hair, and it may have a bluish hue. Their genitals may be slightly swollen. All these strange features are normal and will start to disappear over the next few days and weeks.

WHAT YOUR BABY CAN SENSE

Babies enter the world fully equipped to apprehend and understand their environment. That is, they are in possession of all five senses – sight, hearing, smell, taste and touch – and begin to use them straight away.

Touch. Babies need touch in order to thrive. Your baby is most sensitive to touch around the mouth. Even tiny newborns respond well to gentle stroking, and older babies usually enjoy massage too.

Smell and taste. Research shows that babies have a natural preference for sweet tastes right from the start. They react to smells in the same way as adults: they recoil from bad odours and are drawn to sweet ones. They also quickly learn to differentiate their mother's smell from that of other people.

Hearing. Babies respond to sound in the womb, and may recognize music that they heard regularly before birth. But it is voices that they like best, and they show a preference for their mother's voice above all others. They also show dislike for certain sounds and will jump if they hear a sudden loud noise.

Seeing. Newborns find it easiest to focus on objects 20–30cm/8–12in away – roughly the distance of your face when you hold a baby in your arms or breastfeed. Babies show the most interest in faces, but are also fascinated by simple patterns.

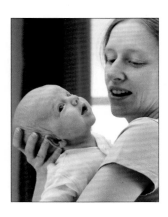

Babies don't have the muscle power to hold up their heavy heads, so you must keep a newborn's head well supported at all times. Gradually, the muscles in the neck grow stronger and they will be able to support the head, but watch out for sudden lapses as the head lolls.

YOUR BABY'S REFLEXES

A newborn baby is entirely dependent on your care, but is born with some instinctive reactions designed to help him or her survive.

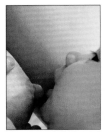

Rooting, sucking and swallowing: If stroked on the cheek, a baby will turn and search for the nipple (this is called rooting). Babies suck when they feel pressure on the hard palate in the mouth, and swallow automatically.

Gripping. If you put a finger in your baby's hand, he or she will grasp it. Your baby will also curl the feet if the soles are touched. These reflexes are left over from our primate ancestors, who needed to cling to their mothers' fur. They gradually develop into a deliberate holding action.

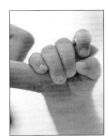

Crawling. When placed on their tummies, babies will curl their legs and arms beneath their bodies and may even produce a crawl-like movement. Gradually your baby's body uncurls from its foetal position and he or she will lie flat.

Stepping. If they are held so that their feet touch a firm surface, newborn babies will lift one foot after another in a stepping motion. This reflex disappears after a few days, and has to be re-learnt many months later when it is time to learn to walk.

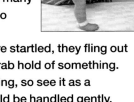

Startle reflex. If newborns are startled, they fling out their arms and legs as if to grab hold of something. Your baby finds this distressing, so see it as a reminder that he or she should be handled gently. The reflex disappears at about two months.

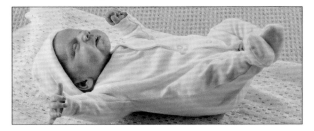

Lifting and putting down your baby

Babies need to be held securely and comfortably in the first few weeks, until their neck muscles have developed enough for them to support their own head. Always lift your baby slowly and gently to avoid startling him or her.

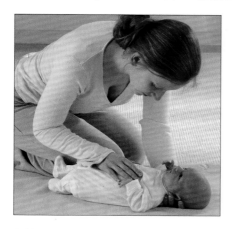

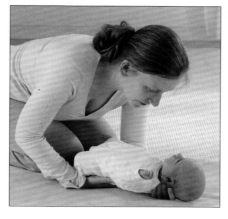

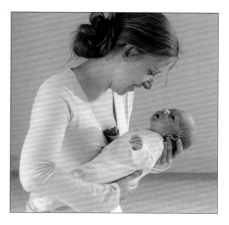

1 Alert the baby to your presence first by speaking softly, and putting your hand on their tummy. Lean over so that your body is close to the baby, and slide one hand under the head and neck.

2 Slide the other hand under the lower back and bottom. Take the baby's weight into your hands, and then bring him or her slowly towards you. When your baby is resting on your chest, begin to sit upright.

3 When putting the baby down, hold him or her close to you as you bend over. This means that the baby doesn't have to travel too far in mid-air. Keep your hands in position for a while before sliding them out.

HOW YOUR BABY COMMUNICATES

As helpless as newborns are, they can communicate in a way that almost guarantees they get their basic needs met: they cry. At first your baby's cries will all sound the same to you. But in time you may notice that he or she makes different sounds depending on what is wrong, and you may learn to distinguish between, say, a cry that means "I'm hungry" and one that says "I'm in pain". After a few weeks, your baby will also start to communicate pleasure, by gurgling, cooing and making other repetitive little noises.

The person who looks after the baby most often – usually a parent – will probably see the first smile, which comes by about six weeks. At first babies will smile at any face – including a picture of one – by three months they smile more readily at the people they know best.

THE FONTANELLE
The bones of a newborn's skull have not yet fused together. The gaps between the bones, called fontanelles, are covered by a tough membrane and can't be damaged by normal handling. The largest one is on the crown of the baby's head, you may be able to see a pulse beating through it. This fontanelle can indicate a baby's state of health. If it is sunken, the baby is dehydrated and needs fluids urgently. A bulging fontanelle is another sign of illness, which also needs immediate medical attention.

Carrying your baby

When carrying your baby, both of you need to feel confident and secure. There are two safe ways to hold your newborn baby: the shoulder hold, which is good for winding and for general carrying around, and the cradle hold, which is a soothing way to nurse your baby.

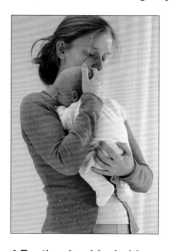

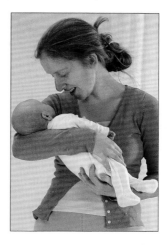

1 For the shoulder hold, support the baby against your chest, so that his or her head leans against your shoulder. Use one hand to support the bottom and back, and keep the other behind the back and head to stop the baby jerking backwards.

2 To use the cradle hold, hold the baby by resting his or her head and shoulders in the crook of your arm, and use your other hand to support the bottom and lower back. Newborn babies will feel most safe and secure held closely against your body.

The first weeks

In many cultures, it is traditional for the mother to stay indoors for 40 days after the birth – one for each week of pregnancy. During this time she is released from the burden of household chores, given special foods to restore her strength and encouraged to stay in bed to bond with her infant. Bedouin Arabs, Jews, Somalis and Latin Americans all observe 40 days of seclusion, while Chinese women "do the month".

Until very recently, western women were also encouraged to rest after giving birth – your grandmother probably spent a week or two "lying-in", either in hospital or at home. But today new mothers are under immense pressure to get back to normal, regain their figures and show the baby off to all their relatives. This makes the first weeks after childbirth more exhausting and stressful than they need to be.

When you are caring for a small baby it is easy to forget to drink enough. Have a jug or bottle of water to hand.

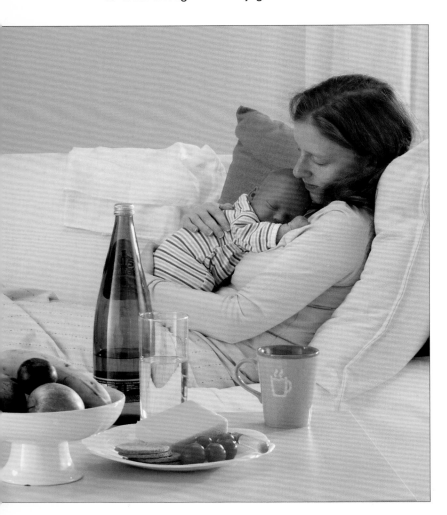

RESTORATIVE TEA

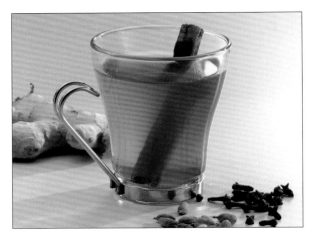

A spicy hot drink can invigorate and energize you. This mixture includes raspberry leaf tea, which encourages the healthy contraction of the womb, and nettle tea, which is a traditional tonic. Drink up to three cups a day.

3 cardamon pods
3 cloves
5cm/2in stick of cinnamon
2.5cm/1in chunk of ginger, sliced
3 tsp raspberry leaf tea
3 tsp nettle tea

Put 750ml/30fl oz water in a small, lidded pan and add the spices. Bring to the boil, cover and simmer for 10 minutes. Add the teas to the spice mixture, steep for 10 minutes then strain into a flask to keep warm. Drink when required.

A MODERN LYING-IN

It makes sense to withdraw from society for a while so that you can concentrate on your new baby. Everyone's idea of lying-in will be different, but it can be helpful to do the following, at least for a week or two.

Stay at home and don't get dressed. Pyjamas or a nightie are much more comfortable to wear than day clothes, and they help to remind you (and any visitors) that you are resting.

Make your bedroom the centre of your existence. Have everything you need close at hand – water, a bowl of fruit, healthy snacks, phone, books or magazines – to make this time pleasurable.

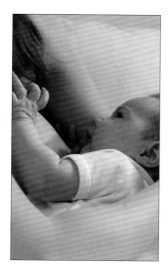

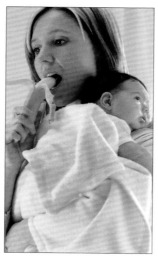

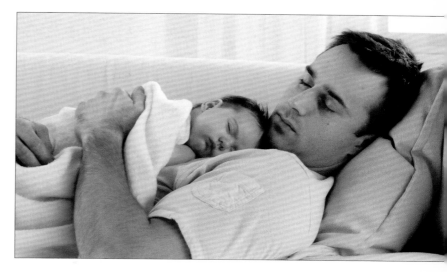

A new baby is happiest cuddled close against the breast. If the contact is skin to skin, even better, as your scent will add to the feeling of security.

If you are going to be on your own at home with a new baby, make sure you have plenty of healthy food that is quick to prepare and easy to eat.

Fathers will also need to get rest whenever they can. It is tempting to fall asleep together on the sofa, but don't, as the baby could become trapped between cushions.

Keep your baby with you all or most of the time. Follow his or her rhythms – feed the baby on demand, sleep when he or she sleeps.

Have another adult around. Ideally, the father will be at home to look after you and share the care of the baby. But if that isn't possible, ask your mother, best friend or another person close to you to stay.

Eat well. Have at least one hot meal a day (cooked by someone else) and lots of healthy, easy-to-prepare snacks at other times – fruit, cereal, yoghurt, oatcakes, smoked salmon, cold meats and so on. Make sure you drink lots of water.

Limit first visitors to close friends and family. For the first few weeks, arrange visits at times that are convenient to you, and keep them short. Ask your partner or supporter to encourage people gently to leave if you start to get tired.

If people offer help, accept it. Ask them to bring you a cooked meal or do some housework, so that you and your partner can concentrate on the baby.

Keep your first outings short and pleasurable. It is quite normal to feel a little strange at first. Many traditional cultures have a celebration at the end of the seclusion period, which serves not only to welcome the new baby but also to help reintegrate the mother into the world.

LOVING CARE FOR YOUR BABY

Looking after a newborn can feel daunting, not least because new parents are inundated with advice. Do ignore suggestions from well-meaning friends and relatives if they don't feel right for you at this moment.

What works for one baby doesn't necessarily work for another, and women who had their babies years ago – including your own mother and mother-in-law – may have ideas that are out of date.

The most important thing is to spend lots of relaxed time with your baby, concentrating completely on him or her, with no distractions, so that you get to know each other. Gradually, you will discover how to tell when the baby is hungry or tired, how he or she likes to be carried and what is most soothing, being rocked or shushed for example. This takes time, and it is important to trust your own instincts as you learn. In the meantime, the following pointers may help.

Babies thrive on physical contact. Cuddle your baby as much as you can, and limit the amount of time spent in a bouncy chair or pram.

Prioritize breastfeeding. As well as meeting your baby's basic needs for food and drink, it brings you physically close and helps with bonding.

Don't spend longer than an hour or two away from your baby. It's natural for mothers to want to be near their newborns, but other people can confuse you by telling you that you need time to yourself, and grandparents in particular may push to "have a turn" at looking after the baby. Don't worry about other people's needs just now, and give in to this kind of pressure only if you really feel that you need a break.

The father is important, too. For the first year or so, the mother is usually at the centre of her baby's world, but the father will develop a much closer relationship with his child if he is involved in day-to-day care: changing nappies (diapers), cleaning, bathing and comforting. Fathers are often better than mothers at soothing babies who are distressed or windy, because the babies pick up on their mothers' anxiety.

Common problems for infants

Even the most beautiful and natural of births is physically gruelling for the baby, who is pushed and squeezed down the narrow birth canal. So it is not surprising that newborns are often bruised and marked and sometimes have bloodshot eyes. These little blemishes will fade in a few days and need no treatment.

If you have had a forceps or ventouse delivery, the baby's head may be misshapen for a while. This too will correct itself naturally. However, a baby who has had an assisted delivery may have a headache for a few days, which can make him or her cry more than normal. Lots of cuddling and nursing will help. If your baby continues to be very fractious, then gentle massage can help. It may also be worth taking the baby to a cranial osteopath, who can gently correct any distortions in the skull.

BIRTHMARKS

Some babies are born with a birthmark that is permanent. Three in every thousand have a pink or purple port-wine stain. This often occurs on the face, and is very occasionally linked to problems such as epilepsy. It can be upsetting when your child has a birthmark of this nature, and it may take time for their parents to come to terms with it. However, port-wine stains can be treated with lasers which can radically improve their appearance. Very occasionally, a baby is born with a raised brown mole. It's important to keep an eye on this and seek medical advice if it changes colour, shape or size: a mole can be surgically removed if there is cause for concern.

Breastmilk has natural antibacterial properties, so it is the perfect cleanser for a newborn's sticky eye.

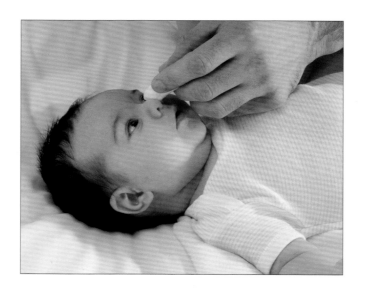

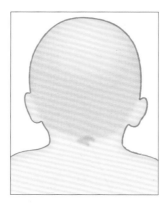

It is thought that stork marks may be the result of pressure on the head once the baby engages.

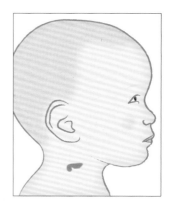

Strawberry marks can be quite prominent, but they usually fade and then disappear in a few years.

TEMPORARY BIRTHMARKS, SPOTS AND RASHES

Stork marks are so-called because it is fancifully said that they are caused by the beak of the mythical stork that delivers babies. They are pink or red marks on the brow, eyelids or back of the neck, which become more prominent when the baby cries. They gradually fade but can take up to two years to disappear completely.

Strawberry marks are red marks that start off flat and gradually become raised, increasing in size. They can be present at birth or develop a few days later. They have usually gone by the time the child is two or three. Mongolian spots are blue or grey patches that can appear on the buttocks or back. They affect black or Asian babies, and usually disappear by the end of the first year.

Most newborn babies develop minor skin problems in their first weeks. Heat rashes (tiny red spots) are very common because babies have immature sweat glands and are unable to control their temperature efficiently. If

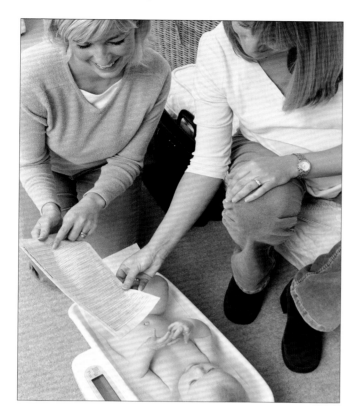

Babies may be weighed often in the early weeks to see that they are growing normally. Frequent checking can feel rather stressful for the parents, but so long as the overall weight gain is steady and your baby looks fit and healthy, there is nothing to worry about.

the sweat glands become blocked, tiny white spots (milia or milk spots) appear. They will disappear of their own accord in a few weeks. Do not pick at them or you may cause infection.

STICKY EYE

The eyes of newborns can produce a sticky, yellowish discharge. If this occurs in the first day or two it usually means they have picked up an infection in the birth canal. Use a cotton-wool pad (cotton ball) soaked in cooled, boiled water, or breast milk, to clean each eye, wiping from the nose outwards. See a doctor if it persists.

JAUNDICE

More than half of newborn babies develop jaundice two or three days after the birth. This is not a disease but a symptom: it means that bilirubin (a pigment produced by the body when red blood cells are broken down) has built up in their system. Usually the liver processes bilirubin, but a baby's immature liver is unable to cope with all the extra bilirubin produced when large amounts of red blood cells are broken down after the birth.

In most cases, the signs of jaundice are a yellowing of the whites of the eyes and the skin (which usually starts on the head and spreads down the chest and stomach).

Your midwife should check for jaundice but do point it out if you are concerned. Usually, no treatment is needed, and the jaundice clears up in a week or two. (In premature babies, who develop it five to seven days after the birth, it can take up to two months to disappear.)

If your baby's jaundice reaches the arms and legs, or there are other symptoms such as difficulty sucking, sleepiness, dark urine or pale stools, see your doctor promptly. Occasionally jaundice can have a serious cause, such as liver problems. The usual treatment is light therapy (phototherapy), which is done in hospital, but very occasionally a blood transfusion is needed.

INFECTED UMBILICAL CORD

It can take up to four weeks for the stump of the baby's umbilical cord to shrink and drop off, leaving a small wound that will heal in a few days. Doctors sometimes advise dabbing the stump with rubbing alcohol to prevent infection, but recent research suggests that it is best left to dry by itself. Clean the area around the stump daily with cooled, boiled water and pat dry with a clean towel. Fold down the top of the nappy so that air can reach the area. This will help it to heal faster. If the stump starts to ooze pus or smell, or the surrounding area becomes red, see a doctor, who will prescribe antibiotic cream.

THE SIX-WEEK CHECK

Babies are checked from head to toe soon after the birth and again six weeks later. At the six-week check, you'll be asked about your baby's feeding and sleeping patterns, as well as what you have noticed about his or her hearing and vision. The baby will be weighed (naked) and measured, and the results plotted on a centile chart to see how he or she compares with the national averages. The baby's vision, head control and muscle tone will be systematically checked and a hearing test may be done. The doctor will also look at your baby's eyes, heart, spine, hips and genitals to ensure all is well.

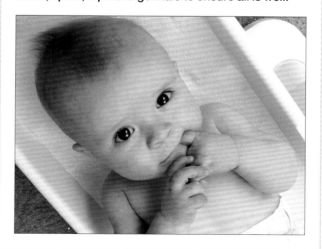

Common problems for new mothers

Every woman needs time to recover from giving birth. Even if you have had a natural vaginal delivery with no tearing, you are likely to feel bruised and tired. You may have aches and pains in odd places, especially if you had an active birth in which you moved around a lot. And, of course, your body is adjusting to the fact that you are no longer pregnant: your womb is shrinking back to its normal size, your hormone levels have dropped and your breasts are producing milk to sustain your new baby.

Much of the discomfort experienced by new mothers can be eased with the help of natural remedies. None of the remedies given will interfere with breastfeeding. However, it is important to see your doctor or midwife if you have severe pain or are worried about any symptom.

Afterpains are often at their most intense when you are breastfeeding, because this triggers the release of the hormone oxytocin, which encourages the womb to contract. Sit in a relaxed position and breathe slowly and deeply and relax your muscles to ease the cramp.

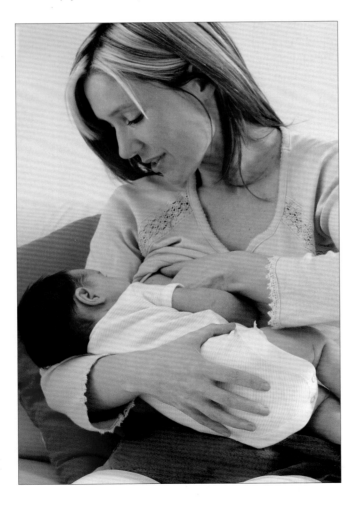

EXERCISING THE PELVIC FLOOR

You probably did pelvic floor exercises while you were pregnant, and it is important to continue after childbirth. Contract the muscles around your vagina and anus and imagine drawing them upwards (as if you were stopping yourself from urinating in mid-flow). Hold the squeeze for a few breaths then release slowly. Try to do this ten times or more, several times a day.

AFTERPAINS

Many women experience cramp-like pains in the abdomen when the womb starts to contract. These start within hours of the birth and usually last three days at most (often less). Afterpains can be intense, particularly during breastfeeding. They also tend to be stronger with second and subsequent children, as the womb becomes increasingly stretched.

There are simple things you can do to ease the discomfort: a warm bath or a warm hot-water bottle held against the abdomen help to relax the muscles. Sipping a soothing herbal tea such as chamomile, or an antispasmodic one such as ginger or crampbark, may also help. Raspberry leaf tea, so useful for strengthening the womb before childbirth, also helps it to readjust afterwards. Some women swear by the homeopathic remedy Mag phos, and Chamomilla can also be helpful.

SORE PERINEUM

If you have had a natural birth, your perineal area will have been stretched, so it will feel sore and bruised. Homeopathic Arnica tablets are excellent for treating the bruising, and will also help with any shock resulting from the birth. Doing your pelvic floor exercises will speed healing, since these encourage blood to flow to the area.

Take one or two warm baths a day to encourage healing and give you a few precious minutes to yourself; dilute a few drops each of tea tree and lavender oil in a carrier oil and add to the water. For immediate relief, apply a pad of cotton wool (cotton ball) soaked in witch hazel. Alternatively, use a home-made icepack (made by wrapping ice in a plastic bag then covering it in two layers of kitchen paper or a cotton cloth), but don't use this for longer than ten minutes at a time.

As you urinate, pour a jug of lukewarm water over the perineal area to prevent stinging. Pat rather than wipe it

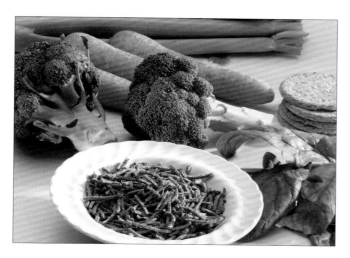

Include plenty of fresh vegetables and wholegrain cereals, including oats and bran, in your diet before and after childbirth to ensure that you get enough fibre and help prevent constipation.

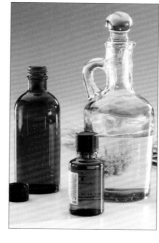

Lavender and tea tree oils can help the healing of tears or cuts. Add 2–3 drops to a warm bath.

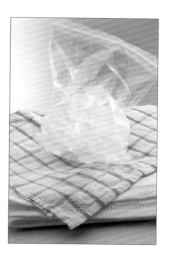

An ice pack – applied for up to ten minutes – can bring welcome relief to a bruised perineum.

dry. Many women worry about how it will feel when they move their bowels for the first time. You may be concerned that your stitches will tear, but be assured that they won't. However, the first bowel movements after childbirth will be more difficult if you are constipated, so drink plenty of fluids and eat lots of fruits and vegetables.

HAEMORRHOIDS

Even if you got through pregnancy without developing haemorrhoids, also called piles, they may well develop when you are pushing down in labour (about one-third of women get them after a vaginal delivery). If you don't have any itching or pain, you can leave them to heal naturally, but taking warm baths and doing pelvic floor exercises will be helpful.

The homeopathic remedy Hamamelis is often recommended for itchy or painful piles. You can apply a pad soaked in witch hazel to the area: this is cooling and

The homeopathic remedy Chamomilla can help with afterpains. You could also try sipping a cup of chamomile tea three times a day.

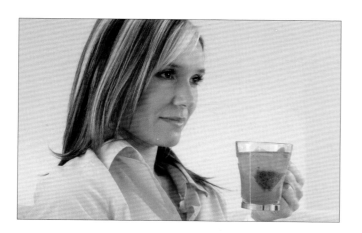

encourages shrinking. You can smooth Calendula cream on the piles between compresses. It's important to avoid becoming constipated (see above), since this will exacerbate the problem. Wash the area with water and pat dry after each bowel movement.

AFTER A CAESAREAN

If you had your baby by Caesarean section, recovery will take a little longer than with a natural birth – you have had major abdominal surgery, after all. You'll be encouraged to get moving as soon as possible in order to start the healing process, and you may be given gentle exercises to practise. But you will have to be careful about how you move and should avoid lifting anything heavier than your baby for at least six weeks. You should not drive for at least a month. Check this with your insurance company.

It is important to keep the Caesarean scar clean and dry. Frequent baths will help with healing; adding lavender and tea tree essential oils may prevent infection. Carefully pat the area dry afterwards, or use a hairdryer on a low setting. Arnica tablets are good for bruising and shock. Once the scar has healed, you can massage it daily with lavender oil and vitamin E oil diluted in a blend of almond and wheatgerm carrier oils.

THE POSTNATAL CHECK

All new mothers are invited to a check-up with their doctor about six weeks after the birth. This is usually done in tandem with the baby's six-week check. You'll be asked about how you are recovering and the doctor will examine you to see if any tears have healed. This is a good time to voice any concerns you have about any aspect of your recovery.

Handling your emotions

Giving birth is an incredible experience, often the most powerfully emotional event of a woman's life. But there is little time for you to reflect on it because there is a tiny, vulnerable baby needing round-the-clock care. Not surprisingly, the first few days after the birth can be a very emotional and bewildering time for both parents. You may feel exhilarated and joyous, exhausted and overwhelmed, proud and fearful, often in quick succession.

As a new mother, it is helpful to remember that your hormones are out of balance, and the physical opening of the body for childbirth has affected you on a deep emotional level. In a way, it would be odd if you felt utterly serene and completely in control as you adjust to the new person in your life.

BABY BLUES

About half of all new mothers get very tearful or anxious a few days after the baby is born, and it is common to experience mood swings. These "baby blues" are probably due to the sharp drop in hormone levels, and they may also be connected with feelings of anticlimax after the intensity of the birth. The most helpful way of dealing with them is to relax, and allow yourself to feel the emotions. Cry if you need to, and be open about how you are feeling to your partner or to a good friend.

A healthy diet, with red meat for iron and oily fish for essential fatty acids, can help you to manage difficult emotions after the birth, and helps breastfeeding too.

EMOTIONAL STRENGTH PLAN

The baby blues are usually temporary, but can sometimes come and go over a few weeks. Prioritize your physical needs – eat healthily and often so that your blood-sugar levels don't drop, drink plenty of fluid and sleep whenever your baby does.

Good nutrition can help with depression. The fatty acids in oily fish help maintain a healthy nervous system; calcium (found in dairy products, green vegetables, nuts and seeds, beans and lentils) and magnesium (nuts and seeds, green leafy vegetables, wheatgerm, sprouted grains, soy beans and whole grains) are also helpful. Check your iron levels – anaemia makes you feel lethargic and one study found that low iron levels could hamper bonding. Liquid iron is more easily digested than tablets, while good nutritional sources are lean red meat, oily fish, pulses, nuts, dark green vegetables and dried fruit. Vitamin C helps your body to absorb iron: citrus fruits are a good source. In addition, doing the following will help keep you in good emotional health and will help you to get through any periods of unhappiness or low spirits.

- Be open about how you are feeling with your partner, close friends and health professionals.
- Talk to your midwife about the birth experience. This can be very useful if you have any ambivalent feelings about your labour or delivery.
- Treat yourself to a postnatal massage or acupuncture treatment. Some complementary therapists will come to your home.

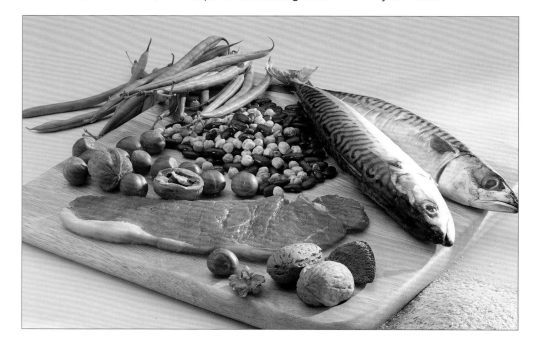

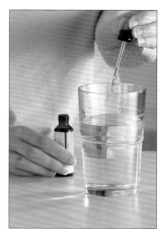

Rescue Remedy is a good instant remedy for any feelings of anxiety, panic or fearfulness.

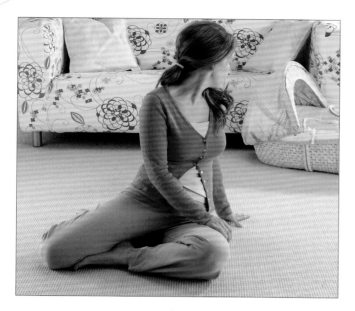

Yoga, or gentle stretching exercises, can have a calming effect and may help to counter feelings of depression.

- If you are on your own with the baby, make sure you see somebody every day. If you feel low, do some physical exercise every day, such as brisk walking and postnatal yoga. After six weeks – provided you get the all clear from your doctor – try a gentle postnatal circuit class or go swimming.

POSTNATAL DEPRESSION

Quite different to the baby blues, postnatal depression (PND) can start weeks or months after the birth, and can be long-lasting. It can make a woman feel so exhausted and lethargic that looking after the baby feels an impossible task, and it may cause anxiety and strong feelings of inadequacy. Fathers can also sometimes suffer from depression after the birth of a child.

Depression is hard to diagnose because it is normal to feel low and inadequate from time to time, but if feelings like this persist for more than a week or so you should seek medical help. There are various treatments for postnatal depression. Practical help, counselling, support groups and, if necessary, medication can all be helpful.

FIRST DAYS AS A DAD

It can be hard to be a new father. You are the parent of a tiny baby, which can feel overwhelming. Your relationship with your partner is likely to feel very different for a while and you may feel excluded by the bond between mother and child, especially if the baby is being breastfed. As new mothers tend to be tired and hormonal, your partner may seem irritable and unappreciative at first. The thrill of fatherhood is no less real or satisfying than the joy of

A new father may feel thrilled with his tiny child, but have moments of feeling overwhelmed or panicked too.

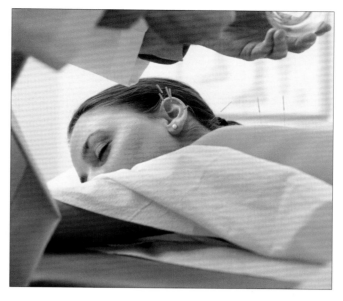

An acupuncture treatment can help you to feel more balanced after the exertion of giving birth.

motherhood, however, and most fathers quickly carve out a role that is all their own, such as taking charge of bathtime or the first change of the day. Such things – however mundane they seem at the time – lay the foundation for the special and unique relationship between a man and his child.

Once the initial month or two are past, you will find that the presence of your child adds a whole new dimension to your relationship with your partner. Your baby is, after all, a tangible and constant sign of your love, a wonderful lifelong link between you.

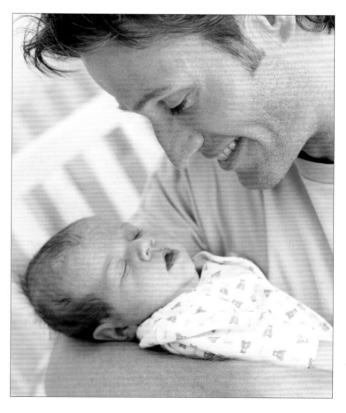

Basic baby care and feeding

" Breastfeeding naturally binds mother and baby together, making them inseparable for the first months of a child's life. "

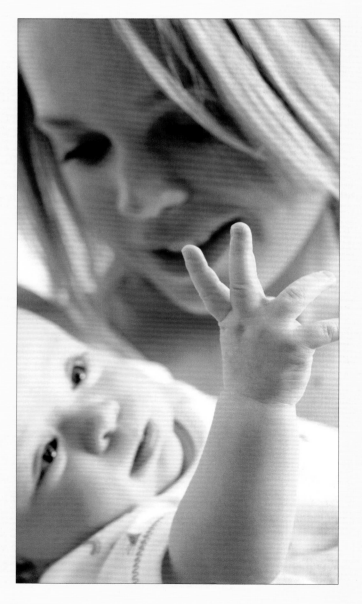

Lots of people talk about the hard work involved in looking after a baby. And it is true that a small baby requires almost constant care and attention. But there is also great pleasure to be had from lovingly attending to your child's needs.

These needs are, generally, pretty straightforward. Babies want feeding, probably more often and more erratically than you can imagine; they need changing when they are wet or dirty; they need to be kept warm; and they need to be held so that they feel safe. All these things are easily done, but the way you go about them can make all the difference between enjoying caring for your baby and finding it a burden or chore.

For instance, changing a nappy (certainly one of the less pleasant aspects of parenthood) is much more than a messy cleaning task. It is, in a strange way, a means of communicating your feelings towards your baby. When you put a towel on the cold changing mat to make it more comfortable, or speak soothingly as you touch and clean your baby, you are

A new arrival brings change and excitement to the wider family, as well as the parents. Siblings will want to be involved in caring for the new member of the family.

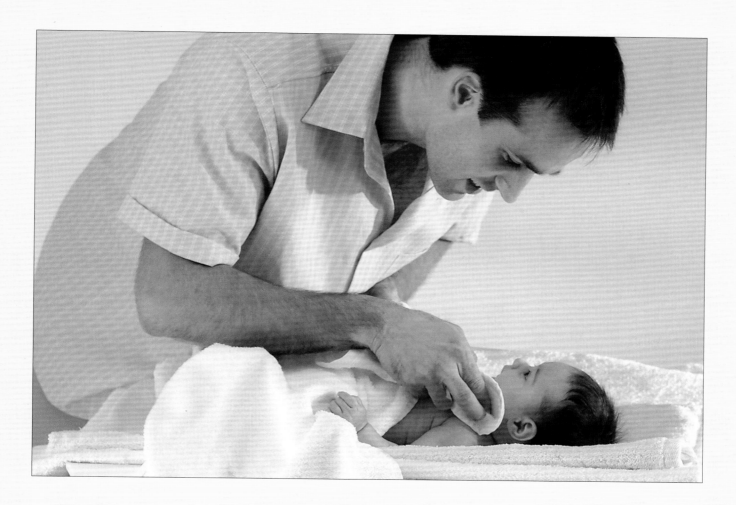

working to make the experience a positive one. Such attentiveness both requires and builds the loving tenderness a parent feels for his or her child.

Nature, through breastfeeding, has provided women with the perfect way to nurture their babies. Breastfeeding naturally binds mother and baby together, making them inseparable for the first months of a child's life. And while this might mean that as a new mother you cannot go out as you used to, it gives you the most wonderful opportunity to give yourself up to motherhood and to forge an unbreakable emotional connection with your child. If you decide to bottle-feed, you can make that connection in the same way, so long as you make a conscious decision to treat feeds as a special time to love and bond with, as well as nourish, your baby.

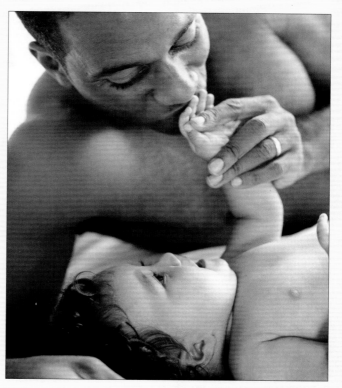

Top: Looking after a baby involves doing lots of small and repetitive tasks – but these can be incredibly fulfilling and enjoyable.

A baby's father will be able to find lots of ways to care for, and bond with, his child, even a breastfed one. Spend as much time as you can with each other.

Changing your baby

It's worth thinking about what type of nappy (diaper) you are going to use for your new baby before you give birth, so you can plan ahead. Parents spend a lot of time changing nappies. Your baby may need anything up to 12 a day at first, and could easily go through 4,000 nappies in the first two years. You should change your baby immediately a nappy is soiled, and at least every three hours otherwise. However, don't wake your baby up just for a nappy change.

WHICH NAPPY?

You can choose between disposable or cloth nappies, or you can use a combination of both. Disposables are convenient and quick to put on, but it's worth considering cloth nappies, especially if you are trying to reduce the amount of waste your family produces. Real nappies are better for babies' skin than disposables because they are

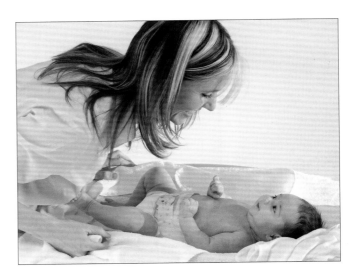

Smiles, eye contact and chat will help your baby to put up with having his or her nappy changed.

REUSEABLE NAPPIES

If you plan to use cloth nappies all the time, you'll need about 24 nappies and three covers. But if you plan to use some disposables, 10 cloth nappies and two waterproof covers should be sufficient. You'll also need two or three booster pads for nighttime, as well as liners. You can get flushable paper liners or reusable cloth or fleece ones.

Terry squares. These are the traditional option and the cheapest. They are good for newborns – a shaped nappy can look huge on a tiny baby. You can now buy plastic fasteners, which are safer than traditional pins.

Prefolds. These nappies are rectangular and have to be folded before use. They come in different sizes, so you will have to buy new ones as the baby grows, but prefolds are generally less expensive than shaped or all-in-one nappies.

Tie-up nappies. These come in one size and are folded in different ways depending on the size of your baby. They are secured using the attached ties.

Shaped nappies. These are probably the easiest to use, because they don't need folding. They come in a range of sizes, or in one size fastened differently depending on the size of the baby, and are secured by poppers or Velcro.

All-in-ones. These are shaped nappies that incorporate a waterproof cover. They are quick to put on, but they take longer to dry after washing and are also more expensive than other nappies. But they can be a good option for when you are out for the day, if you prefer never to use disposables.

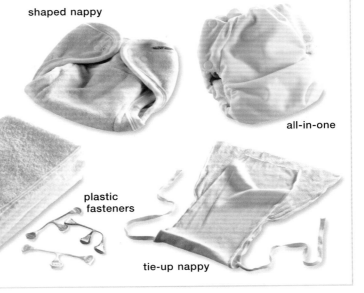

shaped nappy

all-in-one

terry squares

plastic fasteners

prefold nappy

tie-up nappy

Nappy fold for a newborn

Even if you intend to use shaped nappies, it is worth investing in some terries for when your baby is very small.

As with other forms of real nappies, you'll need a waterproof liner to prevent leakage.

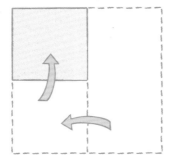 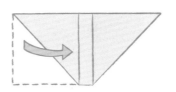 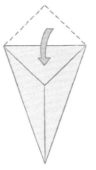 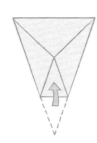

1 Fold the square in half lengthwise to make a rectangle, then again to make a small square.

2 With the four corners of the nappy at the top, pull the corner of the top layer across to make a triangle.

3 Turn the nappy over and fold the square edge over twice, so it forms a pad in the middle of the triangle.

4 Add a liner, put the baby on the nappy, fold up the base, bring one side over the other and secure .

Kite fold

The newborn fold is good for the first few weeks, but your baby will soon be too big for nappies folded in this way.

The kite fold is suitable for larger babies, and will extend the length of time you can use terry squares.

 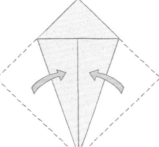 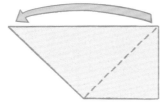 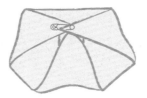

1 Place the square so that one corner is pointing towards you. Fold in the two side corners to make a basic kite shape.

2 Fold down the pointed top, then fold up the point at the bottom, as shown.

3 Place the baby on the nappy so that his or her waist is aligned with the top edge of the nappy.

4 Fold up the base, then fold one side over the other and secure with a nappy pin or plastic fastener.

---

made of natural fabrics and don't contain adhesives or superabsorbant chemicals, which can come into contact with the baby's skin. In the long term, real nappies work out cheaper than disposables, especially since you can re-use them for any other children you have. A local nappy laundering service, which delivers clean nappies and collects your dirty ones, is an alternative costing about the same in the end as using disposables.

If you prefer to use disposable nappies, consider using the eco-friendly brands that are now available from health stores, by mail order, on the internet and in some supermarkets. These have fewer chemicals and bleaching agents than most disposables, and contain more biodegradable materials. However, they tend to be more expensive – and bulkier – than ordinary disposables.

WASHING NAPPIES

You will need a large bucket with a tight-fitting lid to store used nappies, until you have enough to make up a wash that fills the machine. If you want to soak the nappies before washing (it isn't essential), add a few drops of tea tree oil – which has antiseptic qualities – or lavender oil to reduce smells, to the water.

To help keep the nappies free from stains, you can also add a tablespoon of bicarbonate of soda or two tablespoons of white vinegar. It is worth buying a mesh bag for the bucket to make it easier to get the nappies into the washing machine: when you are ready to wash, you simply transfer the whole bag to the machine. Use non-biological detergent, and close any Velcro fasteners to prevent snagging.

CHANGING YOUR BABY

During the day, make nappy changing fun. This is a great time for play – talk and sing to your baby, blow raspberries on his or her tummy, make silly expressions to make the baby laugh. Hang a mobile or mirror above your

Change your baby on a changing station or bed to ease your back and knees. Get everything to hand before you begin, and don't leave the baby alone for a second if the mat is above floor level.

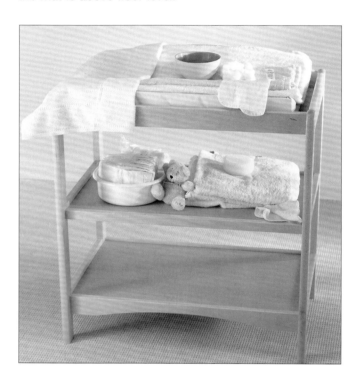

changing area as a distraction. At night, on the other hand, change your baby only if he or she is very wet or has soiled a nappy. Keep the room quiet and dim so that you don't disturb the baby any more than necessary.

CLEARING UP

Put disposable nappies in a nappy sack – you can get biodegradable ones that are made from starch rather than plastic. If you are using cloth nappies, flush soiled paper liners down the toilet and put wet ones in a nappy sack. Hold a soiled reusable liner in the toilet while you flush to rinse it, then place with the nappy in your nappy bucket. Wash your hands with soap and hot water.

PREVENTING AND TREATING NAPPY RASH

Most babies get nappy rash at some point. The best way to prevent it is by keeping your baby clean and dry: he or she is much less likely to get a rash if changed eight times a day or more, and if you leave the nappy off from time to time. It will also help if you use only damp cotton wool to clean the skin, and avoid wipes (especially those that contain alcohol), soap and strong detergents.

If your baby develops any redness, change him or her more often, and leave the nappy off for a few minutes at every change to let air circulate – give longer periods of

CAUTION
Don't use talcum powder on babies: they can inhale the tiny particles, which may be harmful to the lungs.

Cleaning and changing

Get everything ready before you start and have it close to hand. Cover the changing mat with a towel to make it more comfortable and to soak up any accidents. Keep talking to your baby to reassure him or her.

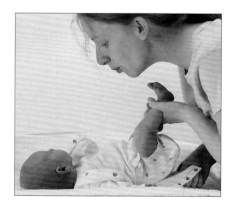

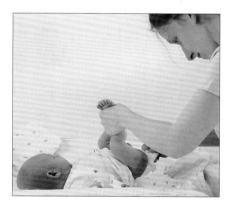

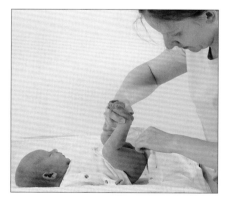

1 Remove lower clothing, and unfasten the nappy. If the stools are very liquid, use some tissue to clean off the worst of it, then clean the baby's bottom using wet cotton wool balls (cotton balls).

2 Lift up the baby's legs, fold the nappy in half and remove. Clean thoroughly, including creases in the legs. Wipe a girl from front to back. Clean under a boy's testicles but don't pull back the foreskin.

3 if there is any redness, apply a thin smear of barrier cream. Lift the baby by the ankles, then lay the clean nappy underneath, aligning the top of the back with the baby's waist. Lower the baby on to it and fasten it.

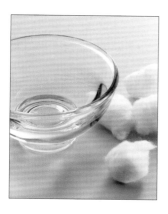

There are lots of nappy wipes on the market, but it is best to use cotton wool (cotton balls) and cooled, boiled water to clean your baby, especially in the first weeks. If you need to use wipes when away from home, use unbleached, chemical-free ones.

bare-bottom time if you can. Use a natural barrier cream, such as calendula nappy rash cream, at every change. See your doctor if the rash doesn't clear up within a few days or if blisters or pimples develop.

A GUIDE TO STOOLS

Babies' vary enormously in the number of soiled nappies they produce. Many will move their bowels at every feed, while some breastfed babies can go for up to a week without having a bowel movement. So long as the stools are normal and your baby is not in discomfort, this is nothing to worry about.

Normal stools. A baby's first bowel movement is black or green and very sticky: this is called meconium and it is passed in the first couple of days after the birth. Subsequent stools are usually yellowish in colour. In breastfed babies, they can be mustard yellow and runny

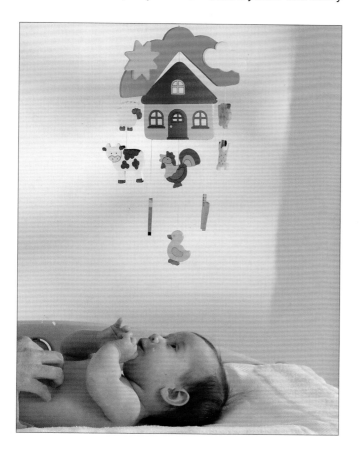

NATURAL SPRAY CLEANER
Bacteria can breed on a changing mat so make sure that you keep it clean. To make your own natural antibacterial cleaner, put two cups of cooled, boiled water in a new, washed, plant-spray bottle. Add 15 drops each of tea tree and mandarin essential oils and shake well before using.

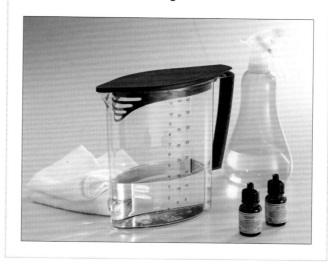

or dark yellow/light brown and grainy. The stools of bottle-fed babies tend to be dark yellow to light brown and firmer than those of breastfed babies.

Green stools. Some formulas can make a baby's stools green, but if they are also slimy, foul-smelling and frequent, then your baby probably has diarrhoea and should be checked by a doctor. A bottle-fed baby may need to drink cooled boiled water instead of formula for a short period; a breastfed baby can feed as normal. A breastfed baby may produce green, watery stools if he or she is getting too much foremilk and not enough of the rich hindmilk. To correct this, make sure the baby has emptied one breast before starting on the other.

Pellet-like brown stools. These suggest constipation. Breastfed babies almost never become constipated because breastmilk is easily digested, but bottle-fed babies may have this problem from time to time. Give cooled boiled water to drink as well as milk and make sure that you are using the correct amount of formula when making up the bottles.

Abnormal stools. Dark brown or black stools (other than meconium) in a young baby may indicate bleeding in the bowel: see your doctor for advice as soon as possible. Dark red or bloody stools may indicate an obstruction in the bowel, this must be checked urgently. Very pale stools may be a sign of jaundice and also must be checked with your doctor.

Hang a colourful mobile above your changing station so that your baby has something to look at.

Bathing your baby

Until a few years ago, mothers were taught how to bath their babies while still in hospital and a bath was seen as an essential part of the daily routine. However, frequent baths are not only unnecessary but also dry out a baby's skin. They can also be upsetting for young babies, who often don't like being naked, and stressful for parents. Handling a slippery infant with a floppy neck can be difficult, especially if he or she is screaming in protest. If your baby screams when you put him or her in the bath, wait a few days and then try again.

If you can, wait two to four weeks before giving the first bath. You can easily keep the baby clean in the meantime by washing his or her bottom at each nappy change, and topping and tailing at least once a day.

NAIL CARE

Most parents find the idea of cutting their baby's tiny nails daunting, but there is no avoiding it. Scratch mittens are useful for the first days, but you can't keep your baby's hands hidden away for long, not least because he or she needs to discover and use them. The easiest way to trim

CAUTION
Never leave a baby unattended in a bath. You should also never leave a baby in the care of an older sibling or any other child, however responsible they may be.

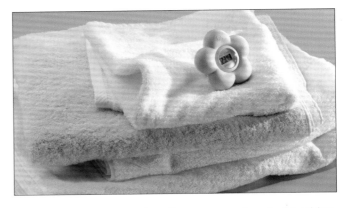

A bath thermometer takes the guesswork out of bathing your baby, but you should still double-check the temperature of the water with your elbow.

Topping and tailing

Clean your baby in a warm room, so that exposed skin doesn't get cold. You can use a changing table, a bed or sofa, or the floor, but cover the surface with a thick towel folded over a few times to keep the baby warm and comfortable. Either undress the baby completely and cover with a towel to keep warm, or remove clothing as you go along. Never leave your baby unattended on a raised surface, even if you think he or she can't yet roll over. Get everything ready before you start: you'll need a bowl of warm boiled water, cotton wool (cotton balls), a facecloth, a small, thin towel and a clean nappy (plus nappy rash cream, if necessary).

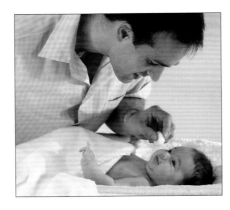

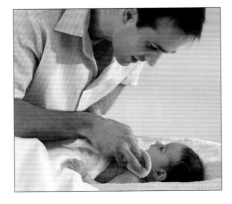

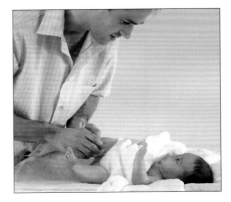

1 Cover the baby's lower half with a towel. Dip a small wad of cotton wool in the water, and wipe the baby's eye from the inner to the outer corner. Use a new piece of damp cotton wool to clean the other eye.

2 Use more wet cotton wool or a clean, damp facecloth to wipe the baby's face, including the nose and ears. Clean the folds of the neck (dried milk can collect here) and pat the baby dry with a clean towel.

3 Move the towel to cover the baby's top half. Now clean the nappy area, make sure you wipe all the folds in the legs and groin. Do not pull back a boy's foreskin or a girl's labia – these areas are self-cleaning. Pat dry.

Bathing

You can bath your baby in an ordinary bath, but using a baby bath is more convenient and uses less water. You can use a baby bath inside an ordinary bath, but it will be less strain on your back if you place it on the floor, or, better yet, on a stand. Make sure that the room is very warm before you undress the baby, and always check the temperature of the bathwater before immersing the baby in it. It's easier to get the right temperature if you fill the bath with warm water and then gradually add cold. Keep baths very short – a few minutes is all that is necessary – and hold the baby firmly to help him or her feel secure. It will be reassuring if you talk in a low, calm tone.

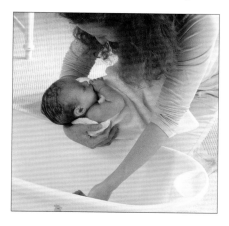

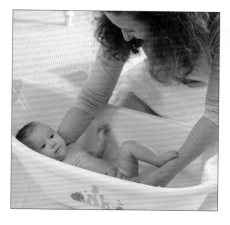

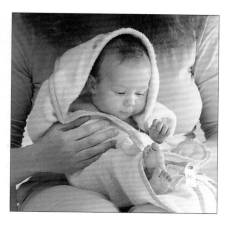

1 Undress your baby and wrap in a towel, leaving the head exposed. Hold the baby over the bath, supporting the back, neck and head with one arm and hand. Use the other hand to wash the baby's hair with water (there's no need for shampoo). Gently pat dry.

2 Remove the towel and lower your baby into the bath, holding under the arm with your hand and supporting the neck and head with your wrist. Support the bottom with your other hand. Continue to support the baby's back and neck while you use the other hand to rinse.

3 Lift the baby out and lay him or her on a towel, quickly wrapping it around him or her, covering the head as well as the body (a hooded towel works best). Dry well, all over, including the creases, and then put on a clean nappy and sleepsuit.

nails is to use baby clippers. Do it after a bath when the nails are softer, or when the baby is asleep. Hold the finger between your thumb and forefinger, and press the pad out of the way while you clip. You can also use a nail file, which doesn't leave sharp edges, or you can nibble your baby's nails short. Fingernails grow quickly, so check them every couple of days. Toenails should be trimmed in the same way, but they grow more slowly so won't need doing so often.

Trim your baby's nails when he or she is asleep, or is at least calm and still. Make sure there is enough light to see by – it is very easy to nick the skin by accident. Use baby nail clippers rather than scissors.

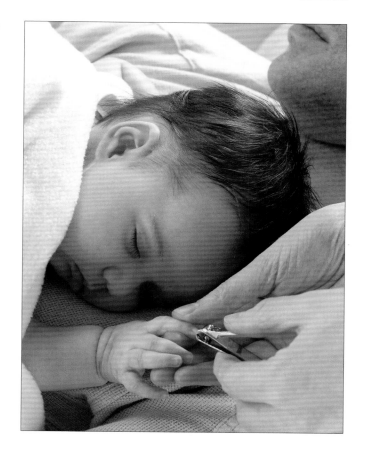

BATH SUPPORT
A framed towelling bath support makes bathing your baby much easier, since it leaves both your hands free and supports the baby's head. When your baby is a few weeks old, it will help to make bath time more enjoyable for you both. The towelling can become chilly when it is wet, so keep scooping water over it.

Caring for your baby's skin

Baby skin is very delicate and can easily become dry. The best way to protect it is to treat it as naturally as possible, and minimize any contact with chemicals. For example, use a soap-based washing powder rather than a detergent (biological ones are definitely to be avoided). Do not use fabric softeners, which can irritate a baby's skin. Always wash new clothing before putting it on your baby, since the fabric may contain chemicals left over from the manufacturing process. Where possible, choose clothes made from organic fabrics, such as cotton. Unbleached, undyed fabrics are the best choice for bedding and clothing that will be next to your baby's skin.

SKINCARE AT BATHTIME
It takes a few weeks for the oils in the skin of a newborn baby to form a natural protective barrier, so it is a good idea to avoid bathing your baby during this time: top and tail instead. Restrict baths to no more than two or three a week and don't use any baby bath products, especially those that contain petrochemicals, alcohol or perfume. Your baby is unlikely to get so dirty that he or she needs washing with soap, and you won't need baby shampoo for months – water will do the job all on its own.

It's fine to add the very gentle essential oils of Roman chamomile and lavender to a baby's bath so long as he or she is three months or more. Use one or two drops, diluted in oil or full fat milk before added to the water.

A baby's skin has a gorgeous natural scent. Perfumed bubble baths and other products aren't necessary.

Bathing in oatmeal
An oatmeal bath is an excellent way to soften and moisturize babies' delicate skin. It can also be used to help relieve the itching associated with eczema, chickenpox or insect bites.

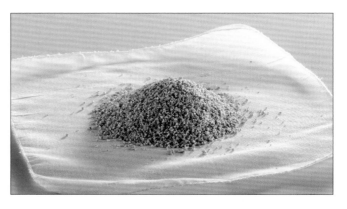

1 Grind two cups of oatmeal in a clean coffee grinder, blender or food processor until it is very fine. Combine the ground oatmeal with four cups of cold water, stirring well.

2 Add the oatmeal solution to a tepid bath – the water should look slightly milky and feel slimy to the touch (if the oatmeal drops to the bottom of the bathtub, it hasn't been ground finely enough).

3 Take care not to get any water in the baby's eyes during the bath since the oatmeal can irritate. You also need to be very careful when holding or lifting your baby because this bath makes skin extremely slippery.

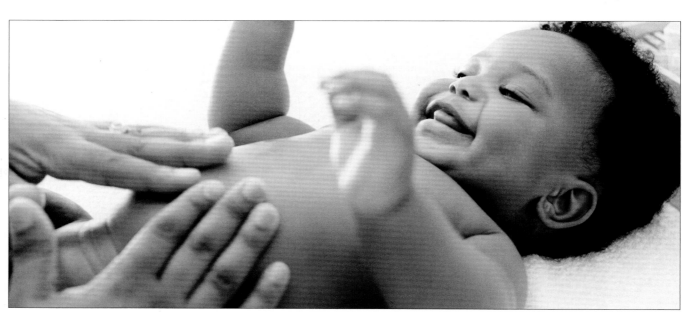

BABY MASSAGE OIL

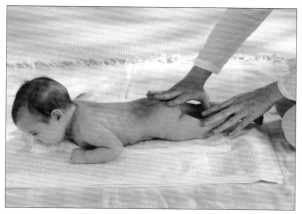

Oiling or moisturizing your baby's skin after every bath will help to keep it soft and hydrated. Using oil will also allow you to massage your baby without pulling the skin. But make sure that all the creases are completely dry before applying oil or you'll be creating the ideal conditions for fungal infection. You can use lavender and Roman chamomile essential oils on babies of three months or older. If your baby was born prematurely, wait until at least three months after your due date.

100ml (3½fl oz) sunflower oil
5 drops lavender essential oil
5 drops Roman chamomile essential oil

Pour the sunflower oil into a dark glass bottle then add the essential oils. Replace the cap and shake well to mix. When using for massage, pour a small amount on your hands and rub your palms together, then smooth over your baby's skin. Add more oil whenever you notice that the skin is starting to pull.

Plain water can be drying, so it is worth adding a little oil to the water to help keep your baby's skin soft and supple. Many parents like to use almond or jojoba oil in their babies' baths. But a few babies can react to nut-based oils such as these, so it may be safer to stick with vegetable oils like sunflower or olive at first. Alternatively, you can use oatmeal in the bath, which is a natural emollient.

CRADLE CAP

Lots of babies develop thick yellowish scales on their scalp. This happens when the sebaceous glands in the skin produce too much sebum, the oily substance that helps to keep skin lubricated. Cradle cap doesn't do any

Cradle cap can last for many months if you don't treat it. Smoothing olive oil into the scalp is a simple remedy.

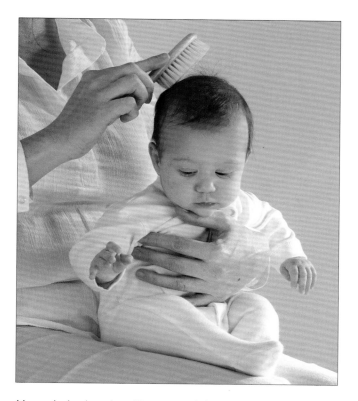

Use a baby brush, with very soft bristles, to help clear off the loose scales of cradle cap.

harm, but it can look unsightly and may persist for months if you don't treat it. To do so, gently rub some olive oil into the area and leave overnight, then wash off in the morning. To help cradle cap on its way, you can brush the scalp with a baby hairbrush to remove loose scales. Never pick off scales with your fingers or you may cause infection. If the cradle cap is very stubborn, try rubbing in calendula cream every night for a few days.

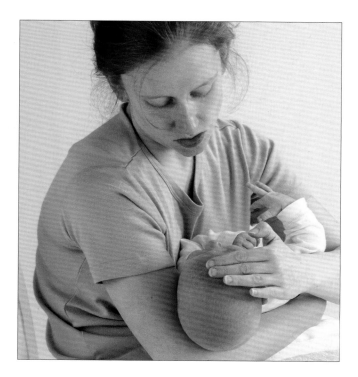

Clothes for your baby

Babies are not good at regulating their body temperature, so they must always be dressed appropriately for the weather. On a hot day, a nappy and perhaps a vest may be all your baby needs. On cold days, a vest, an all-in-one towelling sleepsuit and a light cardigan should be sufficient. Be ready to change your baby's clothing if the temperature changes or you go out.

You can tell if a baby is warm enough by feeling the back of the neck. If it is cold, you need to put on more clothing. But don't worry if the baby's hands and feet feel cooler than the rest of the body; this is quite normal. To check if a baby is getting too hot, feel the tummy or chest. Remove a layer of clothing if the skin is very warm.

Choose clothes made from fabric that is soft, stretchable and machine-washable – cotton is ideal. And make sure that everything is easy to put on and take off. You'll find all-in-ones with roomy necklines and snap fasteners a lot less restricting than denim jackets or party frocks. Shoes may look cute on a baby, but they can cramp the feet and restrict growth if they are too tight. It is much better to let your baby go barefoot so that he or she can wriggle his or her toes freely, or to put him or her in soft socks or tights to keep the feet warm. Make sure there is plenty of "wriggle room" in the socks, and cut the feet off sleepsuits once they get snug in the feet.

BABY BASICS

Some of the most useful basic items of clothes for a young baby that will help you to have what you need whatever the weather are as follows.

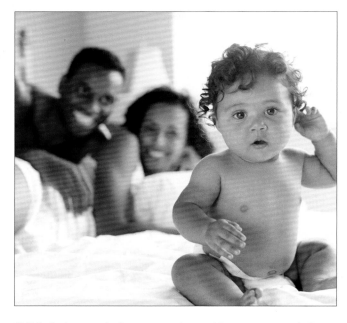

If it is hot, your baby may not need to wear any clothes at all. Some young babies feel insecure if they are naked and prefer to wear a vest, but most soon love the feeling of being bare.

Six short-sleeved bodysuits or vests. These may be all your baby needs to wear on summer days, and they make useful undergarments in winter. Long-sleeved bodysuits are good for winter but are harder to get on.
Six to eight long-sleeved sleepsuits with feet. Great as pyjamas or daywear for young babies, but make sure they are roomy enough in the feet. You'll need fewer in

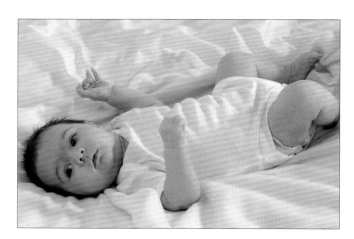

Lots of parents tend to overdress their babies. On a warm day, or in a centrally heated house, a bodysuit or vest on top of the nappy may be all he or she needs to stay comfortable.

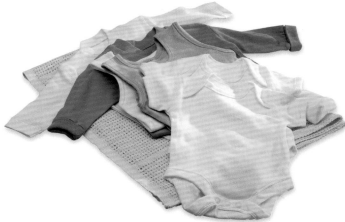

Baby clothes have to be simple and practical. Frills, fiddly buttons and fussy necklines all make dressing your baby hard work, and synthetic fabrics may irritate the skin and cause overheating.

Putting clothes on your baby

Many babies hate having their clothes changed, so do it only when their clothing is soiled or wet – there's no need to put a baby into a different sleepsuit for the night, say, if the one he or she has on is perfectly clean. Make sure the room is warm, especially in the early months, and place the baby on a comfortable surface. Work as gently and as quickly as possible, without getting flustered (it gets easier with practice). If the baby seems worried or distressed when naked, lay a small towel over him or her to give a greater feeling of security.

It will help if you maintain eye contact with your baby and sing or chat as you dress him or her. With an older baby, you can turn dressing into a game – play peek-a-boo as you pull a sleepsuit over your baby's face.

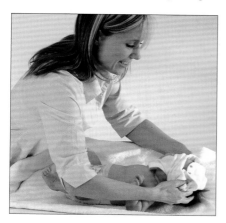

1 When putting on a vest or bodysuit, use your hands to stretch the neck as wide as possible. This will help you to ease it over the baby's head without scraping the nose or ears. Do this as quickly as possible since babies don't like having their faces covered.

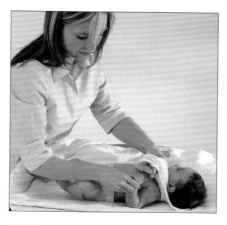

2 If the garment has long sleeves, gather the sleeve fabric as close to the armhole as possible. Put your fingers through, gently hold your baby's hand and pull the sleeve over the arm rather than tugging a tiny arm through the sleeve. Repeat with the other arm.

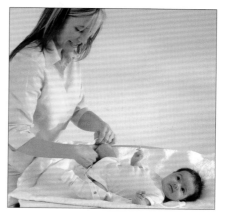

3 To put on an all-in-one sleepsuit, open up all the fastenings and lay the suit on a flat changing surface. Place the baby on top. Gently ease the feet of the suit over your baby's feet. Pull the sleeves over the arms as before. Do up the fastenings from the feet upwards.

---

summer, when it may be too hot for the baby to wear them during the day.

Two to three cardigans. These are much easier to put on than garments that go over the head, but choose the kind that fasten with snaps rather than fiddly buttons.

Baby blanket. Good for wrapping the baby up when you need to go outside, or for use as a cover during naps.

Baby sleeping bag. A great alternative to blankets, which can be kicked off, a sleeping bag is a good way to make sure your baby stays warm. Combine a sleeping bag with a long-sleeved bodysuit, and add a cardigan if it is very cold. You can get bags with lighter tog ratings suitable for summer.

Three to six bibs. Useful if your baby spits up milk after feeds, or is dribbling a lot because of teething.

One or two hats. For summer, choose cotton hats with a wide, floppy brim (especially important if you are using a sling and need to protect the top of the baby's head). For winter, buy hats that are made of fleece or similar, with flaps that go over the ears.

Two to six pairs of socks. Get them all in the same colour, as you are bound to lose quite a few. You won't need many in summer.

Snowsuit with built-in mittens. This is great for keeping a baby cosy when you go out in winter. But you won't need one if you have a warm inner sleeve for the buggy or if you are carrying your baby in a sling; choose a cape or warm coat instead.

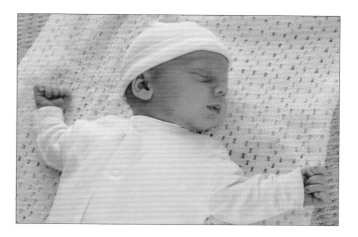

Babies should normally have their heads uncovered when they are indoors, but very small, or premature, babies may need to wear a hat in the first few days. Check with your midwife if you are unsure what is best.

Out and about

Going out with a young baby can feel quite stressful at first, so it is a good idea to keep trips short and relatively simple until you get used to the outside world again. Carrying your baby in a sling will help you both feel secure but can be hard on your back. Sooner or later you will need a buggy. Choose one that lies flat or use a pram for the first few months to avoid putting pressure on the baby's developing spine. A buggy with a seat that faces you will allow you to keep an eye on a young baby, and means he or she has your reassuring presence in view.

When you go out, your baby will need to wear extra layers and a hat (body heat can rapidly escape through the top of the head). To avoid overheating, you should take off any outer clothing and remove blankets and rain covers when you come back indoors or if you go into a warm shop or café, even if it means waking your baby up. Rain

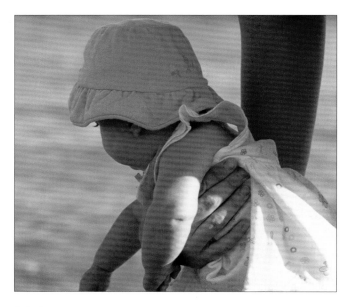

It is important to keep a young baby out of direct sunlight at all times. A wide-brimmed hat will help to shade his or her face.

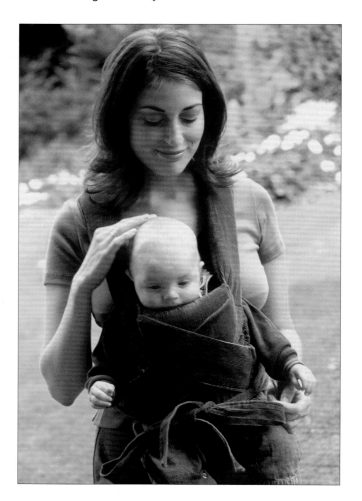

Slings seem fiddly, with lots of straps and buckles to work out, but they are very comfortable and your baby will love being close to you.

CHECKLIST: PACKING YOUR DAY BAG

It is worth investing in a proper changing bag, which is designed to carry everything you need for a day out. Write out your own list and keep it in the bag so that you can check you have everything whenever you go out.

- Nappies (diapers) and cotton wool (cotton balls)
- Flask of boiled water, or alcohol-free wipes
- Nappy sacks
- Nappy rash cream
- Complete change of clothes
- Muslins to protect your clothing and clean up baby
- Bottles of formula or expressed breastmilk, if using
- Bottle of cooled, boiled water, if using
- Snacks for breastfeeding mother
- Comforter or dummy (pacifier), if using
- One or two toys

Take outdoor clothing off your baby when you enter a warm building. If the baby is asleep it is tempting not to do this, but he or she could become overheated.

covers and sunshades trap warm air around your baby, so be sure to open ventilation flaps whenever possible, and put covers and shades down when you go indoors. Using a UV-filter sunshade will keep your baby cooler than the buggy hood, and will give more protection from sunlight.

SUN PROTECTION

Babies under six months old should not be exposed to direct sunlight because their skin is too thin to protect them from harmful UV rays. Put a sunhat with a wide brim on a baby who is being carried in a sling, and cover arms and legs completely with a cool fabric such as cotton. If your baby is in a buggy, get a parasol and adjust it frequently so that your baby is kept in the shade. This is much easier if the baby is facing you; if your buggy faces away from you (as most do), a UV-filter sunshade will be more effective.

CHOOSING A CAR SEAT

It is essential that you use the right type of car seat for your baby, even if you need it only for short trips. A car seat is one baby item that you should definitely buy new, unless it comes from somebody that you know and trust, and you are certain that it has not been involved in an accident. You cannot always tell from the appearance of a car seat whether or not it has been damaged, so it is risky to use one from an unknown source.

For the first nine months or so, babies need a backward-facing car seat. This helps to protect their undeveloped neck muscles from a whiplash-type injury, which would be much more serious than in an adult. Choose one that has high sides to protect from side-impact blows. Once your baby weighs 9kg/20lb or more and can sit unsupported for at least 15 minutes, he or she can go in a forward-facing seat.

A travel cot provides your baby with a safe place to sleep wherever you are.

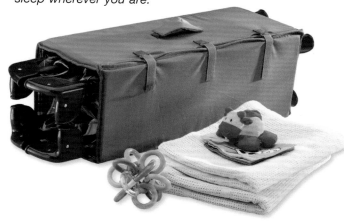

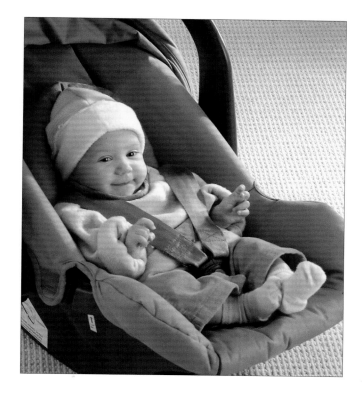

LEAVING HOME

Going away with your baby can be a daunting prospect, especially when you start to think about how much you need to take with you. But it's actually easier when a baby is very small, especially if you are breastfeeding. Here is a list of some of the things you may need.

SLEEPING

- Travel cot or Moses basket (unless your baby sleeps with you)
- Fitted sheet and flat sheet
- Blankets or baby sleeping bag
- Any sleep aids you may have been using (such as CDs or comforters)

CLOTHING

- Three complete changes for each day (fewer if you have washing facilities), and outdoor clothing
- Bibs, if using
- One or two baby towels

FEEDING

- Formula, bottles and teats, if using
- Sterilizer, if using (if you have access to a kitchen, you can boil bottles and teats in a large saucepan instead)

OTHER ITEMS

- Baby bouncer or play mat, if using
- Selection of toys (including any that your baby has grown attached to)
- Change of clothing for you
- Sling or buggy, if using, for going out and about

Why breastfeed?

Breastfeeding involves more than simply giving your baby milk. Snuggled at your breast, your baby enjoys your warmth, your scent and the familiar sound of your heartbeat. He or she can gaze upon your face, which is just the right distance away to focus on. Your baby is blissfully content. Before the birth, lots of women worry about whether they will be able to breastfeed their child. But almost everyone can, provided that they have a supportive environment in which to do it. And although you may experience some difficulties along the way, nursing can be as satisfying and loving an experience for you as it is for your baby.

SUCCESSFUL BREASTFEEDING

One of the keys to successful breastfeeding is simply trusting that you can do it. In societies where breastfeeding is the only safe way to nourish infants, new mothers assume that they can breastfeed – and they do. After all, our bodies are designed to nurture our babies both before and after birth.

Good support boosts your confidence and encourages you to continue through any initial problems. Studies have found that having a partner who is positive about breastfeeding can have a major effect. The support of friends and relatives, particularly women who have successfully breastfed themselves, can also make a big difference. It is well worth seeking out a breastfeeding counsellor or an organization such as La Leche League, who may run a drop-in support group in your area.

WHAT IS BREASTMILK?

Breastmilk is the perfect food for babies. It provides the nutrients they need in exactly the right quantities and it is packed with antibodies to help them fight off infection and illness. It is also completely sterile. Unlike formula milk, breastmilk is a living substance that adapts to your baby's needs. It varies from day to day, and from feed to feed. For example, it may contain specific antibodies to help your baby fight off any germs you encountered that day and it will have a higher water content on hot days. It is usually denser in the morning, after you have rested.

The first milk you produce is colostrum, rich in antibodies and nutrients, and with laxative properties that encourage your baby to pass the sticky first stools (meconium). True breastmilk comes in a few days after the birth. Each feed begins with thin foremilk to quench

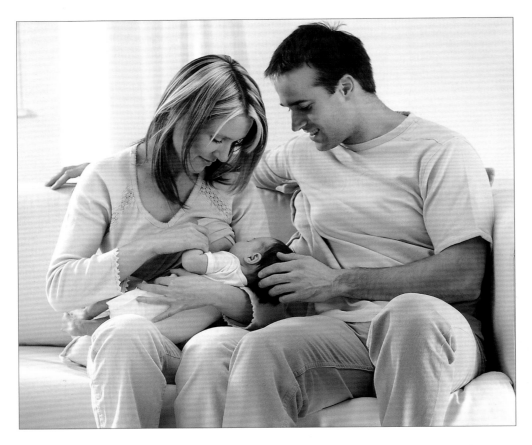

Fathers have a role in breastfeeding too: a supportive partner can be a key factor in successful breastfeeding, as can friends and relatives.

Nursing is an expression of love that only a mother can give. A baby who is upset or ill instinctively turns to you for the comfort of nursing.

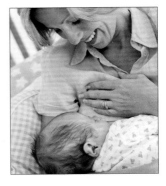

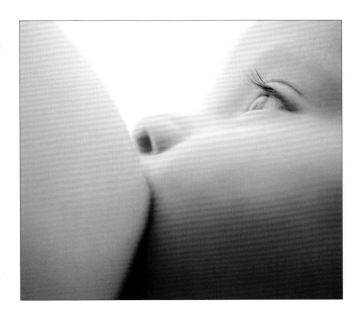

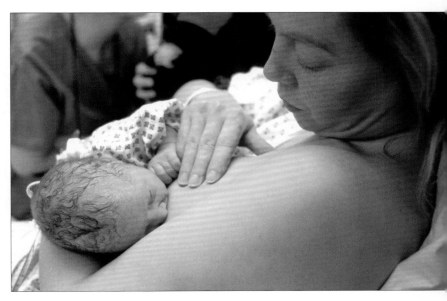

Breastfeeding not only gives a baby a feeling of security and comfort, it also has a soothing effect on the mother, and gives her a reason to relax and rest.

Even if you don't intend to breastfeed for long, nursing your baby for the first few days will give him or her some level of protection from infections.

the baby's thirst. As the baby continues sucking, denser hindmilk is produced. This is high in fat and proteins and gives your baby the energy he or she needs to grow.

THE ADVANTAGES OF BREASTFEEDING

It's more convenient. It is much easier to breastfeed than to prepare and warm a bottle, especially in the middle of the night.

It's better for your baby. Breastfed babies suffer from fewer tummy bugs than bottle-fed ones (one study found that American bottle-fed babies got diarrhoea more than 12 times more often). They also get half as many colds and are less likely to get respiratory diseases and ear and urine infections.

It sets the foundations for good health in adult life. Breastfeeding exclusively for six months helps protect your baby from allergies. Breastfed babies are less likely to be obese in later life, or to develop eczema, diabetes and high blood pressure. There is also evidence to suggest breastfeeding helps with brain development.

It encourages the development of the jaw and teeth. Breastfed babies may have fewer dental problems.

It exposes your baby to a wide range of tastes. The flavour of breastmilk varies depending on what you eat. This may help with weaning.

It is enjoyable. Babies nurse for comfort as well as food, and breastfeeding is the quickest way to calm a baby who is distressed.

It helps you to get back in shape. Breastfeeding stimulates the production of oxytocin, which helps your womb return to its normal size. And the fat stores you laid down in pregnancy are used in producing your milk.

It helps you to relax. You have to sit down to nurse

your baby, which means you rest. Also, nursing mothers have higher levels of the hormone prolactin. This helps you to feel calm, so you can sleep quickly after a feed.

It has benefits for your health. Breastfeeding may reduce the chances of developing breast or ovarian cancer, and lower the risk of osteoporosis.

It delays the return of your periods. Breastfeeding has a contraceptive effect and you are unlikely to become pregnant if you are feeding on demand and do not go longer than four hours between any feeds. But if you need to be certain of avoiding pregnancy, you should use another method of contraception.

VITAMIN D

There is some debate about whether breastfed babies get enough vitamin D, which is important for bone health. It is present in breastmilk in low amounts and is manufactured in the skin when exposed to sunlight. Since we are now advised to protect babies from the sun, they are more reliant on breastmilk for their supply. The American Academy of Pediatrics recommends that all breastfed babies are given vitamin D drops as a precaution, while the UK Department of Health advises vitamin D (as well as C and A) for babies of six months and over who still have breastmilk as their main drink.

Whether or not your baby needs drops may depend on where you live and, to an extent, on the colour of your skin (dark-skinned babies are at greater risk of vitamin D deficiency). It is worth talking to a health professional about what is best for your baby.

Feeding on demand

Your breasts will almost certainly produce as much milk as your baby needs, provided that you feed as often and for as long as the baby wants to. In the first weeks, this may mean you are feeding 10–12 times a day so that it feels like nursing is an almost permanent activity. You may find it hard to believe that your baby can be hungry so quickly after the last feed. But a baby's tiny stomach – about the size of a walnut – can take in only a small amount of milk at a time. Breastmilk is so easily digested that it doesn't remain there for long.

If babies get less than they need at a feed, whether it's because they go to sleep, or feed very slowly, they will want to nurse again sooner. By allowing your baby to nurse as soon as he or she is hungry, your breasts get the message that more milk is needed and will adjust their supply accordingly. It may take anything from a few days to a few weeks, but eventually your baby will start to go longer between feeds.

Every so often, you'll notice that your baby suddenly wants to feed more frequently again. These increases in demand often happen at around two weeks, six weeks

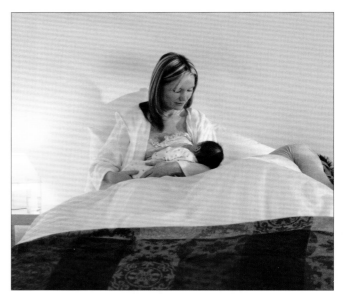

Feeding your baby on demand can be tough at first – most women find that they are nursing four or five times a night. But you get used to going back to sleep quickly, and eventually your baby will wake less often.

Lots of babies come off the breast when they are satisfied, but some like to go to sleep with their mother's nipple in their mouth. You may find that your baby wakes and cries when you remove it. If so, try letting the baby suckle once more and then taking him or her off again. You may have to do this several times before the baby will relinquish your nipple.

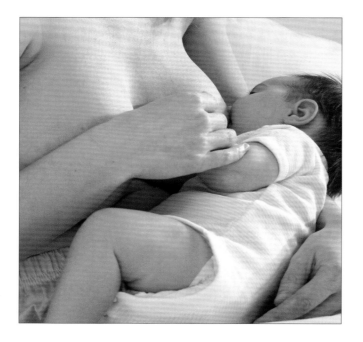

and 12 weeks, and indicate growth spurts. Again, if you let the baby nurse on demand, your milk supply will increase to meet his or her needs. Mothers often wonder how long a feed should last. The answer, annoyingly, is that it varies depending on how your baby feeds. Some babies keep sucking vigorously until they are satisfied, and they may get enough milk in 10–15 minutes. Others tend to feed in short bursts, resting in between. It may take an hour or more for them to feel sated. With slow feeders, it can sometimes feel as if one feed rolls into the next. There isn't a lot you can do about this: just accept that for now you will be spending most of the time nursing. Babies gradually become more efficient at feeding, so your feeds will get shorter.

EARLY BOTTLES

Don't give your baby any bottles of formula early on: if your baby is getting nourishment elsewhere, he or she will feed less often at the breast – and your milk supply won't increase in the way it needs to. Also, it requires less work for a baby to get milk from the teat of a bottle than the nipple, so if you give a bottle, the baby may refuse breastfeeds altogether. If you want to combine breast and bottle-feeding it is still best to breastfeed exclusively for six weeks to establish the milk supply. It is also best to avoid using a dummy (pacifier) during this time.

ONE SIDE OR TWO?

Mothers are sometimes advised to feed from each breast for a specific time. But if you do this, your baby may get only the thin foremilk, so you need to let the baby suckle at one breast for as long as he or she wants. If this empties the breast (which will then feel soft rather than full) but the baby still seems to be hungry, offer the other one. For the next feed, offer the second breast first, so the feeds start on alternate sides. To help you remember which side to start on, try attaching a safety pin or ribbon to your bra strap and moving it to the opposite side at each feed. Some women find that they can tell which breast to start on, because it is heavier.

IS IT WORKING?

The number of wet nappies produced can be the best indicator of whether your baby is getting enough milk: if there are fewer than six a day, you may need to check your latching-on technique or look at ways of boosting your milk supply. Make sure you are resting enough and drinking enough fluids. A baby mustn't be dehydrated, so talk to a health professional if you are worried.

If your baby is gaining weight slowly or in a different way to the development charts babies are measured against, don't assume you are not feeding successfully. It is normal for babies to lose up to 10 per cent of their birth weight in the first week, and to grow less in some weeks than in others. So long as they gain weight steadily over a number of weeks, they are probably feeding enough.

Like any new skill, breastfeeding takes practice and you may want to give yourself privacy at first. But once you and your baby get the hang of it, you can nurse discreetly without other people taking much notice.

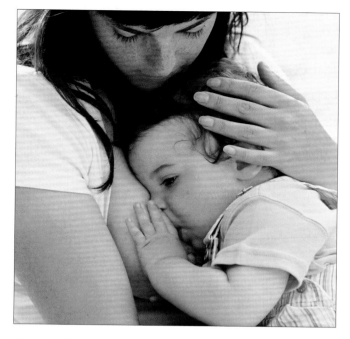

Breastmilk continues to have health benefits even after a baby is on solid food. Many women continue breastfeeding for two years or more.

HOW LONG TO BREASTFEED

Ideally, women would breastfeed their babies exclusively for six months and then continue to nurse for at least the first year, even after solids have been introduced.

Lots of women give up breastfeeding if they suffer from sore nipples or other problems early on. This is a shame, because breastfeeding usually gets much easier, quicker and more satisfying for the mother once the baby is a little older. You may find that you are able to go on longer than you expected, particularly if you get support and seek out other women who are breastfeeding for encouragement.

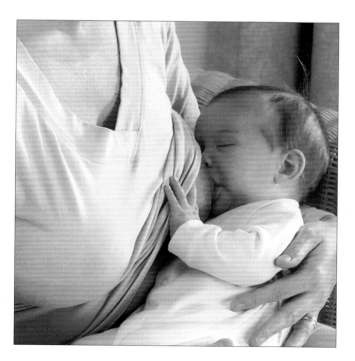

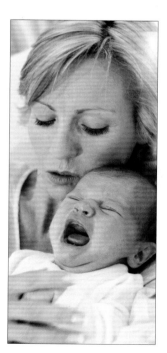

A hungry baby may cry, nuzzle against your breast or make rooting or sucking movements. Try to feed a hungry baby as soon as possible. Any period of breastfeeding will benefit your baby, so it is definitely worth starting, even if you don't think you will want to continue for very long.

Breastfeeding basics

Your baby will instinctively search for your nipple with an open mouth when placed on the breast (this is the rooting reflex that all babies are born with). But you need to give your baby some help to make sure he or she takes your breast in a way that enables him or her to get as much milk as is needed as efficiently as possible. It is also important that the feeding process doesn't make your nipples sore. This can be tricky at first, but with practice you and your baby will achieve the correct latch each time with ease. When a baby is latched on correctly, his or her gums press on the areola (the dark bit around the nipple) and stimulate the milk ducts inside the breast. As the baby sucks, the gums act in the same way as a pump, drawing milk into the nipple. The sucking also sets off the mother's "let-down reflex" in the breast, which pushes milk from the production glands and into the milk glands.

WHAT NOT TO DO

- Don't put your hand behind the baby's head and pull it towards you. The baby will arch away.
- Don't position your nipple opposite the baby's mouth. Make sure that it is in line with the nose, or the baby won't be able to draw it deeply enough into the mouth.
- Don't press on your breast to make an airspace for the baby's nose – you could cause a blockage in a milk duct or move the nipple out of position. If the nose is squashed, try moving the baby's bottom closer to your body to create space.
- Don't continue if you feel pain that lasts more than a few seconds. Take the baby off and start again.

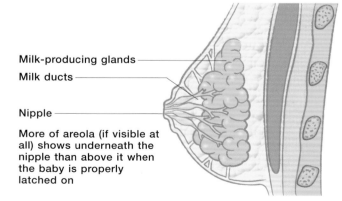

Milk-producing glands

Milk ducts

Nipple

More of areola (if visible at all) shows underneath the nipple than above it when the baby is properly latched on

A baby is properly latched on when the nipple is deeply inside the mouth. The tongue should be beneath the nipple, while the gums clamp down behind it.

LATCHING ON

As the baby sucks you should be able to see the jaw and ears moving and hear swallowing. If you can hear smacking sounds or the baby's cheeks are drawing in, he or she is not latched on properly.

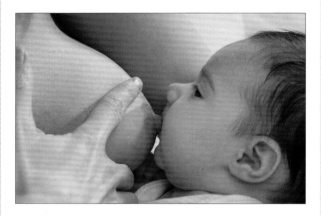

1 Hold the baby close to you, tummy against yours and nose opposite your nipple. Make sure the baby is completely on his or her side, with head, shoulders and back forming a straight line. Support your breast with your fingers, keeping them clear of the areola. Your baby may open his or her mouth and reach towards the nipple. If not, brush the baby's lower lip with your nipple.

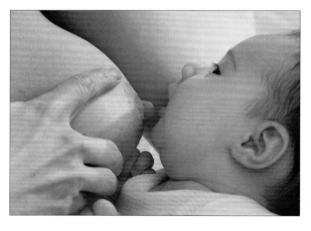

2 As the baby's mouth opens very wide, gently draw the shoulders towards you so that the baby can take the nipple and as much as possible of the areola into the mouth. The gums should close well clear of the nipple. If you feel discomfort for more than a few seconds, wet your little finger and slip it into the side of the baby's mouth to release the suction. Take the baby off the breast, then try again.

YOUR POSITION

You can breastfeed sitting down, leaning back, lying on your side or even standing up. All that matters is that the baby is in the right position for latching on and that you are comfortable and relaxed. You shouldn't have to lean or hunch over in order to get the breast in the baby's mouth – use pillows to support your back and the arm you are using to hold the baby, and put your feet up.

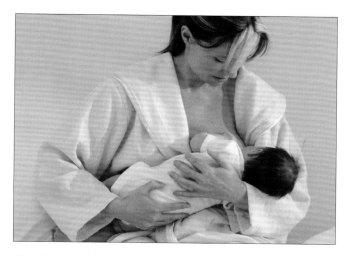

Cradle hold: The baby's head rests on your forearm, just below the crook of your arm, with his or her body supported along your forearm and bottom in your hand. Make sure you are tummy-to-tummy and place the baby's lower arm around your waist. This position is good for women comfortable with breastfeeding.

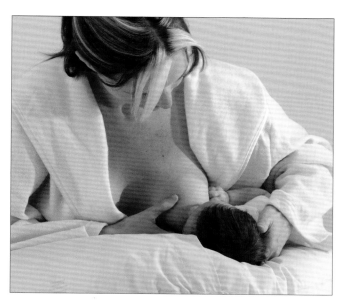

Clutch hold: Tuck the baby under your arm, facing you. The baby's head and shoulders are held in your hand, the back is supported by your forearm and the legs rest on a pillow behind you. This position allows you to guide the baby's head to your breast easily, so it is a good one to start with. It can be used if you've had a Caesarean, and also makes it possible to nurse twins simultaneously.

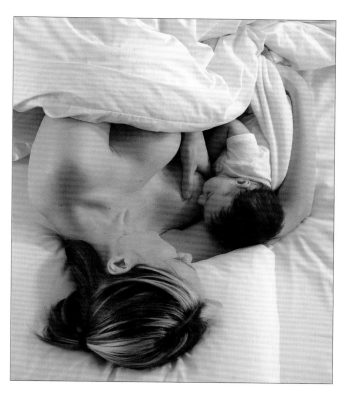

Lying-down position: You and the baby lie on your sides facing each other (put pillows under your head, behind your back and between your knees for extra support). Raise your lower arm above your head or use it to cradle the baby's shoulders and head. This position works well for night feeds but some women find it a bit tricky at first.

BURPING

Babies take in air when they feed and often need to burp afterwards. If your baby has fallen asleep feeding, you don't need to wake him or her to burp, but there may be one later. Some babies don't burp straight away so keep patting or change position, but if your baby doesn't burp after a while, then he or she probably doesn't need to.

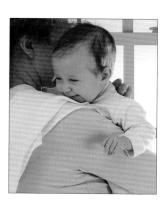

The simplest burping position involves holding the baby against your shoulder and gently rubbing or patting the back for a few minutes.

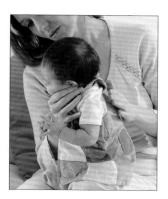

Alternatively, sit the baby on your knee, supporting the chin. Lean his or her chest on one hand and rub his or her back with the other.

Breast care and expressing

Even if you have breastfed a baby before, it can take your breasts some time to adapt to all the extra stimulation that they are getting. There is a lot you can do to prevent discomfort in the early weeks. Make sure you wear a proper nursing bra that fits properly. Most women find their breasts are a cup size bigger when their milk comes in, and a bra that is too small may cause your milk ducts to become blocked. You need three or four bras. Air your breasts often. If they are covered up whenever you are not feeding, warmth and moisture can build up, creating the ideal conditions for fungal infection. So expose your breasts to the air after every feed.

Don't wash your nipples with anything other than water – soap can be very drying and may encourage cracking. After each feed, rub a little breastmilk over the nipple and areola to keep them lubricated. Let them dry naturally. Eat

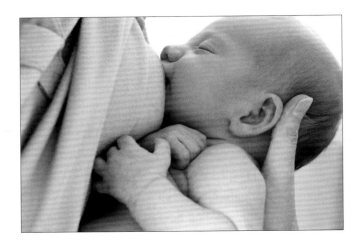

Wear loose, comfortable clothes that can be easily adjusted for feeding, especially in the first few weeks.

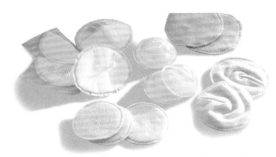

Breast pads protect your bra and clothing from leaking. You can get washable, reusable, unbleached ones, which are more environmentally friendly than the disposable sort. Plastic breast shells to collect the milk are helpful when expressing, or if your breast leaks a great deal when your baby is on the other nipple.

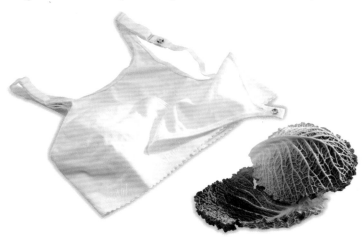

Your breasts may feel hard, hot and swollen when your milk first comes in. To relieve this, place a Savoy cabbage leaf, scored at the stem, inside each bra cup

healthily and frequently. Breastfeeding women need an extra 500 calories a day, more if nursing twins. It is very important not to diet, since this will affect your milk supply and reduce your energy. Drink lots of water. Most women get very thirsty when they are nursing. Have a large bottle of water next to you when you feed, and drink regularly at other times too.

WHAT TO EAT

Both you and the baby will benefit if you have a healthy diet. Your daily requirements for vitamins and minerals go up when you are breastfeeding, but you can easily meet them by eating at least five portions of fruits and vegetables a day, plus whole grains, dairy foods or other calcium-rich foods, oily and white fish, lean meat, pulses and nuts. A balanced diet includes some fat, which you can get from healthy sources such as avocado, olive and vegetable oil, and oily fish.

EXPRESSING MILK

Before you had your baby, you may have assumed that you would express often so that your partner could feed while you rested. In reality you may find that you have neither the time nor the inclination to express. But if your

CAUTION
Do not take any prescription or over-the-counter drugs without checking that they are safe for nursing mothers. Check with your pharmacist or doctor.

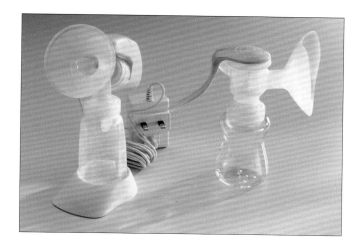

Electric breastpumps tend to be easier to use than hand ones. But expressing is a knack so don't worry if you get only a few drops at first.

baby is in special care, if you develop very sore or cracked nipples or if you have to go back to work, then expressing can be indispensable. There are three methods: by hand, by hand pump or by electric pump. Electric pumps tend to give the fastest results, but some women prefer a hand pump. Hand expressing is much slower, but it requires no equipment and can work very well for women who have a fast milk flow. If you know that you will need your baby to take a bottle, give expressed milk once a week from about six weeks.

STORING YOUR MILK

Expressed breastmilk can be stored in a completely clean, sterilized feeding bottle. Keep the bottle in the middle of the refrigerator (not in the door) for up to 24 hours. If you want to keep it longer, it is best to freeze it. When you are planning to use frozen milk, take it out of

FOOD AND DRINKS TO LIMIT OR AVOID

- Do not eat peanuts or peanut products if you, the father or close relatives of either of you suffer from hay fever, eczema, asthma or other allergies.
- Limit shark, fresh swordfish, marlin and fresh tuna to no more than one portion a week, and canned tuna to two cans a week. These fish contain traces of mercury.
- Cut out any foods that seem to upset your baby. Some babies react if their mothers eat spicy foods, citrus fruit or cows' milk. But don't feel you need to avoid such foods as a precautionary measure since very few babies are affected in this way.
- Avoid or at least restrict your intake of caffeine-rich drinks (coffee, tea, cola), since these can unsettle the baby.
- Do not drink much alcohol. An occasional glass of wine or beer should do no harm, but limit yourself to no more than one glass in a day and avoid drinking just before you feed your baby. The level of alcohol in your milk will drop over time, so if possible wait two hours before feeding again.

the freezer and place in the fridge to defrost for 12 hours. If you need it in a hurry, place the bottle in a bowl of hot water. Do not refreeze defrosted breastmilk.

One of the advantages of introducing a bottle feed is that fathers can take part in the profound bonding experience of feeding their baby.

Expressing by hand

Place warm flannels on your breasts or take a warm shower to encourage your milk to flow. Take a few moments to relax. Think about and look at your baby, or look at a photograph, to stimulate the let-down reflex.

1 Supporting your breast with one hand, use the other to stroke from the top of the breast to the nipple. Do this for 30 seconds or so, and be very gentle.

2 Cup the breast with your thumb and forefinger, placing them at the outer edge of the areola. Use a rhythmic squeeze and release motion, pushing your thumb and fingers slightly backwards (towards the chest wall) at the same time, until drops of milk appear.

3 Lean forward slightly so that you can collect the milk in a sterilized container as you continue to squeeze and release. Move your hand around the edge of the areola, so that you empty the breast. When the flow of milk slows, switch to the other breast. Repeat on both sides.

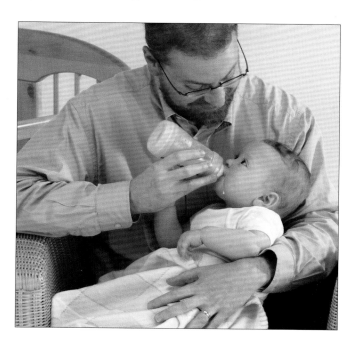

Common problems for nursing mothers

Breastfeeding problems often occur when a new mother is trying to do too much. So the best response is to take yourself off to bed for a couple of days with your baby. Ask someone else to take care of food and any chores so that you can concentrate on nursing. Frequent feeding and lots of rest can do a lot to help.

SORE NIPPLES

The problem new mothers complain about most – and with good reason – is sore nipples. Usually, soreness is due to incorrect positioning at the breast, so the best way to avoid it is to ensure that your baby is latched on properly every time. Rest assured that your nipples won't be sore all the time that you breastfeed – they will adjust and you will find latching on easier. In the meantime, you can help yourself in the following ways.

- Gently rub breastmilk over the nipple area after each feed and let it dry naturally. Airing the breasts regularly will also encourage healing – go topless when at home.
- Use lanolin cream to soften the nipples and heal any cracking. Calendula cream can also be used, but you need to wash off any residue before nursing your baby.
- Take the homeopathic remedy Castor equi.
- Do not restrict feeds, as this can cause the baby to grip the breast and suck harder.
- If all else fails, use nipple shields. These plastic caps cover the nipple while feeding. Some experts advise against using them because they can make it harder for your baby to suck, but they can be a good temporary

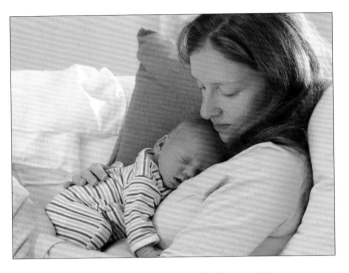

If you get a blocked duct, sore nipples or other breastfeeding problem, it may be a sign that you are doing too much. Spending one or two days in bed or on the sofa with your baby may be all you need to do.

measure if you are in pain, especially if the nipple is cracked. If milk collects behind the shield after your baby has been on the breast for a few minutes, then he or she is probably getting enough.

THRUSH

Occasionally, painful nipples may be due to the fungal infection thrush. If you have thrush, your nipples are likely to be red and itchy, and there may be white patches on them. In addition, you may be able to see white patches in the baby's mouth. You will both need to be treated, otherwise you will keep reinfecting each other.

The pain of thrush can make it hard to breastfeed, so it is important to treat it promptly. See your doctor for some antifungal gel: you spread it on your nipples and in the baby's mouth.

Occasionally, women get thrush in the milk ducts (which causes breast pain). This needs an oral antifungal treatment. It is also a good idea to take acidophilus supplements or eat bio-active yogurt to restore the "good" bacteria in your system: this keeps the thrush fungus naturally under control. You can also get a probiotic suitable for young babies from good health food stores. Some women find it helps to cut out sugar and yeast for a while.

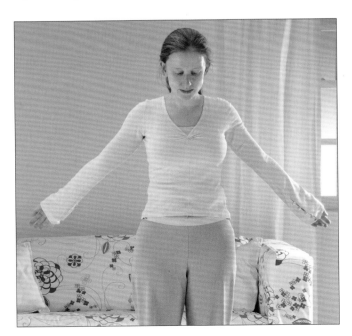

Arm swinging can help with blocked ducts or engorgement because it gets your milk flowing.

Thrush thrives in warm damp areas, so rinse your breasts after feeding (use plain water or a solution of one tablespoon vinegar in one cup of water) and expose to the air until dry. Be vigilant about hygiene: wash your hands with soap after using the toilet, before and after changing a nappy, and after feeding while treatment is ongoing. Use paper towels to dry your hands and discard; wash bath towels after each use in hot water (if possible, add a little white vinegar to the final rinse) Wash any toys or dummies in hot soapy water, then boil for 15 minutes.

BLOCKED DUCTS

If a milk duct becomes blocked, you'll notice a small hard lump in the breast. This may not hurt, but you need to clear it since an infection could develop, leading to mastitis. A blocked duct can be caused by a tight bra or by pressing your breast with a finger to make room for the baby's nose. It is often the result of the baby being latched on wrongly, so that some of the milk ducts are not being emptied. To treat a blocked duct:

- Change your bra or stop pressing on the breast.
- Apply warm flannels to the area before and between feeds. Some women find cold compresses (a packet of frozen peas wrapped in a small towel makes a good one) more helpful.
- Feed often (express if your baby is unwilling).
- Try an alternative feeding position so that your baby drains the breast from a different direction.
- While feeding, very gently stroke your fingers over the area and towards the nipple.
- Try arm circles before a feed, to help the milk flow.

MASTITIS

If a blockage is not cleared, then part of the breast can become inflamed. You will see a hot, red patch on the breast, which will feel hard. This is the early stage of mastitis. If it is left untreated, you will also get a high temperature and feel very ill (as if you have flu). If you

Mastitis starts with a hot, red patch on the breast. If you catch it early on, you may be able to avoid antibiotics.

react quickly enough, you may be able to treat mastitis by resting for a day or two (preferably in bed with your baby) and by following the advice for clearing a blocked duct. It is very important to keep feeding, and it is helpful to express any milk left in the breast after a feed to ensure that the breast is completely drained. A homeopath may recommend Belladonna or Hepar sulph, or you may want to take painkillers such as paracetamol (acetaminophen). See your doctor if you do not start to feel better after a day or so, or if you feel worse despite self-help measures.

If the mastitis is due to an infection in the breast, then it is best to take antibiotics to clear it. If it is left untreated, you may get a breast abscess. Many doctors recommend antibiotics at the first sign of mastitis. Most antibiotics are safe to take when you are breastfeeding, but they may cause your baby to become irritable or to produce stools that are looser than normal. To avoid another bout, be vigilant about positioning your baby correctly at the breast. If you get mastitis more than once you should discuss your technique with a breastfeeding counsellor.

ENGORGEMENT

If the baby goes a long time between feeds, milk can collect in your breasts, making them hard and swollen. Engorgement can also occur if the baby is incorrectly positioned, even for just one feed. To treat it:

- Have a warm bath or shower, or apply warm flannels to the area, then express a little milk before latching your baby on. Be gentle: engorged breasts bruise easily.
- Do some arm swinging before feeding.
- Use a cold compress on the breast to reduce swelling.
- Feed frequently, or express if your baby won't oblige.
- Try drinking fennel or marigold tea three times a day.

It is important that you keep feeding if you suffer from any breast problems. It is quite safe to do so: any bacteria will be destroyed by acids in your baby's stomach.

Herbal teas may ease breastfeeding problems. A fennel or fenugreek seed infusion is said to enhance milk supply, while marigold tea may help with blocked ducts.

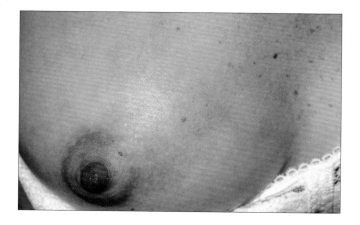

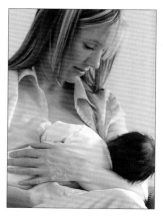

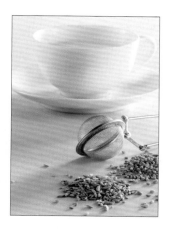

Common feeding problems

Most babies will quickly let you know if they have a problem with breastfeeding. They may cry during or after a feed, keep pulling off the breast or sometimes refuse point-blank to feed. This can be upsetting, but try not to take it as a personal rejection. Often there is a simple cause, which is commonly that the baby is not latching on properly. If it happens often and you can't work out why, a breastfeeding counsellor may be able to help. The following are all possible reasons for difficulty.

• If your breasts are engorged, your baby may find it hard to latch on. Express a little milk before the feed or hold a warm flannel against your breasts to help soften them a little.

• If your nipples are inverted or very flat, your baby may not be able to draw enough of the areola into his or her mouth (see box).

• Your milk flow may be so fast that it shocks the baby when he or she starts to suck. Try lying down or leaning well back (supported on lots of cushions) as you feed your baby. You can also try expressing a little milk just before the feed. Some women with a fast flow find that it helps to wear nipple shields while feeding.

• The baby may be frustrated when your milk flow slows down after the initial rush. Babies have to keep sucking in order to encourage more milk to be released from the production glands. If your baby stops feeding, it can help to switch to the other breast for a while before trying the first one again.

• Your milk supply may be low. There are several remedies you can try to enhance it (see below).

When breastfeeding goes well, it is deeply satisfying for mother and baby.

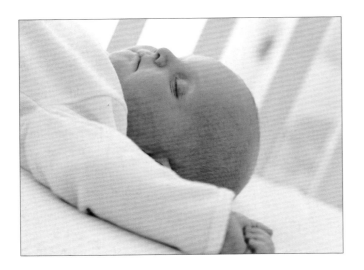

CORRECTING AN INVERTED NIPPLE

To help the baby grasp a flat or inverted nipple, take the areola between your thumb and first finger and gently press them together to push the nipple out. Then bring the baby towards you to latch on. Once the baby is attached, slowly release your fingers. Wearing breast shells between feeds can help to draw the nipples out.

• The baby may be windy. If your baby fusses halfway through a feed, he or she may need to be burped. Reflux, colic, teething or illness can also cause fussing.

• The baby may be distracted, particularly if he or she has just learned a new skill or if you are feeding in a noisy or unfamiliar place.

• You may have eaten or drunk something that the baby doesn't like.

• The baby may not be hungry. It's easy to get into the habit of nursing whenever your baby cries, but the problem may simply be that he or she is tired.

SLEEPY BABY

Some babies fall asleep after nursing for a few minutes, with the result that they need another feed very soon. This doesn't matter from time to time, but if it goes on you may want to encourage your baby to feed for longer.

• Make sure the baby is not too warm – feed in a cool room or remove a layer of clothing to help keep him or her awake.

• Rub the feet or walk your fingers up the back (either side of the spine) to keep the baby awake. Blow on his or her face, and stroke the cheek to stimulate the sucking reflex.

• Check that the baby's nose isn't squashed against your breast, since this can lead to sleepiness.

• Change the nappy halfway through a feed so that the baby is thoroughly awakened.

If your baby continues to be very sleepy and shows little interest in feeding, then he or she may be dehydrated or ill. See your doctor if you think this may be the case.

POOR WEIGHT GAIN

If your baby isn't gaining enough weight, don't be too quick to assume you can't make enough milk for his or her needs. A concerted effort to increase your milk flow can often solve the problem. Make sure you are getting

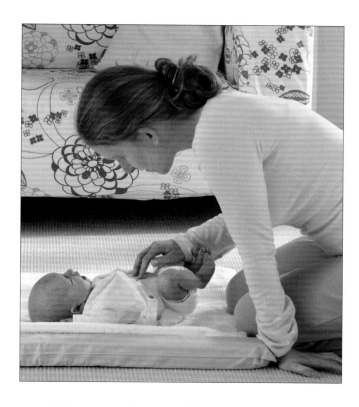

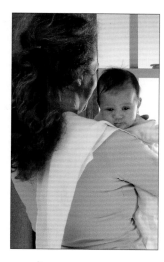

Left: It's hard to wake a sleepy baby. If you feel your baby has fallen asleep before they have enough, changing his or her nappy halfway through a feed will usually wake them up.

Right: There is not a lot you can do to prevent your baby from spitting up, but a cotton muslin will protect your clothes.

enough to drink and to eat – if you are dieting, it will be difficult for you to breastfeed. If you can, take your baby to bed with you for a couple of days; otherwise, spend as much time as possible together and feed frequently. Offer both breasts at each feed (starting on alternate ones each time). As with all breastfeeding problems, it is also worth checking your latching on, since if the baby is not attached to the breast in the right way he or she won't be able to empty it properly. Natural remedies for increasing milk supply include teas made from fennel, caraway or fenugreek seeds, nettle and blessed thistle. Certain foods such as oats and beans are also said to boost milk supply. In addition, it may be helpful to try to increase the fat content of your breastmilk by including more high-fat foods in your diet. Healthy options such as oily fish, nuts and avocados are best, but the odd bar of chocolate could help too.

SICKY BABY

Many breast- and bottle-fed babies bring up some milk after a feed, and some spit up quite a lot. This does not usually indicate a problem, so long as the baby is gaining weight normally, seems well and is producing wet nappies. But a baby who brings up part of a feed is likely to get hungry again quite soon. If the vomiting is frequent or forceful, the baby seems to be in pain or has watery stools, he or she needs to be seen by a doctor.

REFLUX

Some babies suffer from gastro-oesophageal reflux (heartburn). In this condition, the muscle at the entrance to the stomach doesn't close properly, which means that stomach acid can travel back into the oesophagus. The baby often brings up large amounts of milk after feeding and may have poor weight gain. He or she may be distressed during and after every feed.

Try to keep your baby upright during and after feeds – use a sling and feed standing up, or try lying back against pillows and feeding so that the baby's tummy is against yours and he or she is facing the breast. Make sure you are both relaxed during feeds (breastfed babies tend to have less severe reflux at night when there is less distraction). Skin-to-skin contact, warmth and quiet will help. A homeopath may recommend the remedy Chamomilla or Nux vomica to ease discomfort. See your doctor if the symptoms persist.

Holding the baby so he or she is more vertical than horizontal can help babies with reflux or those who struggle with a fast milk flow. Leaning backwards may also help. Keep your baby's tummy against yours.

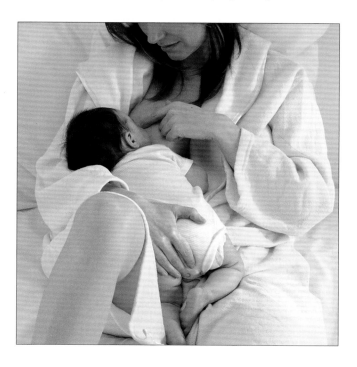

Deciding to bottle-feed

If you decide not to breastfeed, you will need to give your baby formula milk. Babies under the age of one can't have ordinary milk as their main drink because it contains too much salt and protein and not enough iron and other nutrients. Modern formula milks have been designed to resemble breastmilk as closely as possible. Most are based on cow's milk that has been modified to make it easier for babies to digest and to include the minerals and vitamins they need.

WHICH BABY MILK?

There is a huge range of baby milks on offer. Though there are not many differences between them, some do not contain added iron, which is recommended. If you want to use organic formula, the choice is easier because only a few brands are available.

There are two main types of formula: infant and follow-on. These have different ratios of the two main proteins in milk: whey and casein (curds). Infant milks are based on whey, which is more digestible. Follow-on milks are for babies of at least six months and contain more casein, which is denser and more satisfying. Some manufacturers also offer a casein-based milk for younger babies – often marketed as being for "the hungrier baby". It is best to start with an infant milk and to switch to a denser formula only if your baby seems to need it.

Formula milk is available in powdered form or ready-made in cartons. Ready-made milks are convenient if you are out and about, but they are expensive, so most

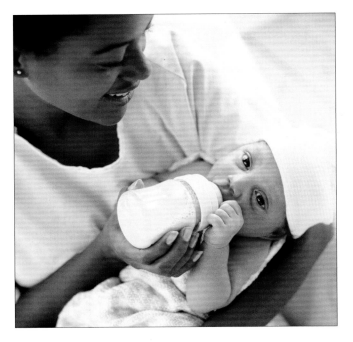

When possible, give your baby skin-to-skin contact during a feed and concentrate on your baby to replicate the nursing experience.

people use powdered milk, which needs to be mixed with boiled water. Most organic milks are available only in powdered form, though this may change as they become more popular.

ALTERNATIVE FORMULAS

If your baby proves to be allergic to baby milk (see box), he or she may be able to tolerate a special cow's milk formula called protein hydrolysate formula. In this milk, the proteins have been broken down into smaller particles to make them easier to digest. Health professionals can advise you on this.

Another alternative is soy-based formula, the only vegan option. Soy-based formulas contain high levels of the plant chemical phytoestrogen, which can have an adverse effect on thyroid function, so you should not use them before discussing the implications with your doctor.

If you are going to bottle-feed your baby, then you will need to sterilize the bottles to prevent tummy upsets. An electric sterilizer does the job quickly.

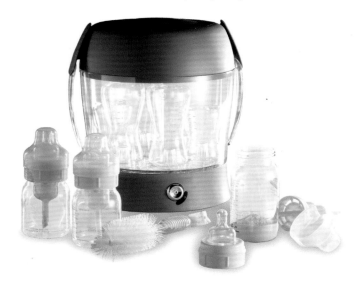

ALLERGIC TO FORMULA?
Signs of a true allergy include frequent diarrhoea, regular and forceful vomiting, excessive tiredness and skin rashes, but any of these symptoms should always be checked with a doctor since they may have other causes.

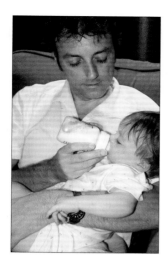

Left: Feeding time is a wonderful opportunity to sit quietly and cuddle your baby. Remember that sucking is a pleasure for the baby – concentrate on what you are doing together.

Right: Bottle-feeding allows the baby's father, or another person close to you to feed and bond with the baby.

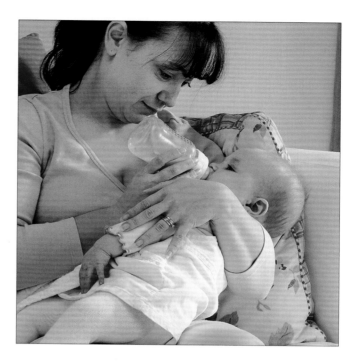

Some parents prefer to give their baby a formula based on goat's milk, which can be easier to digest than cow's milk. However, it contains some of the same proteins, so a baby who is allergic to cow's milk formula may also react to goat's milk formula.

BONDING OVER A BOTTLE

Drinking milk is not only nourishing for your baby, it is pleasurable too. So take your time with feeding, and make it a loving and relaxing experience. When possible, loosen your baby's clothing and place him or her on your chest so that you are skin-to-skin. Look at and talk softly to your baby during the feed. It will help mother and baby to bond if she is the one to give most of the bottles for the first few weeks, with the father or one other close person lending a hand.

Make sure you are comfortable and put a pillow under the arm you are using to hold the baby. You will need to hold the baby slightly upright (at a 45-degree angle), with

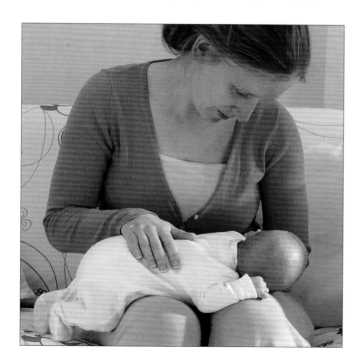

head well raised, so that the milk doesn't flow too fast. This will also help the baby to burp if necessary. To prevent the baby taking in too much air with the milk, hold the bottle up so that the teat is completely full. Never prop the bottle up and leave the baby to feed alone. Not only does this make feeding a rather lonely experience, it could lead to choking.

After the feed, help to release any air taken in with the milk by placing your baby against your shoulder and patting or rubbing the back until he or she burps. Sitting the baby on your lap, supporting the head with your hand or laying the baby on his or her tummy across your lap may also help. If any milk is left in the bottle you can keep it for up to an hour in case the baby wants more; after that it should be discarded.

HOW MUCH, HOW OFTEN?

Don't be in a hurry to put your baby on a feeding schedule. For the first few weeks, it is best to respond to the baby's needs and feed whenever he or she seems hungry. Babies' appetites vary and it will make both of you miserable if you restrict feeds or try to force the baby to accept more milk than he or she naturally takes. Offer the bottle whenever you think your baby wants it, and let him or her decide how much to drink – some babies will take a lot at one go and and then wait three to four hours before the next feed, others like to take less but feed more frequently. Over time, the gaps between feeds will get longer and you'll be able to plan your day around your baby's natural feeding pattern.

Experiment to find the best way of winding your baby. Try laying the baby across your lap, keeping the head slightly higher than his or her body.

Bottle-feeding basics

You will need at least six bottles and teats. You can reuse another baby's bottles, so long as they are not scratched, but you should always buy new teats, and there are lots of different ones on the market. Teats have different flow rates: slow, medium and fast. Generally, if your baby empties the bottle in just a few minutes, the flow rate may be too fast; if the feed takes half an hour or longer, the flow rate may be too slow.

If your bottles have wide necks, you can mix up the feed in them. If not, you will need a measuring jug and a plastic fork or knife (of a type that can be sterilized) for mixing the formula. You'll also need a bottlebrush and sterilizing equipment.

KEEPING CLEAN

Bacteria multiply quickly in milk, so it is vital that any bottles you use are scrupulously clean and sterilized to protect your baby from gastroenteritis and tummy upsets. Always wash bottles in hot water and washing-up liquid, and use a bottlebrush to clean around the rim of the bottle and the screw top. Squeeze washing-up liquid into the teat and use your fingers to clean it, turning it inside out to ensure that no residue remains. Rinse in hot water and then sterilize.

You should always wash your hands with soap and water before giving your baby a feed, and before making up the milk. Don't keep milk at room temperature for more than an hour or so, and always throw away any milk left over at the end of a feed.

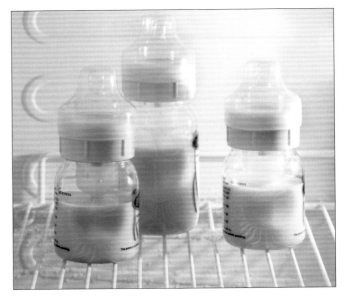

Always keep bottles of formula in the refrigerator once you have made them up. It is important to keep them cold to prevent bacteria from multiplying. If you haven't used the bottles within 24 hours, discard the milk.

WHICH STERILIZING METHOD?

Steam sterilizer units are the easiest and quickest way to sterilize feeding equipment, and don't use any chemicals. You simply add a little water, close the lid and switch on.

Boiling needs no special equipment except a large, lidded pan, which you should keep just for sterilizing. Fill with cold water, add the bottles and lids and submerge completely (making sure that no air is trapped in them), then boil for ten minutes with the lid on. Don't take the lid off until you need the equipment: once you remove the lid the water is no longer sterile, so you must take everything out (wash your hands before doing this).

Chemical sterilizing can be a useful method if you are away from home, but it is probably too time-consuming for general use. You can buy a cold-water sterilizing unit or use any large container, such as a bucket, with a lid. You will also need sterilizing solution or tablets. Make up the solution according to the manufacturer's instructions, and add to the bucket. Immerse the bottles, lids and teats

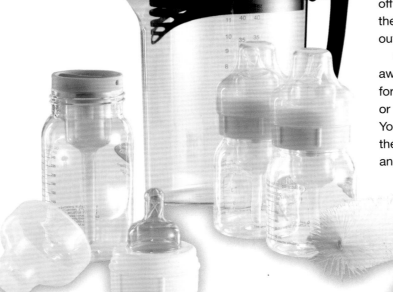

Before you embark on bottle-feeding, you need to have all the necessary equipment, including enough bottles to see you through 24 hours, a bottle brush, measuring jug, and plastic cutlery that can be sterilized.

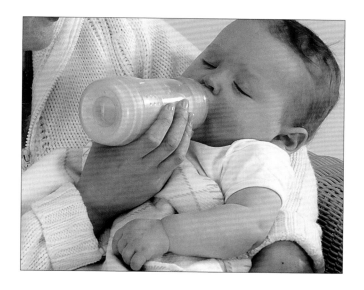

WHICH BOTTLE?

Many plastic baby bottles are made from polycarbonate plastic, which contains the hormone-disrupting chemical Bisphenol A. Minute amounts of this chemical may leak into the baby's milk, especially when the bottle is heated, or if the surface is scratched. Although the risks are very small, as a precaution you may want to buy bottles made from heat-resistant toughened glass (which can also be recycled) or from polypropylene plastic, which does not contain Bisphenol A. Check on the internet for manufacturers of suitable brands.

Some babies don't mind drinking milk cold, but most prefer it to be the same temperature as breastmilk.

completely (making sure that no air is trapped in them) and use a plate to weigh them down. Leave for at least two hours, or as specified by the chemical manufacturer. Wash your hands before taking out the bottles. If you want to rinse off the chemical solution, use boiled, cooled water, not tap water (which isn't sterile).

When your baby is ready for a feed, take the bottle from the fridge and heat in a bowl of hot water, keeping it out of children's reach. Shake the bottle, then test the temperature with a few drops on your wrist.

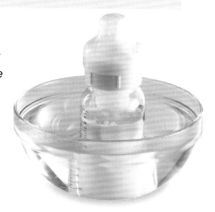

Making up a feed

You can make up each feed as you need it, but it will save time if you prepare all the bottles your baby will need for 24 hours in one go. It also means that if you've got a furiously hungry baby you have the vital feed ready at hand.

Put the caps on the bottles and store them in the fridge until required. Make sure everything you use for making up the feed – bottles, tops, teats, measuring jug, plastic knife and fork – is clean and sterile.

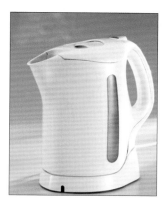

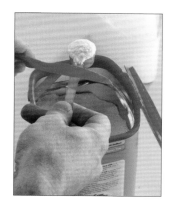

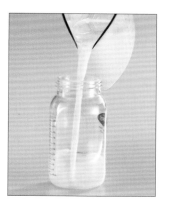

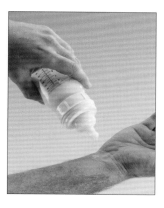

1 Always use freshly boiled water: empty the kettle, rinse it and fill with cold water. Boil, then leave it to cool. Wash your hands. Pour the correct amount of water into a measuring jug, or directly into bottles.

2 Add the exact number of scoops of formula recommended by the manufacturer (usually, one level scoop per 30ml/1fl oz water). Overfill the scoop and then level off the powder using the back of a sterile knife. Do not pack the powder down.

3 If you are using a jug, stir with a fork to mix, then pour the formula into the bottles. If you are mixing in the bottle, add the teat, the disc and the cap and shake well to mix. When all the bottles are full, put them in the centre of the fridge so they chill quickly.

4 Before a feed, warm the milk in a bowl of hot (not boiling) water. Don't use a microwave oven, which heats unevenly and can cause hot spots. Test it is at blood temperature by shaking a few drops on to your wrist; it should feel neither hot nor cold.

Crying, responding and sleeping

> ❝ As babies get older they are more interested in noise, colour and movement, and will respond to your efforts to entertain them. ❞

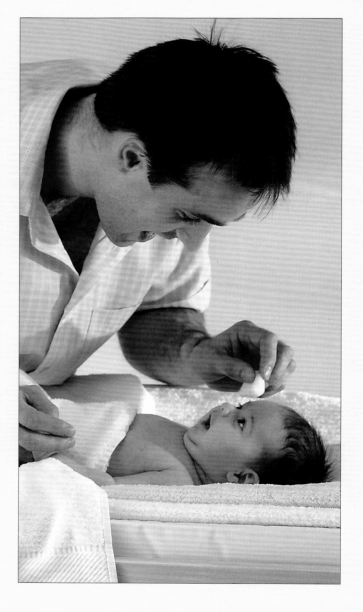

I t's normal for babies to cry. It is the only way that they can communicate with us, to let us know when they are hungry, cold, uncomfortable or lonely. But some babies definitely cry more than others. A British study, conducted in Manchester, found that the amount young babies cried over the course of a day could be as little as a few minutes or as much as five hours.

Many babies are naturally easy-going. They cry only for obvious reasons, such as hunger or when they are startled. They may also be easy to soothe, once you have worked out what they like best: being rocked or sung to perhaps.

If your baby cries a lot, it is very easy to feel that you are doing something wrong. It is true that there is sometimes a clear cause for frequent crying, such as illness or persistent hunger, which obviously needs to be addressed. But often babies who cry a lot are highly sensitive, and simply find it hard to cope with all the stimuli that they are bombarded with in a normal day. If this is the case with your

There is no doubt that some babies are easier to care for than others. If you have a high-need baby, the calm moments can be all the more special.

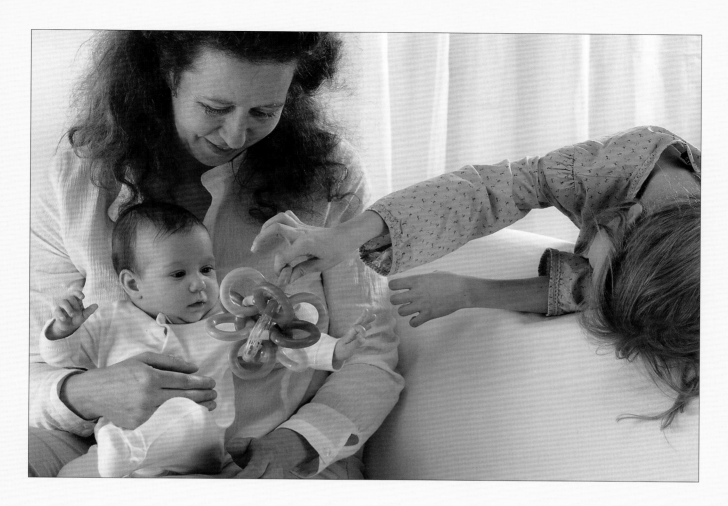

baby, you will have to call on all your reserves of compassion and patience to nurture him or her through this tricky stage. It can be very helpful to remember that it won't go on forever: sensitive babies often settle down after three or four months. This is also the time when you can expect your baby's sleep pattern to begin to coincide more with yours. Very young babies don't distinguish between night and day and, if anything, they tend to be more wakeful at night.

There is a lot you can do to help your baby sleep better right from the start. But, like so many aspects of parenting, having a relaxed attitude and realistic expectations is important and will help you to cope with the inevitable disturbances and disruptions to your painstakingly established routines.

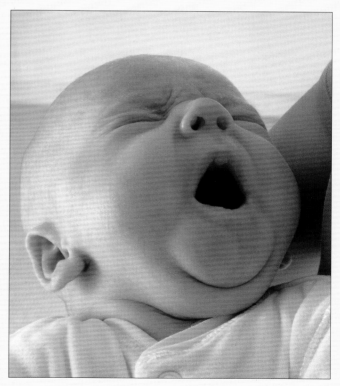

Top: As babies get older they become more interested in noise, colour and movement, and will start to respond to your efforts to entertain them.

Babies have all sorts of new things to look at and experience in a day. It's not surprising that they can become overwhelmed in these early months.

Why babies cry

Crying is the only way a very young baby can communicate. And it is a very effective method for the baby to get attention: when you rush to soothe your crying baby, you are doing what comes naturally to parents all over the world. Babies cry in different ways depending on what is wrong. In time you will learn to distinguish between cries, and recognize the different sounds your baby makes when hungry, uncomfortable or overtired. You may also start to pick up on certain gestures – for example, arching the back when windy – or you may become more aware of what triggers your baby's distress – such as too much handling by visitors.

CHECKLIST: WHY IS MY BABY CRYING?
In the early days, discovering why your baby is crying is a matter of trial and error. It's helpful to have a mental checklist of possible causes that you can run through to help you pinpoint the cause.

Is the baby hungry? Young babies can get hungry more quickly than you would think possible. They go through growth spurts, which means they suddenly need to feed more than usual. So even if you have fed your baby very recently, crying may mean he or she is hungry.

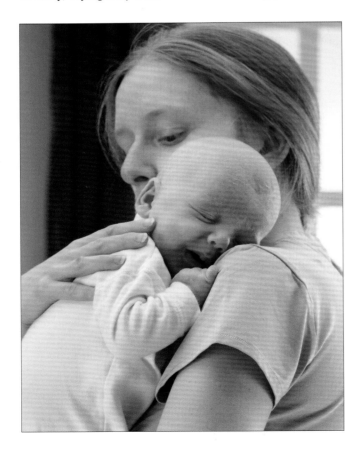

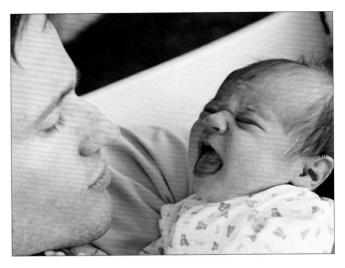

Don't worry that you are teaching your baby bad habits by attending to his or her cries. You are showing that you can be relied on to be there when needed.

Is the baby wet? Some infants hate feeling wet, and will scream when their nappy is dirty or a cloth nappy is damp. Others don't mind it at all.

Is the baby uncomfortable? Babies cry if they are too hot or cold, if their clothing is tight or uncomfortable, and sometimes when they are having a bowel movement. Check that the room is warm enough and that your baby is dressed appropriately. Make sure that clothing isn't rubbing, scratching or pressing against the skin. Check fingers and toes, too – perhaps a hair is wound tightly around a tiny digit. Have a look at the nappy (diaper) area – the cause may be a painful rash.

Has the baby been startled? New babies often jerk around a lot, especially when they are dropping off to sleep. A baby who is frightened – by a loud noise, say – will cry. All the baby needs is to be held close until he or she calms down. Swaddling or holding close can help your baby to feel secure and prevent any sudden movements that will be disturbing.

Does the baby dislike being naked? Some babies cry whenever they are changed or washed. If this is the case with yours, be as quick and gentle as you can. Laying a small towel over a naked baby's chest and tummy may help him or her feel more secure. Making eye contact, talking and singing may also be reassuring.

At difficult moments, focus on calming yourself down – if you are tense, you will find it harder to soothe your baby. Relax your shoulders and breathe slowly.

Has the baby got wind? Babies cry during or after a feed if they need burping, and some may need burping again later on when the milk is being digested. Sometimes they need to pass wind: it can help your baby to do this if you pat his or her bottom rhythmically. Your breastfed baby may also cry if you have eaten a particular food that he or she is sensitive to.

Is the baby ill? Babies who are crying in a different way than usual may be unwell. Check the baby over: is there a rash, a temperature, a runny nose or other signs of illness? Call a doctor if your baby is crying strangely or persistently, or looks or behaves unusually.

Is the baby overstimulated? Babies can become irritable if they get too much stimulation; they cry as a way of shutting out external noise. If your baby is tired and overstimulated, he or she will find it hard to drop off.

AM I SPOILING MY BABY?

Young babies are not capable of crying in order to manipulate you – their brains don't work that way. They cry because they have a need that isn't being met; making a noise is the only way that they can signal that something is wrong. It's important that your baby learns he or she is safe and can rely on you. Don't hesitate to pick the baby up for a cuddle whenever he or she is upset. In this way, you help to establish a relationship based on trust and love.

Researchers have found that the more quickly their carers respond to their cries, the more quickly and easily babies are soothed. In other words, if you leave your baby to cry for ten minutes in the hope that he or she will settle, it may take you much longer to calm him or her down. Other studies show that babies whose cries are quickly and consistently responded to in the first months will develop into more independent toddlers than those who are often left to cry. So don't worry that you are teaching your baby bad habits by attending to his or her cries. You are letting the baby know that you can be relied on to be there when you are needed.

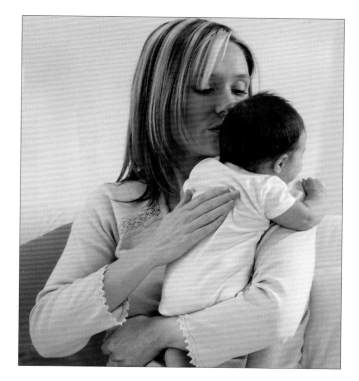

You will soon learn how to comfort your baby: some like to be held upright, others prefer being cradled.

Being held, rocked, or patted on the back is a good way to settle an overtired baby, but some seem to prefer being laid down in a quiet, dark place and allowed to cry for a minute or two, after which they will go to sleep.

Is the baby lonely? Babies need lots of physical contact, and will cry if they want to be picked up and cuddled. If you find it hard to hold your baby as much as he or she seems to want, take it in turns with a partner, enlist the help of a grandparent or friend, or use a sling to carry the baby while keeping your hands free.

You will often hear parents say that they are happy to leave their babies to cry so long as they know they are fed, burped and changed. But a baby may be crying simply because he or she feels fearful or lonely and needs your comforting presence.

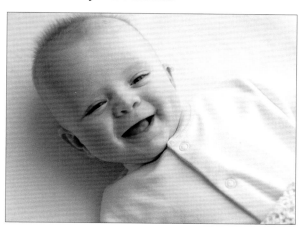

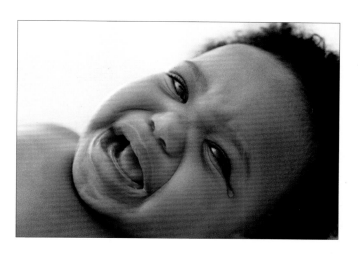

Soothing your baby

If your baby is crying, check the basics first: offer a feed and check for a wet or dirty nappy. Try burping to release any trapped air. If your baby is clean, fed and burped, but still crying, one or a combination of the following methods may be soothing.

GETTING PHYSICAL

Bear in mind that no one method works for all babies – finding out what calms your baby is a matter of experimentation, and nothing will work every time.

Hold the baby close. Physical contact has a calming effect, especially if you place your baby naked on your bare skin. Try shutting out any other stimuli by going into a dark, warm room. You may find that changing the way you hold the baby is also soothing – try an upright position or the colic hold (see Coping with Colic).

Try rocking. Most babies love to be swayed from side to side – it's the same movement they experienced in the womb. Researchers have found that parents automatically rock their children approximately in time with a heartbeat. If rocking doesn't seem to work for your baby, try upping the tempo a little – about 60 rocks a minute is good. Rocking your baby in a pram can also be very soothing, or you can use a sling and walk around.

Dance. If your baby is agitated, playing music or singing while you dance rhythmically with the baby in your arms

may help to soothe him or her. You can gradually slow the pace as the crying subsides.

Let the baby suck on something. Some babies are very "sucky" and like to nurse for comfort for long periods. If you are not breastfeeding – or if you are but your baby doesn't seem to want the breast – your clean little finger makes an excellent temporary pacifier. Dummies can also work well or you can try guiding your baby's own fingers to his or her mouth to suck on.

Keep the baby warm. A baby who feels warm and cosy may calm down more quickly. Heat the room to a comfortable temperature and wrap your baby in blankets or try swaddling (see Coping with Colic).

GOOD NOISE

Before birth, babies are exposed to constant noise from their mother's heartbeat, her muted voice and the low rumble of the womb. So similar kinds of noise can be comforting for distressed infants.

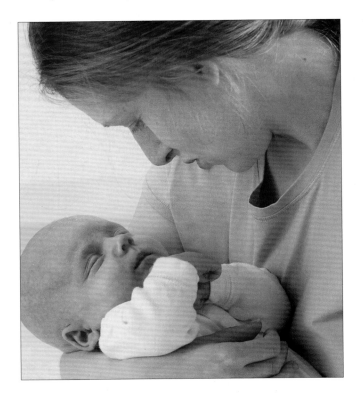

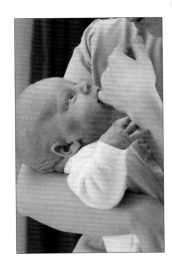

Left: Shushing helps to shut out extraneous noise and also relaxes the baby as it recalls the noise of the womb. This is why we instinctively use this sound to soothe babies.

Right: Holding your baby close for a while may be soothing, but you may also need to rock a crying baby, or offer your little finger to suck.

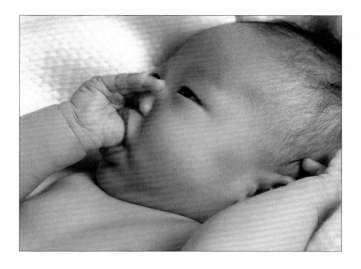

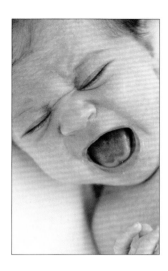

Left: Babies have been seen sucking a thumb in the womb – it is a great way of self-soothing.

Right: Long bouts of crying are rare in cultures where babies are carried all day, so it may just be that your crying baby wants to be held. Using a sling and more cuddling or nursing may reduce your baby's crying.

Shush. Shushing is a traditional and effective way to quieten a baby – simply place your mouth a little distance from your baby's ear and say "ssssshhhhhh". Do long shushes, increasing the volume if your baby doesn't seem to be responding.

Sing. The other sound traditionally used to soothe a baby is singing. It doesn't matter whether you have a good voice or not – your baby will appreciate your singing. It's worth learning a couple of lullabies for this purpose.

Use white noise. The roar of a vacuum cleaner, the hum of a washing machine or untuned radio static can all quieten a baby, sometimes in an instant. You can buy CDs of these sounds or record your own. It's not a good idea to operate a vacuum cleaner near your baby for long periods since this will affect the quality of the air that he or she is breathing.

Play music. Classical music has been shown to have a soothing effect on babies, and Mozart has been shown to be particularly good (no one knows why). But try light concertos rather than, say, operas.

CHANGE THE ENVIRONMENT

Consider your surroundings. If it is noisy and bright, with lots of activity, the baby may feel overwhelmed.

Take the baby somewhere quieter. Sometimes a change of place is all a baby needs to calm down.

Get some fresh air. Going outdoors will often stop a baby crying – and it can help you to relax too. Many babies fall asleep when driven around in a car for a while, even if they wake up the instant you stop the car.

Pass the baby to somebody else. If you haven't been able to soothe your baby, ask your partner or another close person to take a turn. Don't take it personally if the crying stops – it may just be that the change of company has distracted the baby.

A crying baby may be distracted from his or her distress by something new – an interesting toy, a funny noise or even a comical expression.

Try diversion. Offer a toy, walk in front of a mirror so that the baby can see his or her reflection, or walk around the house. Some babies find a warm bath very soothing; others don't.

AND FINALLY...

If all else fails, just stop trying to calm your baby down and accept the fact that for some reason he or she needs to cry. Continue to hold the baby close, but make a positive effort to release any tension that you might be feeling. Let your shoulders drop downward, take a long slow breath in and then out. Sit quietly for a few minutes, holding your crying child, controlling your breathing, and allowing yourself to accept the difficulty of the situation. If you can be relaxed about what is happening, you may well find that the baby stops crying in response.

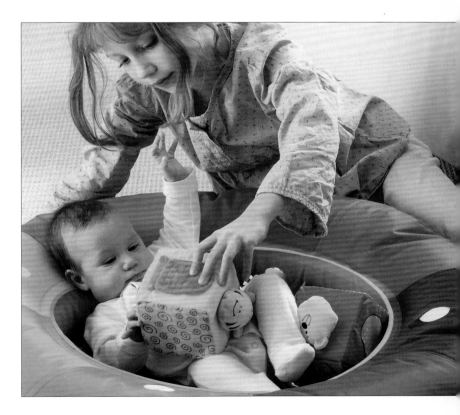

Baby massage routine

Massage is a wonderful way to build a loving bond of trust between parent and child, and can be a useful part of a bedtime routine. It has practical benefits, too: it can stimulate your baby's circulation and immature immune system, and it helps to improve the digestion. Massage is best done when your baby is already relaxed and calm, so aim to do it between feeds – a massage may be uncomfortable immediately after feeding, and if the baby is hungry he or she won't want to lie still. Don't try to do anything else, like watch TV, while you are

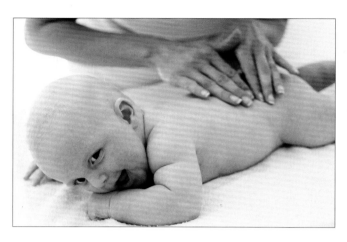

As your baby grows and becomes more robust, you can increase the pressure slightly, but never be firm or probing. Newborns should simply be gently stroked.

WHEN NOT TO MASSAGE
Check with your doctor or health adviser if your baby has health problems or if you have any doubts about the suitability of massage. Do not massage if your baby is ill or has a skin condition, and wait for 48 hours after immunization – longer if the baby has been adversely affected. Stop the massage if your baby doesn't enjoy it, and drop or adapt any movements that he or she does not seem to like.

massaging your baby – make this a quiet and precious time that you can both enjoy: go to a quiet place and switch off any bright overhead lights. As you massage, keep looking at your baby – smiling, chatting and singing will help to maintain his or her interest.

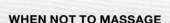

Massage techniques

You can massage your baby clothed or naked. A naked massage gives the skin-to-skin contact that babies enjoy, but use oil so your hands glide over the skin without pulling. An ordinary vegetable oil such as olive or sunflower is ideal. Make sure that the room is warm, and lay your baby on a thick towel so that he or she is comfortable (you can place a clean nappy under a naked baby). Take a few slow breaths to help you relax. Use light strokes that are just firm enough not to be ticklish – this routine is for babies of about one month or older. Do each stroke several times.

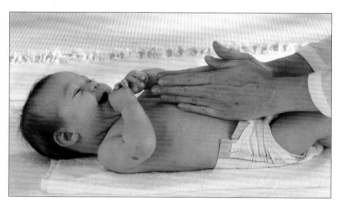

1 Lay your baby on his or her back and look into his or her eyes. Place your palms together and gently lay the sides of your little fingers on the centre of the baby's chest. Slowly open your hands, keeping the thumbs together and sliding the little fingers apart until your hands are flat on the baby's body. Stay like this for a few moments.

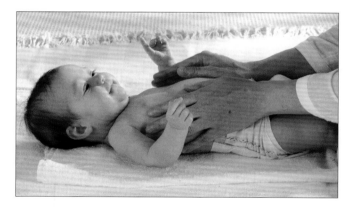

2 Tell your baby you are going to give him or her a massage. Slowly stroke down the baby's torso. Start by using both hands then turn your hand so that it covers the top of the baby's chest. Gently stroke down the torso. As you do so, place your other hand at the top of the baby's chest. Stroke one hand after the other in a smooth action.

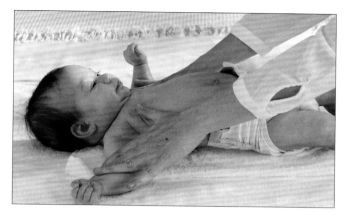

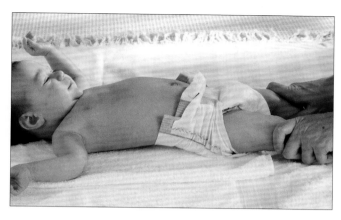

3 Rest your hands on the baby's chest and stroke upwards and outwards so that your hands pass down the baby's arms and hands.

4 Now stroke both hands all the way down the torso, gradually lengthening the strokes to include the baby's legs. Take the left leg in one hand, using the other to support the ankle. Work your way down the leg using a gentle squeezing action.

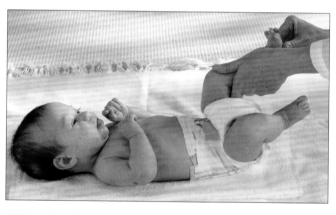

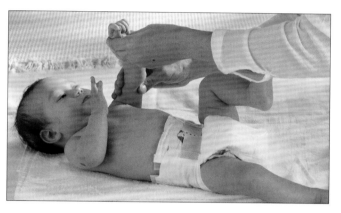

5 Take the left foot in your hand, supporting the heel with one hand. Use the thumb of your other hand to stroke over the sole, from the inner to the outer edge, and from the heel to the toe. Do the same on the right foot.

6 Now take the left arm in one hand, holding the baby's hand or wrist with your other hand. Work down the arm to the wrist, gently squeezing, then change hands so that you maintain a continuous action. Do the same on the right arm.

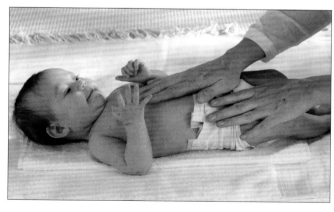

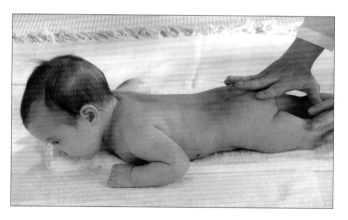

7 Gently rest your hand on the baby's abdomen and trace an arch from the bottom right of the trunk to the bottom left – this follows the digestive path. Take care not to press down.

8 Turn your baby over, remove the nappy if you want to. Place your hands over the shoulder blades and draw your hands all the way down the spine and over the back of the legs. Using the flat of your hand, trace an arch from the right buttock to the left one, then stroke down the back of the body again.

Coping with colic

A young baby who has regular and long bouts of inconsolable crying with no apparent cause is said to have colic. About one in five babies are affected. Nobody knows exactly what colic is or what causes it, but there are many theories. In a few cases, it may be caused by a cow's milk intolerance or, in breastfed babies, by a reaction to something in the mother's diet. The crying could also be due to discomfort from reflux or wind. However, in many cases, colic may simply be a sensitive baby's reaction to all the stimulation received during the day. The immature nervous system becomes overloaded and the baby expresses this through crying.

Colic is hard for parents to cope with, but it is important to remember that it does stop in time. Try to arrange for help at the time of day when your baby is likely to cry. If you find the crying unbearable, don't hesitate to get support: your doctor or health visitor should be sympathetic, or you can call a voluntary organisation such as Cry-sis. Remember that you can place the baby in a safe place – such as the cot – and go into another room if you need a breather.

IS IT COLIC?
Colic usually starts when a baby is two to four weeks old and lasts for up to four months. Babies are said to have colic when:
- they have lengthy bouts of crying on most days
- there is no obvious cause

Many colicky babies:
- have crying bouts at the same time each day, usually in the late afternoon or evening
- draw their knees up to their chest and clench their fists, as if they are in pain, and are red in the face
- may pass wind or have difficulty passing stools

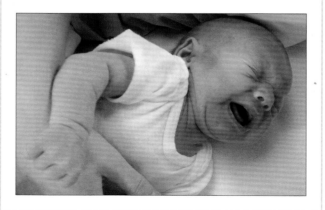

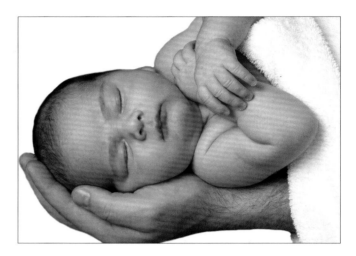

A small study of 28 babies found that cranial osteopathy reduced crying and improved sleep in colicky babies.

SOOTHING A COLICKY BABY
Reduce external stimuli – turn off overhead lights, music and the television. Then try doing all of the following, one after the other, or use the techniques separately.
- Swaddle your baby in a light blanket or shawl (see box)
- Hold the baby close so that you place gentle pressure on the abdomen: hold the baby along your forearm in the colic hold (see picture)
- Shush in the baby's ear or play white noise.
- Rock the baby in your arms.
- Give the baby something to suck on, such as your little finger or a dummy (pacifier).

USING A DUMMY OR PACIFIER
Babies love to suck. You can sometimes encourage a baby to suck on his or her own fingers or thumb by guiding them to the mouth. Alternatively you can give the baby a dummy (pacifier), which, used wisely, is useful if your baby needs to suck a lot.
- Never dip a dummy in sugar or honey.
- Don't use a string or ribbon to tie a dummy around the baby's neck.
- Don't use a dummy in the first six weeks if you are breastfeeding.
- Don't give your baby a dummy whenever he or she is upset (it will become a hard-to-break habit).
- Ideally, restrict use to sleep times and colic.
- Wash and sterilize dummies between each use.
- Throw a dummy away if it shows signs of damage.

SWADDLING YOUR BABY

Some babies prefer to be wrapped so their arms and hands are free. You will need a stretchy, light blanket or cotton sheet about 90cm/3ft square.

1 Place the sheet diagonally on a flat surface and fold down the top corner by about 15cm/6in. Place the baby so that his or her neck rests on the folded edge.

2 Straighten the baby's arm at the side, then pull one side of the blanket over the arm and across the body. Tuck it under the back at the opposite side.

3 Fold the bottom of the sheet over the feet and the baby's body. Tuck it into the first fold to secure it. Straighten the free arm, then pull the other side of the sheet over it and across the baby's body, as in step 2. Tuck it under the back on the opposite side.

WORTH A TRY?

One common over-the-counter remedy is simethicone. However, studies have shown it to be no more effective than a placebo. The following are proven to help some infants with colic, so may be worth trying with your baby.

- If you are bottle-feeding and think your baby may be allergic to formula, ask your doctor about using a hypoallergenic formula.
- If you are breastfeeding, take note of what you eat and see if certain foods seem to make your baby's colic worse. Tea, coffee and colas, dairy products, alcohol, spicy foods, citrus fruits, onions, garlic, cabbage, broccoli and cauliflower may all have an effect. If you notice a correlation, cut out the offending food for a few days to see if your baby cries less. If you cut out dairy products, make sure you get enough calcium from other food sources or a supplement.
- Consider taking your baby to a cranial osteopath for treatment. Sometimes the pressure of the delivery can cause slight misalignments in the way the flat bones of the skull join together, causing headaches and distress. A cranial osteopath will very gently manipulate the bones to relieve any pressure, and this can sometimes have a miraculous effect on a previously colicky baby.

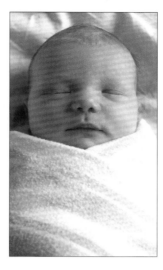
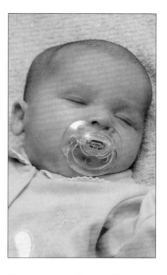

Many hospitals advise against swaddling at night because of the risk of overheating, but wrapping can be very soothing when you are awake and can keep an eye on your baby.

Some parents can't imagine life without dummies, others think they are an abomination. But, used wisely, they are useful if you have a baby who wants to comfort-suck a lot.

- To prevent wind and help with reflux, feed in an upright position and make sure you burp after every feed. If you are breastfeeding, get an expert to check your technique. If bottle-feeding, try using a teat with bigger holes; if they are too small, your baby may be swallowing lots of air with the milk.

For the colic hold, support the baby's crotch with your hand while the tummy rests on your forearm and the head is near your elbow. For the reverse colic hold, support the head with your hand; the baby's front rests on your forearm and the crotch on your elbow.

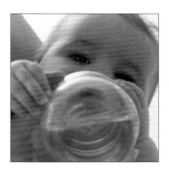

Cool, diluted chamomile or fennel tea can help to soothe a gripy tummy. Be very wary of other herbal remedies for colic – star anise used to be recommended but it has caused poisoning in some infants.

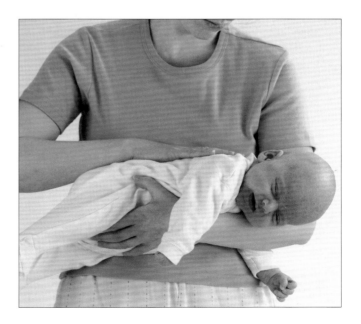

A place to sleep

Young babies sleep when they are tired, and they stay asleep as long as they need to. It doesn't matter to them whether they are in a cot or being carried through a crowded shopping centre. If your baby needs sleep, he or she will drop off without your help.

It is inevitable that your baby will fall asleep often when you are holding him or her, and cuddling a sleeping newborn is one of the silent joys of parenthood. But if this happens every time, your baby will associate sleeping with being held. As a rule, it is a good idea to put babies down when they are looking tired or yawning so that they learn to drop off in bed. It's impossible to do this all the time, especially if you are breastfeeding. But letting your baby fall asleep on his or her own sometimes will help establish good sleep patterns for the future.

If your baby protests at being put down, try stroking or patting him or her in the cot. Singing or playing soothing music can also help the baby to relax. A musical mobile can distract and lull the baby to sleep.

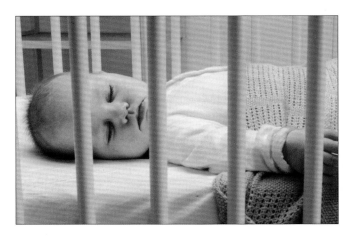

Putting your baby to sleep on his or her back is the best way to reduce the risk of SIDS. Some babies don't like this, but they will get used to it in time if you always put them on their backs. However, if you decide to let your baby sleep on one side, make sure the lower arm is to the front to prevent the baby from rolling forward.

CHECKLIST: SAFE SLEEP

All parents worry about their babies, and most find themselves checking on sleeping infants from time to time. The following steps reduce the risk of a baby suffering SIDS (sudden infant death syndrome).

- Always put your baby to sleep on his or her back.
- Put your baby to sleep on a firm mattress (not a sheepskin or pillow).
- Do not let anyone smoke near your baby (if possible, ban smoking from your home).
- Do not let your baby get too hot (or too cold) – keep the room temperature comfortable. Never put the cot next to a radiator or heater, or let your baby sleep with a hot-water bottle or electric blanket.
- Put the baby's feet at the base of the cot (the feet-to-foot position) so that he or she cannot wriggle down under the covers.
- Keep the baby's head uncovered. Make sure that covers reach no higher than the shoulders and are tucked in securely.
- Use sheets and thin blankets only (cellular blankets are ideal). Don't use duvets, pillows, wedges or bedding rolls.
- Don't use plastic sheets, cot bumpers or anything with strings or ribbons in your baby's bed. Keep toys out of the cot when your baby is sleeping.
- Seek medical advice promptly if your baby is ill.

A SNUG BED

Some babies happily sleep in a cot from birth, but most seem to prefer being in a cosier space (which is what, after all, they have been used to in the womb). A Moses basket, rocking crib or the carrycot from a pram are all suitable, and your baby can sleep in one until he or she gets too big for it, or is starting to roll over.

Your baby's mattress should be firm and clean – it is best to buy a new one for each baby. Choose one with a removable, washable waterproof covering or a complete PVC covering, and clean and air it regularly. Check that it fits well – there shouldn't be any gaps between the edges of the mattress and the sides of the cot.

A PLACE FOR NAPS

Opinions vary on whether it is best for your baby to be in the same place for every sleep, or whether it is helpful to differentiate between daytime naps and nighttime sleeping. Like many aspects of baby

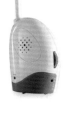

You don't need a baby monitor unless your baby's room is out of earshot. If you do get a monitor, choose one that monitors sound only – a breathing monitor can just increase your anxiety levels, which is counterproductive.

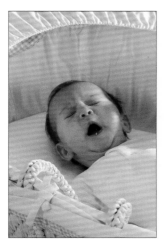
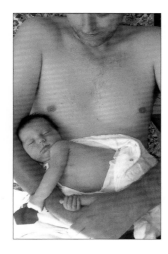
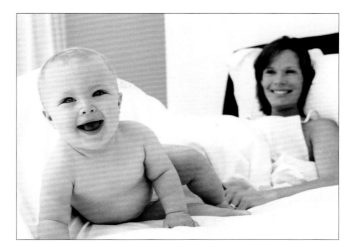

There is no need to keep everyone quiet while your baby naps. Young babies can sleep through normal household noise, and it is a good idea to get them used to this from the beginning.

care, it is down to what suits you and your baby best. You will probably find it easier to go out and about if your baby takes daytime naps in a pram. But some babies settle better when they are placed in their own cot in a darkened room. Experiment to see what works for you.

SLEEPING WITH YOUR BABY

It is recommended that your baby should share your room for at least six months. A baby who sleeps near his or her mother may be better able to regulate breathing. However, it is best for a young baby to sleep in a cot. An adult bed is not designed for a baby, who could become trapped between the mattress and headboard, or suffocate if a sleeping adult rolls on him or her.

Although a cot is the safest place for a baby to sleep, many mothers find that they do end up sharing their bed with their baby for part or all of the night. Bedsharing also makes breastfeeding easier – women who co-sleep tend to breastfeed for longer. A bedside cot can give you the best of both worlds. But ultimately you will make your own decision about what is right for you and your baby. If you decide to bedshare, there are some extra safety precautions you need to take into account.

WHEN NOT TO SLEEP WITH YOUR BABY
It may be inadvisable to bedshare with a premature or small-at-birth baby or a baby with a fever.
Never sleep with your baby:
• If you smoke.
• If you have drunk alcohol or taken drugs, or if you are ill or so tired that you may find it hard to respond to your baby.
• On a sofa or armchair.

Even if you don't sleep with your baby, you'll certainly enjoy spending time on your bed together.

• Sleep on a firm, flat mattress – not a sofa, armchair, waterbed, beanbag or soft and sagging mattress.
• Do not place the baby between you and your partner – fathers are less aware of their babies and so may be more likely to roll on top of them.
• Make sure that your baby cannot fall out of bed or be wedged between the side of the mattress and the wall. A guard rail is useful.
• Dress your baby in no more clothing than you would wear in bed yourself. Use lightweight covers for your baby, not the duvet.
• Make sure that the covers cannot cover the baby's head and that he or she can't wriggle under a pillow.
• Don't leave the baby alone in the bed.

If you have twins, you may like to put them in the same cot. A study by the University of Durham showed that putting twins in the same sleeping space was safe, provided all the safe sleep guidelines were followed.

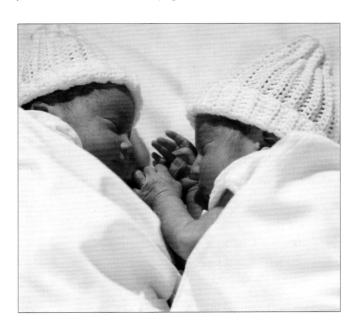

How babies sleep

Babies spend a lot of their time asleep, but they don't go about it in a way that is convenient for their parents. Small babies have lots of naps – an hour here, two or three there. This is because they have tiny stomachs and need feeding frequently. Bottle-fed babies tend to go longer than breastfed babies because formula milk takes longer to digest.

Unlike adults, young babies don't operate on a 24-hour cycle, and they don't distinguish between day and night. In the early weeks, there is very little you can do about this. So there is little point in trying to establish a sleep routine early on.

Gradually, your baby will adapt to the daily rhythm of light and dark. By the age of three or four months, most babies are sleeping about twice as much at night as during the day. Some babies may even sleep through the night at this stage, but most still wake up at least once a night to feed.

BABIES' SLEEP CYCLES
Like adults, babies sleep in cycles of active (dream) sleep and quiet sleep. A baby is more likely to wake at the end of one of these cycles, which usually last between 45 minutes and an hour. An adult cycle lasts up to two hours, but we usually don't remember waking up because we have learned ways of putting ourselves straight back to sleep.

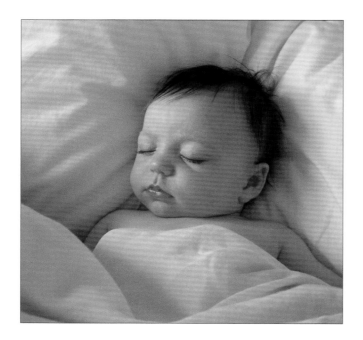

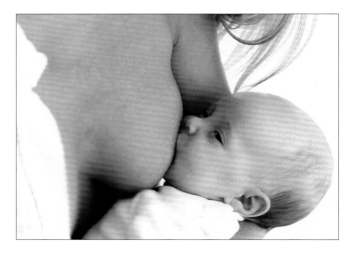

A good feed at bedtime will help to lull your baby into a long and restful sleep.

CREATING A GOOD SLEEPING ENVIRONMENT
You can encourage a young baby to get as much sleep as possible at night by providing a good sleeping environment for them.
- Keep the room warm (16–18°C/60–65°F). Make sure that your baby's cot isn't positioned in a draught.
- Darken the room. Use a low lamp to tend to your baby at night.
- Position the cot somewhere quiet. If it is near a window, outside noises may wake your baby up.
- Change your baby at night only when it's really necessary. Even then, keep activity to a minimum – speak as little as possible and only in a low voice.
- Similarly, make night feeds quiet and functional.

STRUCTURING THE DAY
Giving a baby a good daytime routine can help to improve nighttime sleep. If your baby tends to sleep late to make up for a restless night, try waking him or her up earlier to help the baby's body clock adjust to yours. Prioritize daytime sleep even if it means missing out on some activities or going for long walks in order to get your baby to drop off.

Young babies nap several times a day. Once they reach the age of three or four months, and start sleeping longer at night, they have longer periods of wakefulness during

The average newborn sleeps for about 16 hours a day – but yours may not need this much sleep, or may sleep much longer. Some babies get by on as little as eight hours a day.

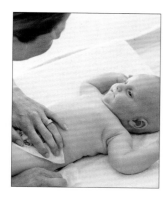

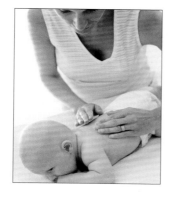

A set bedtime routine might be a warm bath, then being dressed before you do any final winding-down activities such as a feed.

A very gentle, soothing massage might be what your baby enjoys as part of the bedtime routine, but only if he or she finds it soothing.

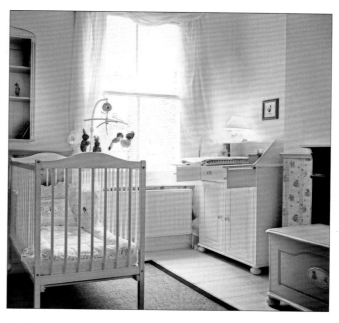

Babies need a quiet room to sleep in without too much stimulus. Keep toys hidden in cupboards and out of the cot, so that there is nothing to distract them from sleep.

the day. But they still need at least two naps. It is important to realize that babies get tired very quickly. Most need a nap about two hours after they wake up, and another longer nap in the early afternoon. So if they wake up at 7.00 am, they will need a sleep around 9.00 am and again at about midday. Young babies also need another sleep in the late afternoon (as may some older babies). It is best if this nap is kept short, though, or nighttime sleep will be affected. It's helpful to put your baby down for a sleep after a feed, which has a naturally soporific effect. Don't restrict daytime sleep in the hope that your baby will sleep better at night – it is likely to have the opposite effect. An overtired baby is likely to sleep fitfully at night.

Some babies take only short naps. If this is the case for yours, it may be worth noting the times when the baby wakes after first dropping off. Then try going to the cot a few minutes before the usual wake-up time and stroking or singing your baby back to sleep if there are signs of stirring. This may help the baby to sleep for longer, and eventually he or she should do this without you going in.

Schedule plenty of activity in the afternoon, then have extended calm-down time in the run up to bedtime. Most importantly, feed regularly. Some older babies are hard to feed during the day because they are distracted – and they then need to feed more at night. Feeding in a dark, quiet room can help them to concentrate.

A GOOD BEDTIME ROUTINE

Babies respond well to repetition, and an evening routine can help your baby to settle well at night. Three or four months is a good age to institute a bedtime routine, but you can start it earlier if you like. Try to stop boisterous play (such as tickling) at least an hour or so before the

Give your baby plenty of kick-around time. An active day can help a baby to sleep better at night.

baby's bedtime. Make this a quiet wind-down time, with gentle play. Your bedtime routine could include some of the following. It will help if you stick to the same elements in the same order each evening. But don't make a bedtime routine too complicated or it will take you ages to put your baby to bed.

• Warm bath
• Massage
• Being dressed in nightclothes
• Story or song
• Lights out
• Breastfeed or bottle
• Kiss and cuddle
• Time alone in the cot, perhaps with a musical mobile, a ticking clock, radio turned down low or a CD of lullabies to help lull the baby to sleep.

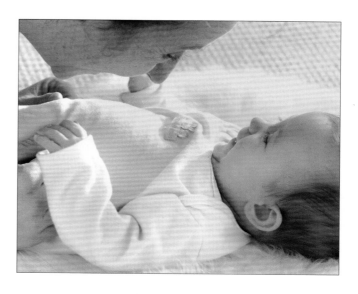

Helping a wakeful baby sleep

Most parents want their children to sleep through the night, but it is important to realize that in the early months most babies are unable to sleep for longer than five hours at a stretch. If your young baby goes from midnight to 5.00 am without waking, you can consider that to be sleeping through the night. By the end of the first year, your baby may sleep for 10–12 hours at a stretch. But many babies continue to wake up at least once at night. All babies will have wakeful periods from time to time, especially if they are teething or ill.

IMPROVING SLEEP

If your baby is still waking up several times a night after the age of three or four months, it may be that something is preventing him or her from sleeping longer. It is worth going through the following checklist to see if you can encourage a better sleeping pattern.

Is your baby getting enough fresh air? Research shows that babies who go out in daylight after 2.00 pm get a better night's sleep.

Is your baby having enough daytime naps? If a baby doesn't sleep much during the day, he or she may well have more disturbed sleep at night.

Is he or she sleeping too much during the day? Don't let your baby sleep for more than three hours at a time during the day, or night sleep may be affected. Keep naps in the late afternoon to no more than 30 minutes.

Is he or she getting enough stimulation? It is important to let your baby have a good kick-around on the floor and for you to provide new experiences to enjoy. Babies tend to be most alert in the afternoon and early evening, so this is a good time to take them out.

Make sure your baby has plenty of opportunity for stimulation and movement during the day.

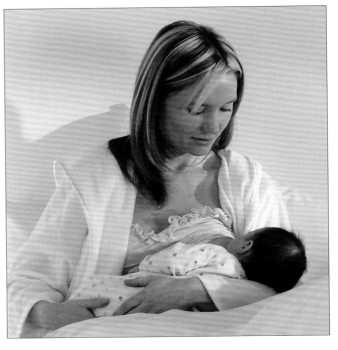

A study of English babies in 2003 found that fewer than a quarter of them were sleeping through the night by the age of ten months.

COMFORTERS

If your baby wakes in the night a comforter can help him or her get back to sleep. Provide the same soft toy or piece of cloth every time the baby goes to sleep. It will help if you imbue it with your scent – place it between you and the baby every time you breastfeed, or wear it next to your skin for a day or two. If your baby takes to the comforter, make sure you have at least one spare for when it is in the wash or in case it gets lost.

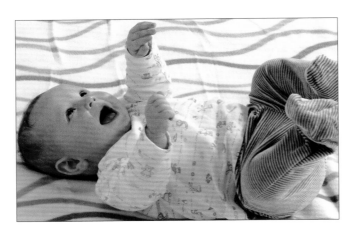

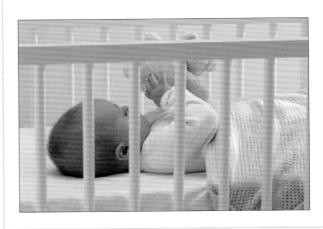

Is he or she getting too much stimulation? If your baby is being distracted when he or she is getting sleepy, it may be harder to drop off at night. Be alert to signs of tiredness: yawning, turning the head away, rubbing eyes.

Is he or she getting enough milk? A hungry baby may often be lulled back to sleep temporarily but will keep waking up until he or she is given milk. Both bottle-fed and breast-fed babies benefit from being given a feed at about 10.00 pm, or at the parents' bedtime, to help them sleep through the main part of the night.

Is bedtime early enough? Most babies like to go to sleep at 6.30–7.30 pm. If yours is getting to bed much later, try putting him or her to sleep 15 minutes earlier each evening until you reach this time.

Is the baby warm enough? If a baby is too cold, he or she will wake up. A baby sleeping bag is good if covers tend to be kicked off.

Is the room too light? Invest in blackout blinds if light from the street or the sun is waking your baby up.

Are your expectations too high? It is unrealistic to expect a young baby to sleep for many hours without a feed, especially if you are breastfeeding, because breastmilk is digested more quickly than formula.

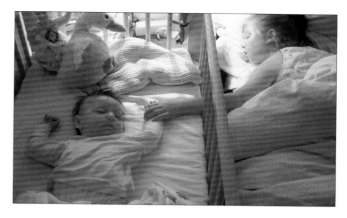

Your baby might settle more easily if he or she sleeps in the same room as an older sibling.

SHOULD YOU LEAVE A BABY TO CRY?

If you have a wakeful baby, then somebody may advise you to leave the baby to cry. But young babies are not old enough to assume that you are nearby. All they perceive is abandonment, so being left to cry may have a negative psychological effect. Even advocates of controlled crying say that sleep training shouldn't be tried with babies under the age of six months.

Gentle persuasion

If your baby tends to cry when put back down to sleep after a feed, he or she may want your company. If you want your baby to settle in the cot, try the following routine. You can also use this method to institute a regular bedtime. If the baby starts to cry at any point, revert to the previous action. You may find you have to run through the routine many, many times before your baby goes to sleep, but stay calm and persevere. Use the yoga exercise on the next page if you find yourself getting wound up, or let your partner take over. Don't feel you can't try again if you give up from time to time – if you repeat this routine regularly, your baby will eventually settle more easily.

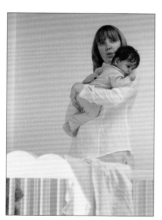
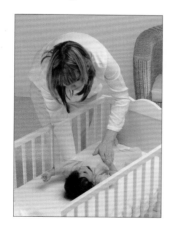
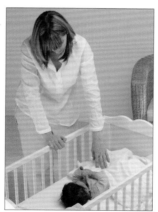
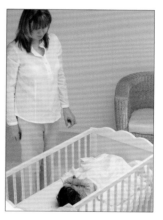

1 When your baby cries, go in to the room, don't put on the light. Pick the baby up and soothe him or her with quiet shushing noises. As soon as the baby is calm, lay him or her gently in the cot again.

2 Keep one arm under the baby. Stroke the baby's tummy with the other hand still shushing. If you use a dummy (pacifier), give it to the baby. Slowly slide the arm out from under the baby, with the other hand on the tummy.

3 Continue shushing. Gradually decrease the stroking, but leave your hand resting there for a few moments longer. Slowly take away your hand, and gradually reduce the volume of your shushing.

4 Move slowly away from the cot, still quietly shushing, until you are out of the room. If your baby protests, go back and put your hand on his or her tummy. Repeat the process if you need to stop the baby getting upset.

Coping with broken nights

Sleepless nights are probably the hardest aspect of parenthood. Every parent feels tired at some point, and some find the first weeks and months disappear in a blur of exhaustion. Accept that you will get less sleep than before you had your baby – disturbed nights can be easier to deal with if you are relaxed about them. Some breastfeeding mothers say that they come to enjoy night feeds as a quiet time to share with their babies. Many parents feel pleased to see their baby, whatever the time. The following techniques can all help you to deal with being woken at night and minimize sleep deprivation.

- Have everything you may need in the night to hand: nappies, cotton wool (cotton balls), warm water in a flask, a spare sleepsuit for the baby; a bottle of water for you. You'll get back to sleep more quickly if you haven't had to go hunting around the house for these.
- Wear nightclothes so that you don't get cold if you get up and you don't have to scrabble around for a T-shirt when the baby is crying.

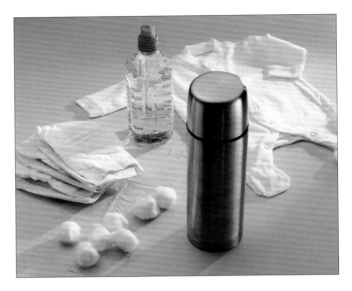

Being woken several times a night by your baby is hard. Keep fuss to the minimum by having everything you need to change the baby nearby.

Yoga relaxation exercise

This is a simple yoga pose that induces deep relaxation. You need at least ten minutes to relax fully. So it is best to do this exercise either when the baby has just gone down for a nap and is definitely asleep, or – better still – when there is somebody else in the house who can attend to the baby if he or she wakes.

Before you begin, make sure the room is warm and quiet – turn off any music, switch off the phone, close the curtains and ask anyone else in the house not to disturb you. Lie on a rug, yoga mat or large towel. You may like to cover yourself with a light blanket, and to put on some socks, to keep warm.

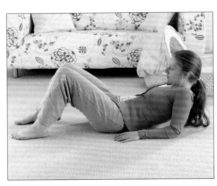

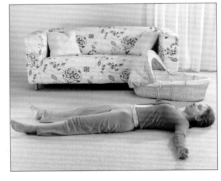

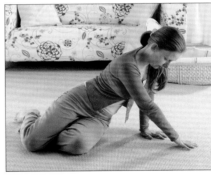

1 Sit on the floor, feet together and knees bent. Put your hands on either side of your buttocks. Slowly lie back, supporting your weight on your hands then elbows until you are lying flat, knees still bent. Lengthen the back of your neck as you put the back of your head on the floor. Stretch out your legs, feet apart.

2 If you feel discomfort in your lower back, place a cushion under your knees or leave them bent. Let your arms move comfortably out to your sides, palms upwards and fingers slightly curled. If your shoulders feel hunched, slide them down slightly. Close your eyes, relax and breathe for about ten minutes.

3 When you are ready to get up, bend your knees and roll over on to your left side. Come to a sitting position – taking your time – then get up slowly. Try to maintain slow steady breathing and a quiet frame of mind for a while. At the very least, don't instantly start to rush about.

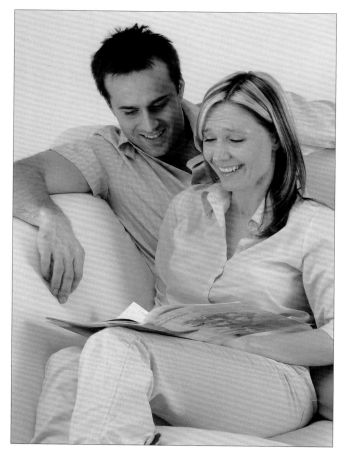

- Make yourself go to bed earlier than you might otherwise, even if you don't feel sleepy. If you find it hard to drop off, institute a nightly routine for yourself as well as for the baby. Have a warm bath, with a few drops of lavender or chamomile essential oil added to the water. Have a milky drink. Don't watch television in bed or read for long before sleep.
- During the day, grab a nap whenever the baby sleeps. Don't use the time to catch up on chores or phone calls if you are really tired; go to bed and rest. Even if you don't sleep, lying quietly will help replenish your energy.
- Eat well and healthily. Tiredness is harder to cope with if you are hungry.
- Practise deep breathing to calm the nervous system. Whenever you get a minute or two to yourself simply sit up straight, relax your shoulders and breathe.
- Consider taking time out to go to a yoga or pilates class. Check that the class is suitable for new mothers – ideally, go to a specialist class (you may be able to take the baby along or you may prefer to ask a friend, relative or your partner to babysit so that you can concentrate on your practice).
- Get out of the house at least once a day, even if you are feeling really tired. Fresh air and some kind of physical activity will do both you and the baby good and you may find the baby sleeps better at night if you provide plenty of stimulation during the day.

DEVELOPING A NIGHTTIME STRATEGY

It's a good idea to have a strategy for dealing with broken nights. Discuss this with your partner in advance. It's much better to decide beforehand who is going to do what than to try and negotiate in the middle of the night when neither of you is likely to be feeling very reasonable.

Be realistic. Some partners may not be able or willing to do any nighttime parenting, especially if they have to get up early to go to work, and if you are breastfeeding, most of the night care will inevitably fall to you. Whatever strategy you have, there will be times when you need to be flexible. A father or helper can help at night in the following ways.

- If you are bottle-feeding, by giving a feed last thing at night. That way, you can go to bed earlier and get a few hours of unbroken sleep.
- By rocking or walking around with a baby who is ill or can't settle after being fed.

It is easy to get irritable when you are very tired, so take time to connect with your partner. Ask someone to take care of the baby to allow you to spend an hour or two alone together.

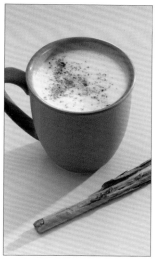

A drink of warm, cinnamon-spiced milk before you go to bed will help to relax you and encourage sleep.

- By getting the baby up in the morning so that you can get an extra hour's sleep.
- By taking care of the baby in the early evening, to give you a break.

Some new fathers opt to spend nights sleeping in the spare room or on the sofa. This can help both of you in the short term – your partner gets a full night's sleep (which may make him better able to help you at other times) and you may sleep better if you have the bed to yourself. But obviously it is not something either of you will want to do for long.

Development and play

" Every baby is an individual: each one develops at his or her own pace and in a different way from any other. "

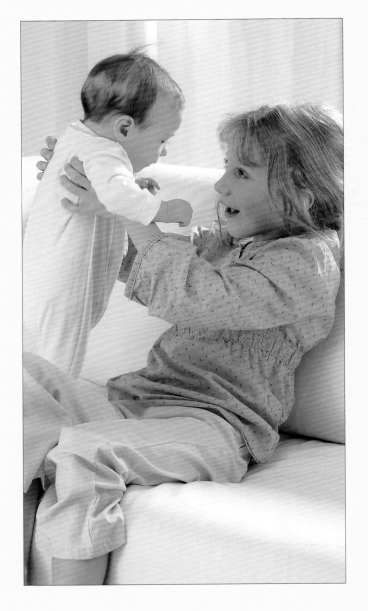

One of the real pleasures of parenthood is to watch your baby grow and develop. The tiny wriggling bundle you start with very soon becomes a fascinating child who sits up, laughs, babbles, and is curious about the world. Some changes happen suddenly – one day your baby is content to lie on a playmat, staring at a hanging toy; the next day he or she hits out at it. Other milestones, such as sitting up, take weeks of practice. And there are plateau periods, when your baby seems content simply to be. Doctors divide a baby's development into four key areas.

- Social development is about how your child interacts and responds to you and others, with smiles and little noises.
- Language development relates not only to how quickly and well a child learns to speak, but also to how much he or she understands what others say.
- Large motor development covers major physical actions such as sitting up, rolling over, crawling and walking.

The budding relationship between a baby and a sibling can be wonderful to watch. Babies often reward older children with the biggest smiles and belly laughs.

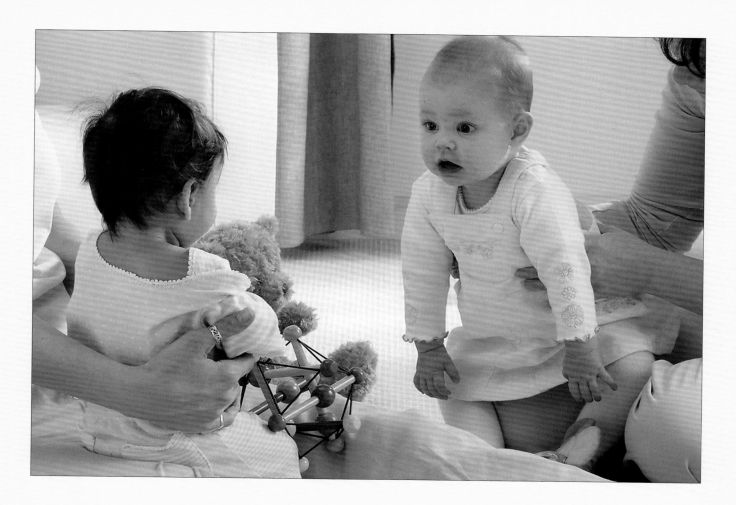

• Small motor development concerns more precise skills, including hand-to-eye coordination and the ability to hold and manipulate objects.

Health professionals will evaluate your baby's key achievements from time to time, to check that all is progressing normally. But if your child is late in developing certain skills, this doesn't necessarily mean there is something wrong. Every baby is an individual: each one develops at his or her own pace and in a different way. Some babies seem to learn new skills very easily, while others take longer to acquire them. Often a baby will be advanced in one area but late in others, and will forget about one skill for a while as he or she concentrates on learning something new.

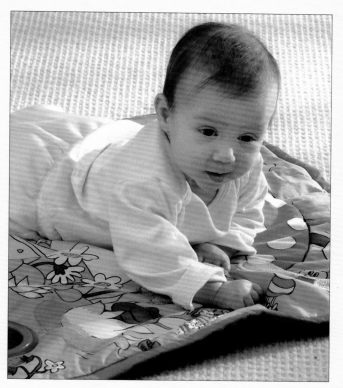

Top: Babies can be transfixed by other young children. At just a few months old, your baby may find another child much more fascinating than a new toy.

Your baby is preset to develop all the skills he or she needs. All you need to do is to provide him or her with a safe environment to explore.

Helping your baby to learn

Babies acquire new abilities when they are ready. As a parent, there isn't much that you can do to speed up this process. Pushing a child to learn a new skill before he or she is ready is at best pointless and at worst frustrating for you and potentially harmful for the child. However, you can make sure that your baby has a good environment for learning – one that is loving, stimulating and encouraging.

Babies are born with a drive to explore the world around them. The way they learn best is through human interaction, so lots of love and attention is what a baby needs most. Talk directly to your baby, sing to him or her, explain what is going on. Describe what you are doing as you, say, change a nappy, and point out interesting things when you are out together. Your baby won't understand the words you are using, of course, but will pick up on your interest and respond to it.

Until your baby can walk around and explore, you have to bring the world to the baby. Offer interesting things to look at and let the baby touch them. If you are looking at a plant in the garden, say, hold the baby close enough to reach out and grab it. Gently brush different materials – silk, cotton wool, corduroy – across the baby's skin to help him or her learn about texture.

Give your baby interesting things to smell, such as a citrus fruit or a lavender bag. Let the baby hold your watch or a sturdy necklace when sitting on your lap. From a few months old, your baby will start to put everything in his or her mouth: this is not an attempt to eat things, but an infant's primary mode of investigating physical objects.

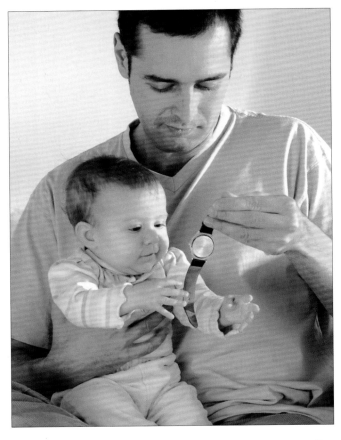

Babies need human company in order to develop well. A baby who spends hours each day in a cot or bouncy chair, without anything interesting to look at, will become bored and understimulated.

Sometimes a baby doesn't need a toy or other entertainment, he or she will be quite happy just watching you and following your movements.

While babies love to play with their parents, siblings and other close people, they don't need to be actively entertained all the time.

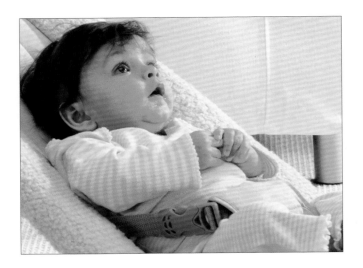

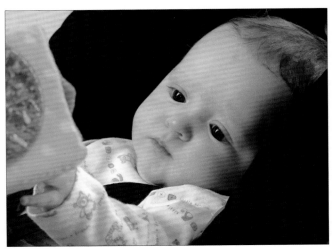

DEVELOPMENTAL MILESTONES

Keep a relaxed attitude to your baby's development. Most parents look at developmental charts at some time or other, and it is very easy to worry if your baby hasn't achieved a so-called "milestone" at the usual time. If your baby seems to be very late, or has missed several milestones, then discuss this with a health professional. But don't get too hung up on whether your child is "advanced" or "behind". The ages given for developmental milestones are simply statistical averages of certain easily observable behaviours. They are not an exam your baby has to pass. Reaching the stages early does not mean your child is phenomenally clever, and reaching them late does not imply anything about future academic achievement. Albert Einstein, one of the most incisive and original minds of the 20th century, was a "slow" child who did not start to talk until he was three.

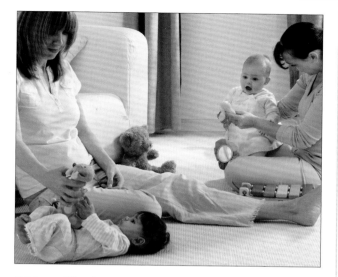

Mixing with other parents and babies gives you a good idea of how babies develop at different rates.

Lots of cuddles help babies to feel secure, and give a sense of a "base" from which to explore their surroundings. But that doesn't mean they have to be held all the time. In fact, it is good to let your baby see things from different positions. Put the Moses basket or pram in a variety of places where there are interesting things to look at. Lay the baby on his or her front sometimes, so that he or she gets a new viewpoint and can practise different movements such as lifting the head.

FOLLOW THE BABY

Tailor playtime to your baby's temperament, likes and dislikes. Some babies are very active from a young age and enjoy being tickled, say, or bounced up and down. Others are more nervous and prefer gentler play. It is important to be sensitive to your baby and not to persist with games that make him or her unhappy or scared. Similarly, don't let anyone else play with your baby in this way – it is quite common for men, in particular, to play rough games with baby boys in the mistaken belief that this will toughen them up. If your baby doesn't seem to be enjoying a game, put a stop to it.

Always follow your baby's lead. If he or she is enjoying a particular toy, don't try to introduce another one. Let the baby explore this one fully, show him or her what it does, and join in the game.

Try to pitch activities at your baby's level, or just above it. This makes playtime stimulating but fun. If your baby is

Introduce your baby to different textures by stroking fabric over his or her tummy or palm. Try something soft such as a square of velvet or a furry soft toy, and see how the baby reacts.

taking an interest in a particular toy, say, you could play peek-a-boo with it. The baby will appreciate the surprise and will soon learn that things are still there even when they can't be seen – a key human attribute. If the baby likes to hold a particular rattle, next time try offering one that is a different shape, size or colour to explore.

Be aware of your baby's moods. If he or she is hungry it is time for a feed, not playtime. And even when happily enjoying a toy, a baby won't want to play with it for more than a few minutes. Starting to cry, turning away or getting a glazed look are signs that the baby has had enough: follow these cues.

Above all, mark your baby's tiny successes with enthusiasm. Babies, like the rest of us, like to be encouraged. Use exaggerated facial expressions and a joyous tone of voice. Your smiles, claps and exclamations of "Clever baby!" will delight your child and make him or her want to try new things.

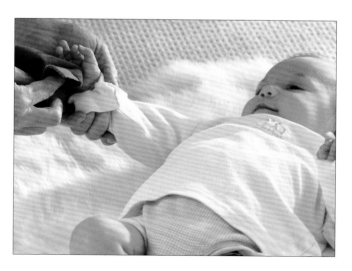

Seeing and hearing

People used to think that newborns were deaf and blind, but we now know that babies can see and hear from birth. Their vision is poor at first, but they can see almost as well as adults by the time they are eight months old. Hearing is the most developed sense in a newborn and is almost perfect by the time the baby is a month old.

SIGHT

The vision of newborn babies is limited and blurred, but they can focus on things that are 20–30cm/8–12in away. Faces are what interest babies most at this stage, but they will also be transfixed by simple patterns that have good contrast – try showing your baby simple black and white geometrical designs.

By two months, babies are able to track a moving object with both eyes. They are just starting to be able to distinguish colours at this point – they may show an interest in bright primary colours as well as more complicated patterns. This can be a good time to begin to show a baby colourful board books.

Babies start to get a sense of perspective by about four months, and this helps them with their new-found grasping skills. They are now able to focus on small

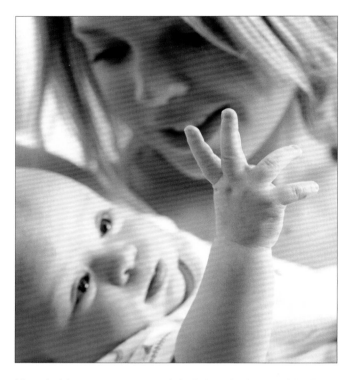

New babies are unaware of their hands, but suddenly they discover these fascinating things belong to them.

Check it out

Your baby's vision and hearing will be checked at routine developmental reviews, but it is important to see a doctor if you think your baby is not responding to sound or that there may be a problem with his or her sight. Many problems are easier to correct if they are picked up early on. You can check your child's hearing in the following ways, but don't panic if your baby doesn't respond: he or she may just be absorbed in something else, or be tired and distracted. Don't keep going; just give up and try again another time.

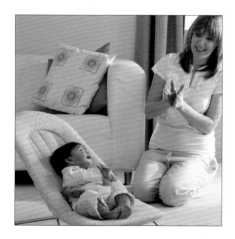

0–3 months: Clap your hands behind a baby's head (not by an ear). If the baby reacts, hearing is normal.

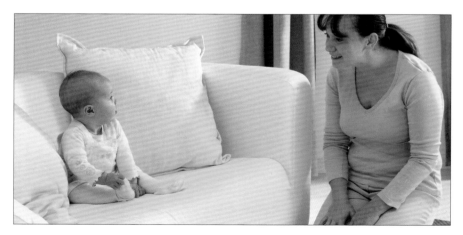

4–6 months: Call your baby's name to see if he or she turns to you. Babies of this age should also turn towards the source of an unusual sound – try tapping on a glass with a fork or making a squeaking noise.

Babies are born with perfect pitch and enjoy listening to all manner of soothing sounds – such as a ticking clock or a set of wind chimes.

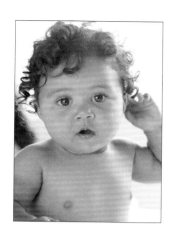

Babies are fascinated by shiny objects that catch the light. Try holding up a length of foil and watching your baby react.

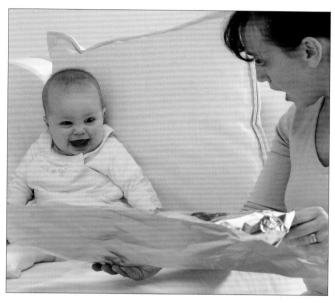

objects as well as large ones. Over the next month or so, they begin to spot small items from farther away, and get better at tracking moving objects. They also find it easier to distinguish between different colours.

HEARING

The sense of hearing develops in the womb, and there is evidence to suggest that babies can hear sounds outside the womb as early as 25 weeks. One study found that newborns could recognize the theme tune of the Australian soap opera *Neighbours* if their mothers had watched it regularly while pregnant.

From birth, babies are interested in human voices: they show a preference for their native language and they prefer their mother's voice to anyone else's. They also respond more keenly to high-pitched tones than low ones – most people sense this and automatically assume a higher pitch when they talk to babies. But even though your baby is listening intently to you, he or she may not turn towards you when you speak until the age of about three months. Babies also show an innate appreciation of music; they enjoy soothing music from birth, and they seem to prefer songs to purely instrumental music.

FIVE GOOD TOYS FOR YOUNG BABIES

Newborns babies don't need toys, but by three or four weeks old your baby will be able to appreciate some of the following.

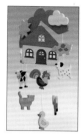

Mobile. A mobile makes a wonderful amusement. Hang it within easy focusing distance – ideally, about 25cm/10in away – and to the baby's right or left (babies usually lie with their head pointing to one side rather than upwards). Babies can't distinguish between colours until they are three months old, so choose one that has sharp contrasts – either black and white or bold colours.

Mirror. Babies are fascinated by their own reflection – although they don't understand that they are looking 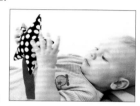 at themselves until they are well over a year old. Choose soft toys or books that have a special unbreakable mirror attached.

Black-and-white patterns. A new baby will be fascinated by geometric black-and-white patterns, and you should be able to find cloth books or soft toys that use these designs. Alternatively, draw some simple designs on paper and stick these to the wall next to the Moses basket.

Rattle. Babies are interested in noises so they like playing with rattles. Moving a rattle around helps to make the connection between cause and effect, as the baby learns that shaking the rattle makes a noise.

Baby gym. A baby gym can give your child months of pleasure. When lying on his or her front there are different textures, colours and sometimes sounds to enjoy. Lying on his or her back, the baby has space to kick around and toys to look at, swipe and grasp. Hang the toys in different places so that there are different ones to reach for.

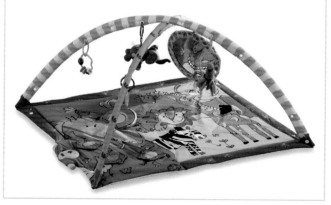

How movement develops

Newborns aren't able to control their movements, and any seemingly purposeful movements they make – such as sucking or grasping – are due to survival reflexes. However, both before and after birth babies will kick, fling out their arms and twist their bodies. These simple random movements strengthen the muscles and stimulate the nervous system. Gradually, your baby learns how to lift and move different parts of his or her body.

The development of motor control follows a set pattern in all babies: it moves from the top downwards and from the centre outwards. So, babies will learn to hold up their head long before they can move their legs. And they will use their arms to hit out at an object before they can close their hand in order to hold it.

HEAD CONTROL

In very young babies, the neck muscles are too weak to hold up the heavy head, so you need to support it whenever you hold your baby. By six weeks, there is some degree of head control: when held, babies start to lift their head up for a few seconds at a time, and may move it from side to side. They can keep their head steady when sitting in an infant carrier or a bouncy chair.

When they lie on their tummy, three-month-old babies will lift their head off the floor and turn it so that they can look around – a few babies are strong enough to do this when they are just a few weeks old. They won't do it for long at first, but as their strength grows, they'll start lifting up on their hands so that their shoulders come up too. This is an important precursor to crawling.

By four months, your baby will be able to keep his or her head up as you carry him or her around (though you may still need to support the head if you are performing an awkward manoeuvre, such as getting the baby into a

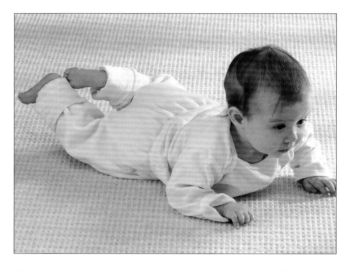

Head control develops very slowly, so you need to support your baby's head for several months. But he or she will try to lift the head from an early age.

car seat). And by six months most babies have developed neck muscles strong enough to keep themselves upright if their lower bodies are supported. Soon they will be able to sit up by themselves; some already can at this age.

ROCKING AND ROLLING

The first independent movement babies make is rolling (usually from their front on to their back). Instead of lying wherever you have placed your baby, he or she discovers how to get a toy that is just out of reach or change his or her viewpoint. It's hugely exciting for both of you, and once your baby has mastered the skill, he or she will roll at every opportunity. Babies sometimes roll from front to back as early as two months, but rolling from back to front takes greater control of the head and arms. It usually happens between five and seven months.

Because rolling sometimes happens without warning, it is essential that you never leave a baby unattended on a high surface (such as a bed or changing table). Don't turn away for a second.

TRYING TO SIT

Babies start trying to sit up from three or four months, once they have some head control. If you lay babies of this age on their back, they may lift up their head so that

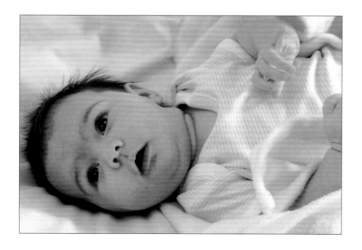

The first step towards rolling over is when a baby starts to crane the head while lying on the back. It takes many practice goes before he or she manages to flip over.

Encouraging rolling

Like all physical skills, rolling happens when your baby is ready. But you can encourage back to front rolling with a toy that they reach for. Make sure he or she is lying on a flat surface – a crumpled blanket will impede movement.

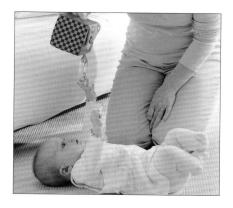

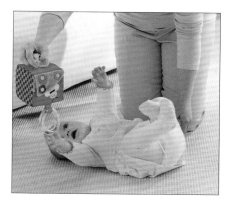

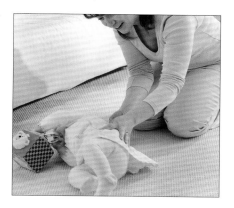

1 Lie your baby on his or her back. Attract your baby's attention by holidng a favourite toy above him or her, just out of reach.

2 Hold the toy away to one side to encourage the baby to stretch towards it, and begin to rock on to his or her side.

3 Gently hold the baby on his or her side for a few moments. Then slowly turn the baby on to his or her front, making sure he or she is happy.

Encouraging Sitting

Babies start trying to sit up from an early age. But they have to develop neck muscles strong enough to support the head. When this happens, your baby will enjoy being pulled to a sitting position.

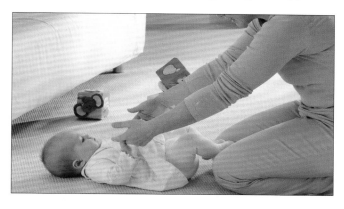

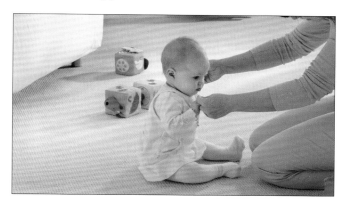

1 Wait until your baby is lying on his or her back. Offer the baby your hands and see if he or she tries to rise up. If so, you can gently help him or her come to a sitting position. Make sure that the neck stays in line with the body.

2 From a sitting position, you can slowly lower your baby back onto their back. Again, make sure that the neck is in line with the body. A few well-judged sound-effects – "dooooown", "uuuuuuup" – will make it more fun.

they can look around. If you give them your hands, they'll try to pull themselves up to a sitting position.

Babies enjoy being propped up so that they can see what is going on around them. A bouncy chair is ideal for this, especially one that can be adjusted from an almost reclining position to a more upright one as the baby's head control improves. When the neck and back muscles have strengthened to the extent that your baby is nearly sitting up (usually at about five or six months), you can use an L-shaped breastfeeding cushion or ordinary pillows to support him or her. Make sure that there are cushions all around so that the baby isn't hurt if he or she falls forward or sideways.

As soon as they master some head control, babies love to sit up and watch what is going on around them. Prop your baby up on some cushions for brief periods, but as he or she will inevitably slip gradually downwards, you'll have to be there to make sure he or she stays upright and doesn't topple over.

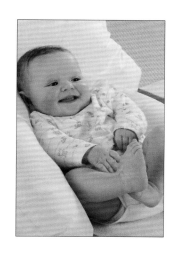

Fun with movement

All babies really need for the development of large motor control is a safe space to move about in. If they are always in a bouncy chair, sling or pushchair, they won't be able to learn how their body moves. So, give your baby plenty of time on the floor where he or she can enjoy a good wriggle around.

You can help your baby to practise his or her new-found muscle control by playing physical games. Always

From about six weeks, put your baby on his or her tummy often to practise lifting his or her head, which will strengthen the neck muscles. A few minutes a day is all that is needed. Sit on the floor close by and chat to encourage your baby to look up at you.

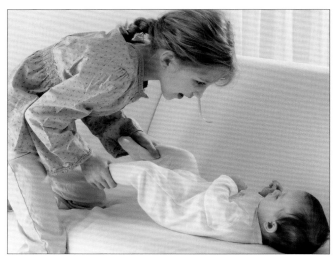

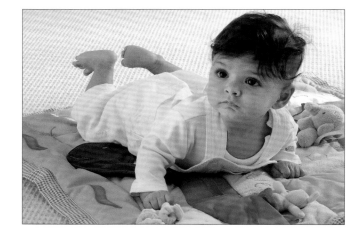

Babies love using their bodies. 'Bicycling' is a great way to help them experience a different movement.

be gentle and do what your baby seems to enjoy. When the baby is lying on his or her back, try bicycling: move the legs alternately towards the body, bending them into the chest and then stretching them out towards you. Lift the baby up into the air and move him or her around before bringing him or her back to the safety of your lap.

Give your baby lots of tummy time so that he or she can practise lifting up the head and upper body. Some babies don't like going on their tummies, but there are lots of ways you can make this fun. Get down there too,

Ball play

This little game of catch will keep your baby amused during his or her tummy time. It is also good exercise for the neck, arm and leg muscles, making it a good preparation for crawling. Stop as soon as your baby seems uncomfortable.

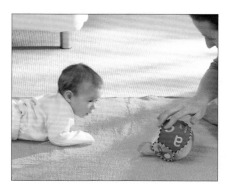

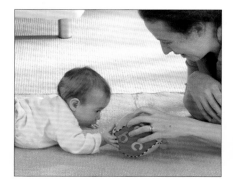

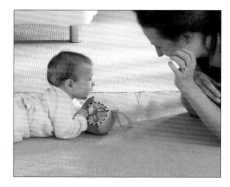

1 When your baby lifts his or her head, roll a ball about 60cm/2 ft in front of him or her. At first the baby will be content just to watch it move.

2 As he or she gets stronger, the baby will reach out to grab the ball as it rolls. Give lots of praise whenever this happens.

3 Always end the game by giving your baby the ball to play with. He or she is more likely to stay interested in a game than ends in success.

Baby yoga: wind-relieving posture

This aptly named yoga pose works on the digestive system and helps a baby to release any trapped wind. If your baby is windy or colicky, it is a good one to include in a massage routine, or you can just do it by itself.

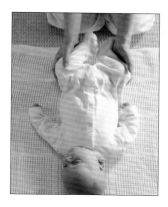 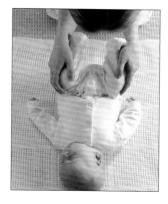 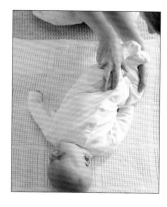 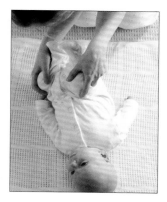

1 Place your baby on a blanket on the floor. Holding the baby's knees, open his or her legs out so that the knees are wider than the hips.

2 Slowly bring the knees to touch the body. Make the movement smooth and relaxed. Release the pressure, and then repeat twice more.

3 Keeping the baby's knees bent, bring the legs over to the left. Hold for a moment, pressing the knees gently into the side of the abdomen.

4 Release the pressure and slowly return the legs to the centre. Move them to the right and hold against the side of the abdomen. Repeat twice.

so that your baby doesn't feel scared: make eye contact, talk or sing, and make silly expressions to keep him or her amused. Use a playmat that has different textures and colours to explore. Place a mirror in front of the baby so that pushing up is rewarded by his or her own face.

Hold your baby under the arms so that he or she can "stand" on your lap; the baby will push down to straighten his or her legs and may enjoy bouncing up and down. Once he or she has good head control (at about five or six months) the baby will probably appreciate being in a baby bouncer for short periods. Some babies who can raise themselves up on their arms when lying on their front enjoy the "wheelbarrow" position: try lifting your baby's legs, then lowering them back down and repeating. Show the baby you are excited by these achievements by exclaiming, smiling and making plenty of eye contact.

BABY YOGA

Yoga helps babies to learn about and enjoy their bodies. If you are interested in baby yoga it is worth going to classes, but you can also do some simple movements at home. Babies are naturally flexible, so the postures are more like massage techniques than exercise, and you can easily incorporate them into a baby massage routine. But it is very important to be gentle; never force a movement or persist with the poses if your baby seems unhappy.

Baby yoga; butterfly pose

This is an adaptation of another favourite yoga pose, which works on the hips and pelvis.

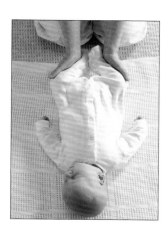

Babies have very flexible hip joints so they love this movement. Hold both your baby's ankles with your hands. Move the feet together so that the soles are touching. Gently push the feet into the abdomen, hold for a moment and then release. Then try pushing the legs slowly in and out in a rhythmic way.

CLASSES FOR BABIES

Baby classes of some kind are available in most areas. You could easily sign your baby up to a curriculum that involves baby yoga, baby gymnastics and baby swimming, as well as baby signing and baby music. All these can be fun. But be selective: cramming lots of classes into your baby's schedule may make him or her tired and cranky.

If you do choose to go to a class, pick one that feels relaxed and fun. Avoid any that make excessive promises about baby development, or that seem to foster a competitive spirit. Above all, don't feel that you are depriving your baby if you don't join any classes. Your baby can learn just as much at home, on simple outings and in parent-and-baby groups.

Handling and chewing

Newborn babies are born with the grasping reflex but it takes months before they can reach for an object and pick it up. During the first weeks of life, babies' hands are curled into fists. They may hold a small toy if they are given it, but won't really explore it for some weeks to come. At about eight weeks, your baby may start to hit out at objects, such as the items hanging on a play gym, or toys attached to the bouncy chair or pram. It is a good idea to make sure they are within arm's length, so that the baby doesn't become frustrated. At this stage, babies play with their own hands from time to time, but they don't yet realize that they actually belong to them – they won't look at their hands unless they happen to be in their line of vision.

From about eight weeks, babies start to open their hands. If given a small toy to play with, they will instinctively grasp it and may finger it for a little while. A noisy toy, such as a rattle, is ideal because the sound it makes will draw a baby's attention to his or her hands. By three months, babies' hands are their favourite playthings. They examine them intently, put them in their mouth, bring them together and apart again. They also enjoy batting toys within reach, and occasionally manage to grab hold of one.

All this activity helps to develop hand-to-eye coordination. By three or four months, babies can pick up large objects they see and will deliberately grasp a toy

A small wooden toy with moving parts like this one is perfect for fingering, and will keep your baby entertained for several minutes at a time.

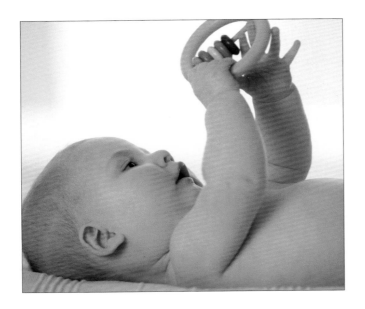

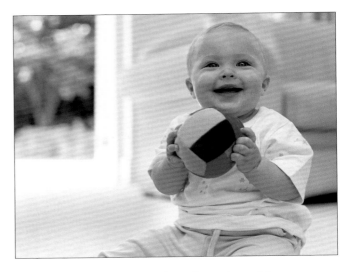

A soft ball can be grabbed easily and provides an interesting texture to explore. If it has a bell inside, then the amusement factor is even greater.

that is held out to them. Make sure that you give your baby the time he or she needs to reach out, though, as it can take a baby a little while to respond. Try using a squeaky toy to add to the fun.

Once babies can hold objects, they will put them in their mouth. The mouth has more nerve endings than the fingertips, so it is the best tool for exploration. This means that everything within reach of your baby should be safe for sucking. Don't give a baby anything that could be toxic or allow him or her to handle anything small enough to choke on (such as a string of beads).

By six months, babies can pass a toy from one hand to the other and reach for an object without looking at their hands as they do so. And they can work out whether a toy is within reach or not – they won't try to grab it if it is too far away.

GOOD TOYS FOR GRASPING

When your baby is at the swiping stage, hang an interesting mobile so that the items are within batting distance. A play gym is excellent for this, especially if you can move the toys around to keep up the baby's interest. Your baby can play with other things besides toys, of course. Household objects that have no sharp edges – such as a whisk, a set of measuring spoons or some plastic pots – are ideal for your tiny explorer. Once your baby can take hold of things, provide a range of toys to explore, including different sizes, textures, sounds and shapes, such as the following.

- Toys that have small protrusions for easy grabbing.
- Toys with two handles for passing from hand to hand.
- Toys that a baby can safely put in his or her mouth – this is good for teething.
- Toys that are brightly coloured with sharp contrasts.
- Toys that are interesting to feel – squishy fabric blocks, smooth plastic objects, soft toys, toys that have contrasting textures.
- Toys that make any kind of a noise, such as rattles and squeaky toys.

GRASPING GAME

A good game you can play to encourage grasping is to attach a brightly coloured soft toy to a piece of string or ribbon. Prop your baby up in a sitting position and then dangle it in front of him of her. When the baby reaches for it, say "Well done," with lots of smiles. Always end the game by giving the toy to the baby to play with, but detach the string or ribbon first.

TOYS AND SAFETY

Make sure that anything your baby plays with is safe. In particular make sure you follow these guidelines:
- A toy should not be small enough to fit completely into the baby's mouth.
- There should no detachable parts that are small enough to choke on.
- It should be lightweight, so that it will not hurt if your baby drops it on to his or her face when lying down.
- It should be made of non-toxic materials.
- A soft toy should be machine- or surface-washable. Check that the seams are securely sewn and make sure there are no trimmings, such as eyes, noses, buttons or ribbons that can be pulled or bitten off.
- All toys should meet the recognized safety standards.
- Don't give a toy that is intended for an older child to

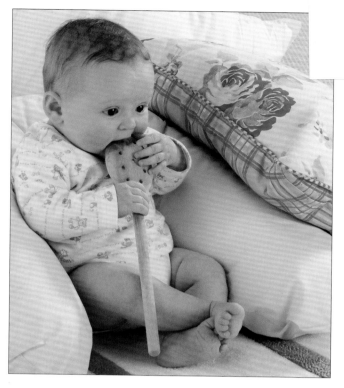

From two or three months, babies can hold objects and will lift them up to their mouths to suck. Small items of kitchen equipment hold as much fascination as any toy – try giving your baby a set of plastic measuring spoons, or a wooden spoon to explore.

your baby. Toys are labelled with recommended ages for safety reasons.
- Don't give a balloon to a baby. It may burst, which will be frightening, and if a small part of the balloon is swallowed it may cause choking.
- Don't attach a toy to a cot or pram with string or ribbon.
- Remove mobiles and other hanging objects once a baby begins to push up on hands or knees.

Once your baby can sit, he or she will enjoy knocking down a tower of bricks that you have built.

Encourage your baby to grasp by holding out a toy. If he or she reaches for it, give it to them.

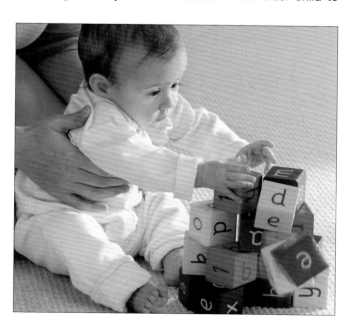

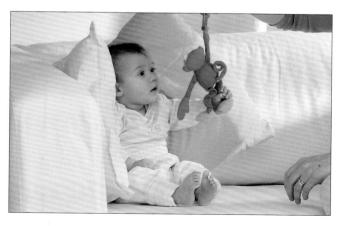

Sociability and language

Babies are social beings. Right from the start they need company, and are happiest when they are getting plenty of cuddles. Young babies don't have a sense of being a separate person – they don't know their hands are their own, for example, and they can't tell where their mother's body ends and theirs begins. They just instinctively know that it is good to be around people.

Young babies like to look at faces more than anything else, but they can't at first tell the difference between a real face and a picture, and they cannot recognize expression: a scary face is just as interesting and enjoyable to a tiny baby as a smiling one.

By about three months babies can recognize individuals, and will smile more readily at those they know well – their mother, father, siblings and so on. Over the next weeks and months, they become increasingly attached to their main carer. This is usually the mother, but if both parents share the care – or if a grandparent or childminder is very involved in the child's life – then the baby will naturally develop strong attachments to those people too.

But babies are also interested in new people. It's a good idea to give your baby plenty of opportunities to meet people, and to let him or her engage with relatives, friends and people that you come into contact with when you are out. This helps to foster the notion that the world is a friendly place – which is good for socialization skills.

First smiles are a response to a familiar voice. It's not until about eight or nine weeks that a baby will smile when you smile. When he or she realizes that smiling gets attention and cuddles, the baby does it a lot more.

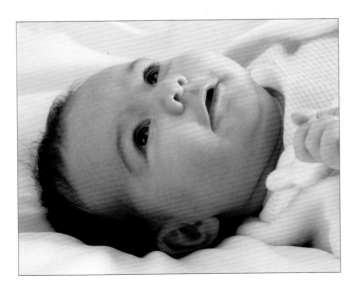

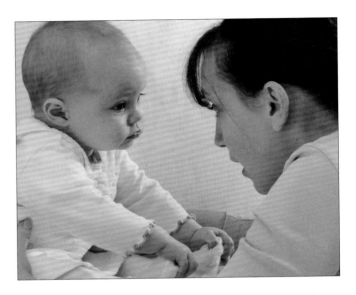

Your baby will learn to speak by listening to your voice and copying you. It will help if you make eye contact, and give him or her a chance to respond.

BABY TALK

At first your baby communicates only through crying, but after the first weeks, he or she will start to coo and gurgle. The first sounds – "aah", "eeeh" and other vowel sounds – will be random at first. But soon you will notice that the baby coos at you or at a particular object that has captured his or her attention.

Your baby will also start making easily articulated consonant sounds – "ma", "da" and "ba". Some babies do this as early as three months, some not until six months. Whatever age they start, they enjoy practising their new sounds. They also love it if you make the same sounds to them – try it and see how your baby reacts. Gradually babies start babbling: practising strings of consonant sounds such as "babababa", "dadadada", "mamama", over and over. Six months is an average age to do this – but many babies will do it considerably later.

By now, you'll be waiting for your baby to say "Mama" or "Dada". Lots of babies can do this at about eight months, and "Dada" usually comes first. But they won't use these words to mean their parents for another few months to come.

As well as practising sounds, babies start to laugh at about three and a half months. They also learn to screech to attract your attention. Don't worry that you are teaching bad habits when you respond to a deliberate scream – your baby will adopt different ways of calling you as soon as he or she is able.

GOOD WAYS TO TALK TO YOUR BABY

• Read to your baby from a young age. Look at a brightly coloured picture book together and make up your own words. Read the same story again and again. Give your baby cloth and tough board books that can safely be chewed.

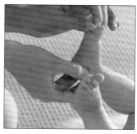

• Play games – count your baby's toes and play "This little piggy" on them, play "Round and round the garden" on his or her palm and "Incy-wincy spider" on the baby's tummy.

• Recite nursery rhymes. If you have forgotten the words, buy or borrow a children's book.

• Sing to your baby often. Play lots of music too – classical music helps to stimulate areas of the brain that deal with literacy and numeracy.

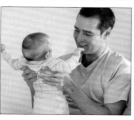

• Have "conversations". Even very young babies move their mouths, as if trying to speak. Respond to this with "How interesting", "That's a good story" and so on.

• When your baby starts to makes sounds, copy them – you'll get a smile when you do. Remember to pause so that the baby can "answer" you.

• Point out things of interest when you are out and about. Name common

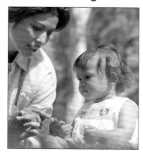

objects – "cow", "car", "flower" – as the more often your baby hears words in context the more quickly he or she will learn them. Talk about whatever you are doing – changing or bathing your baby, say.

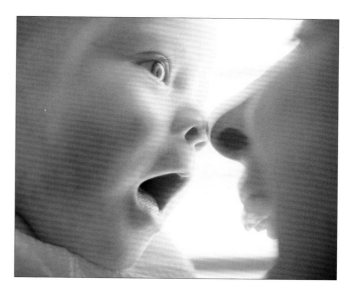

A baby will observe your face closely, so make exaggerated expressions when you talk to him or her. Try opening your mouth and sticking out your tongue – even a very new baby may copy you.

repetition are helpful: they serve to reiterate the main sounds of the words, giving babies a second chance to hear them and commit them to memory. Diminutive endings – "teethies", "doggies" – are another universal element of baby talk: this way of speaking is also helpful, as "framing" the consonant sound between vowels makes it easier to hear and learn. So don't feel embarrassed about lapsing into baby talk when you chat to your child – you are just doing what comes naturally.

BILINGUAL BABIES

Learning to speak is a fantastic intellectual achievement – one that all babies accomplish by the age of three. Strange as it may seem, it is no harder for a baby to learn two languages than one. So, if you and your partner speak different languages, each of you should stick to your own. Your baby will assume that there is a mummy language and a daddy language and will rise magnificently to the challenge of acquiring both.

HOW TO TALK TO YOUR CHILD

Some people find it very easy to chat to their babies; others think it is pointless talking to a baby who cannot understand them. But talking gives babies emotional stability, and it helps with language development and learning. Children learn their native language because they hear other people using it, so you have to give them the "raw data" to work with.

Most people naturally adopt a pitch higher than normal when talking to babies, as they are more responsive to this. "Baby talk" also includes lots of rhymes – such as "milky-wilky" and "itty-bitty" – and repetitive elements – "night-night", "bye-bye". Both rhyme and simple

It's great if your baby is happy to go to other people for a cuddle, but he or she will always want to come back to you. You may also notice that your baby grabs at your face and pokes his or her fingers in your mouth with great gusto, but is a lot more restrained when held by someone less familiar.

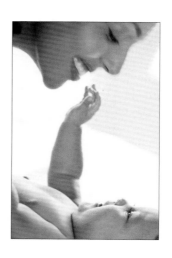

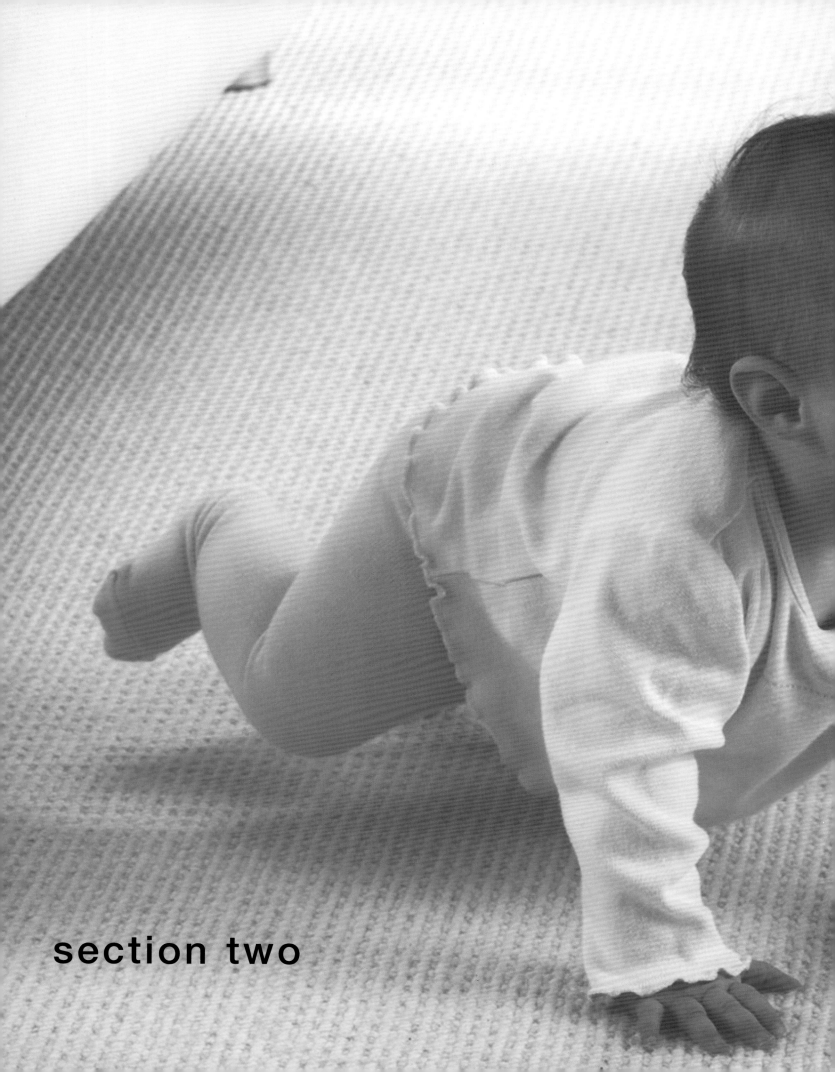

section two

your older baby

six months to one year

The experience of caring for a small baby is a mixture of anxiety and joy. But gradually, as you become seasoned parents, the joy starts to predominate and everything seems much easier to accomplish. You will be astonished by the rate at which your baby changes during his or her second six months. You can almost literally see him or her grow and develop before your eyes, and little by little a distinctive and individual personality begins to emerge.

General care and feeding

" It is immensely satisfying to know that you are training your baby's palate, laying the foundations for a lifetime of healthy eating. "

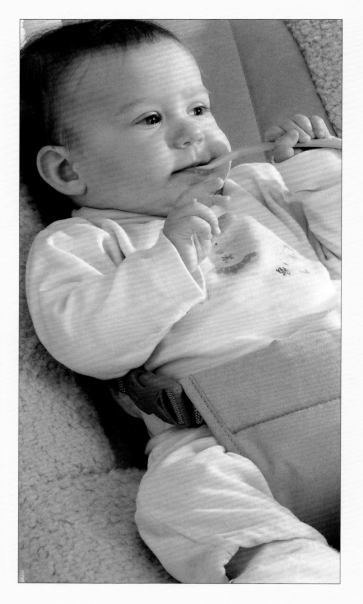

By now you will be better accustomed to caring for your baby and will be able to meet his or her basic needs with a more practised ease: long gone are the days when you struggled to get that sleepsuit over tiny arms and legs.

But babies grow fast and parenthood brings with it an ever-changing set of challenges. Around the six-month mark, your baby will start to cut his or her first teeth. Some babies do this without seeming to notice it; others feel a lot of pain and require lots of gentle aid to help them through the teething process.

The advent of teeth is a sign that your baby is getting ready for real food. Don't be surprised if you find it hard to give up the deep connection that comes with breastfeeding: this is a normal feeling. It is one of the many acts of letting go that are integral to parenthood. If you are committed to providing your baby with natural food, you will find that the changeover to solids involves a great deal of work at first: there are all those fruits and vegetables to cook, purée and pour into ice-cube trays for freezing. But it

Your baby may find a first experience of solid food strange, but he or she will soon get the taste for it and may grab the spoon out of your hand.

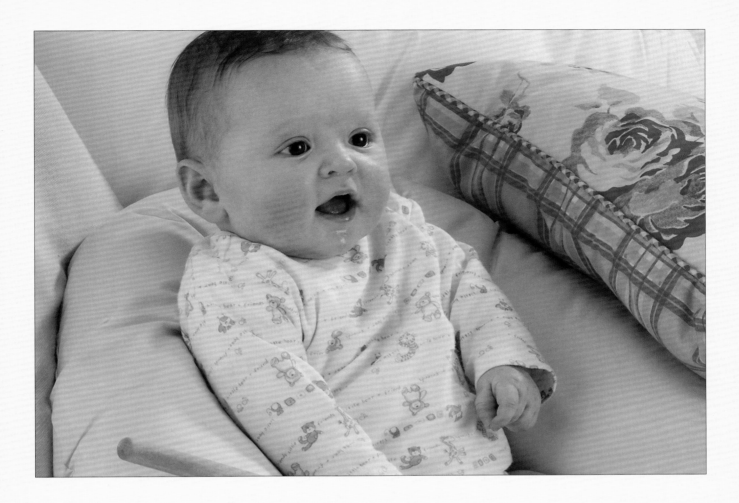

is also immensely satisfying to know that you are helping to train your baby's palate, laying the foundations for a lifetime of healthy eating. And, like all aspects of childcare, feeding your baby gets much easier with practice.

Many women return to work in their baby's first year, for perfectly good reasons, but if you find that you cannot bear to leave your baby after all, you are not alone. It's worth considering whether you can extend the time you spend together by negotiating more flexible working hours, for example. But if you do need to go back to work, for whatever reason, you will naturally want to choose your childcare carefully. Leaving your baby is much easier once you are confident that he or she is being looked after lovingly by someone you trust.

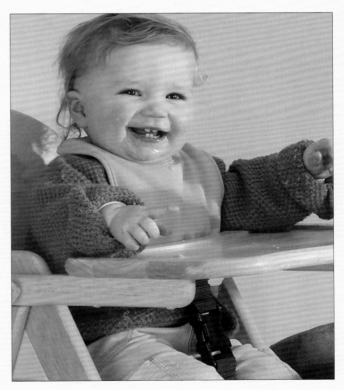

Top: Your baby will be much more aware of, and entertained by, his or her surroundings, and will watch your face and activities with absorbed interest.

Weaning is fun. There is huge pleasure to be had in introducing a baby to new flavours and seeing his or her growing enjoyment of good food.

Teething and tooth care

Spotting that tiny white line on your baby's gum is an exciting event – the first tooth is on its way. This can happen at any time in the first year, but teeth usually start coming through when a baby is around six months old.

WHEN THE TEETH COME THROUGH

Baby teeth tend to come through in pairs in a set sequence. But your baby's teeth may emerge in a slightly different order to the one described here, and they may appear earlier or later than the average ages given. They will look crooked when they are coming through, but will soon straighten out. Eventually your baby will have 20 milk teeth (compared to an adult's 32 permanent teeth).

TEETHING PAIN

The first teeth are sharp, thin incisors, so they usually cut through the gum quite easily. But if your baby is cutting more than one tooth at once, or if one of the large flat molars is emerging, this can cause a lot of discomfort.

To help your baby cope with the teething process, try rubbing the gums with a clean finger or a finger-toothbrush. You may be able to feel a bump on the gum before a tooth comes through. Something cool to bite on can help: a smooth hard toy or a clean facecloth dipped in cold water both work well, or you can use a teething ring that's been cooled in the fridge (not the freezer). Some people find that a stick of peeled carrot, a breadstick or a sugar-free teething biscuit helps; stay close by in case your baby manages to bite off a bit. You

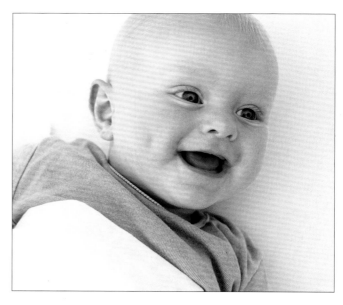

A few babies are actually born with teeth, while others don't develop any until after they are a year old.

can also breastfeed for comfort. Teething babies often want to nurse more frequently and need lots of fluid.

Many babies find homeopathic teething granules (Chamomilla) very soothing. But if natural methods don't seem to work, try rubbing teething gel on the gum. This numbs the area and can help a baby get off to sleep, but it is suitable only for babies over the age of about four months. You can also give your baby infant paracetamol (acetaminophen) to help with pain and reduce any fever.

This is a general guide to when you can expect which of your baby's teeth to appear.

Get your baby a toothbrush as soon as the first tooth comes through.

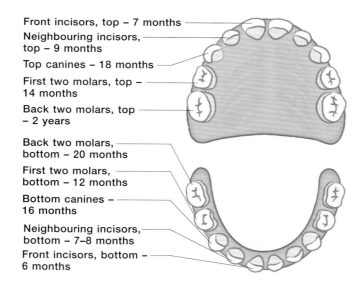

Front incisors, top – 7 months
Neighbouring incisors, top – 9 months
Top canines – 18 months
First two molars, top – 14 months
Back two molars, top – 2 years

Back two molars, bottom – 20 months
First two molars, bottom – 12 months
Bottom canines – 16 months
Neighbouring incisors, bottom – 7–8 months
Front incisors, bottom – 6 months

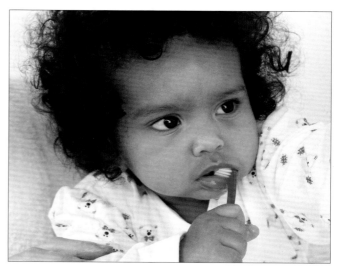

PROTECTING YOUR BABY'S TEETH

- Don't give your baby any sugary foods.
- Limit dried fruit to an occasional treat.
- Limit drinks to water and milk only.
- Always use sugar-free medicines.
- Take your baby with you when you go to the dentist for your own check-ups, so that the surgery becomes familiar. Always talk about going to the dentist in a positive and enthusiastic way.

TOOTH CARE

Start cleaning your baby's teeth as soon as the first ones come through. You'll find this easier if you lay the baby on your lap so that you are looking down at his or her mouth. If your baby doesn't like you using a baby toothbrush, try using a piece of damp gauze wrapped around your finger. Put a tiny smear of toothpaste on the gauze and clean the teeth very gently using circular movements, twice a day.

Don't worry if your baby won't let you brush his or her teeth at all; just give the brush to the baby to chew on. So long as you are using a fluoride toothpaste, this will help to strengthen the teeth and protect them from decay. It is important not to let tooth cleaning become stressful. At this stage it should be enjoyable and fun; but once several teeth are through they will need to be cleaned.

THE RIGHT TOOTHPASTE

Most dentists recommend that you use a specially formulated children's fluoride toothpaste for your baby. Adult toothpaste contains higher levels of fluoride, so it is not suitable: too much fluoride can cause discoloration of

Babies are fascinated by toothbrushing. Try giving your baby his or her own brush at the same time as you use yours, to copy you. Let your baby have a go at "brushing" your teeth while you are cleaning his or hers.

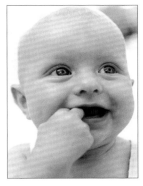

CHECKLIST: IS YOUR BABY TEETHING?

Be careful not to confuse real illness with signs of teething. If your baby seems to be in real pain, has a high temperature, a rash, diarrhoea or other symptoms, see a doctor. The following are the classic signs of teething.

Dribbling: More saliva is produced, so your baby is likely to dribble a lot more than usual. Many babies get a runny nose as well.

Distress and irritability. Pain will make your baby fractious and possibly more clingy than usual.

Biting and gnawing. Pressure on the gum relieves the pain so your baby may want to chew on everything (including you). The baby may bite his or her bottom lip before the first teeth come through.

Swelling on the gum. The gum may look red, bumpy or sore.

Flushed cheek. One or both cheeks may be red.

Fever. A slightly raised temperature is common with teething, especially at night.

Nappy rash. Many babies produce runny stools and are prone to nappy rash when teething.

Wakefulness. The baby may wake up more than usual at night.

the teeth. Fluoride is a mineral found in water. Additional fluoride is added to the water supply of some British regions and almost all US states to improve dental health. If there are only low levels of fluoride in your water, you may consider giving your baby a fluoride supplement, but you must take advice on this from a dentist: you could damage your child's teeth if you give too much fluoride.

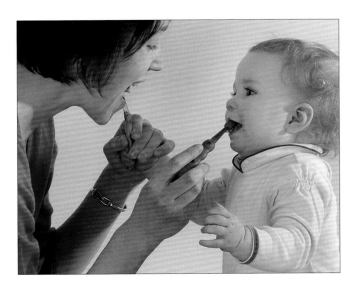

Bikkie pegs are natural, rock hard, teething chews that some babies enjoy gnawing on.

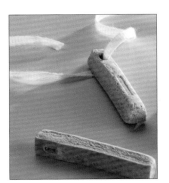

Homeopathic teething granules don't ease pain, but have a soothing effect on any fretfulness.

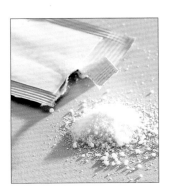

Bathing and dressing an older baby

Bathtime is a lot more fun once your baby is old enough to enjoy toys, games and lots of splashing in the big bath. Most older babies love having a bath, and a soak in warm water can be an excellent way of calming them down before bedtime. But having a bath straight after a meal can make a baby sick so leave a gap.

Make sure the bathroom is very warm and have a towel ready so that you can wrap your baby up as soon as you lift him or her out of the water. Until your baby is a confident sitter, you will have to lean over to support him or her throughout bathtime. This is hard on your back: make sure you are facing the bath squarely so that you are not twisting it.

BATHTIME GAMES

The best way to get your baby enjoying water is by playing in the bathtub.

- Lay your baby down on his or her back in the water, supporting the head and bottom, and swoosh him or her up and down the bath. Then turn the baby over and do the same, this time with your hands under the chin and tummy.
- Scoop water up in a beaker and pour it gently over the baby's tummy. Hold the beaker high and pour water into the bath in front of the baby so that it makes a glistening stream. He or she will reach out and touch it.

If your baby stops wanting to go in the bath, try getting in too. Take extra care when you are getting in and out, or have someone else there to lift the baby out for you.

BABY BATH OIL

To give your baby a beautifully aromatic and calming bath before bedtime, add a few drops of oil scented with mandarin orange to the water. Combine ten drops of mandarin essential oil with 100ml/3½fl oz sunflower oil, and store in a dark glass bottle out of direct sunlight. This oil will keep for 12 months.

- Gently trickle water on the baby's face using a facecloth or a scoop toy. This should help your baby to cope with any splashing in the pool if you go swimming together.
- Get some bath toys to play with. A natural sponge is great fun, and your baby will enjoy filling and emptying stacking cups or plastic bowls and beakers.
- If you have an older child, let them take a bath together – your baby will love playing in the water with a big brother or sister.

WASHING YOUR BABY

It is best to avoid baby bath products that contain chemicals, since these strip the natural oils from your baby's skin. You don't usually need to "wash" your baby at this age anyway: you can do without shampoo, soap and bubble bath. If your baby has some grubby patches, you can use an oatmeal "sponge": simply put a handful of oats in a muslin square, and twist to make a pouch. Water dries out the skin, so add a little oil to the bath. And of course, you don't have to bath your baby every day; a daily sponge bath of face, neck, underarms, hands, nappy area and feet is enough to keep a baby clean.

Babies love water games, and a natural sponge and a few simple toys add to the fun of bathtime.

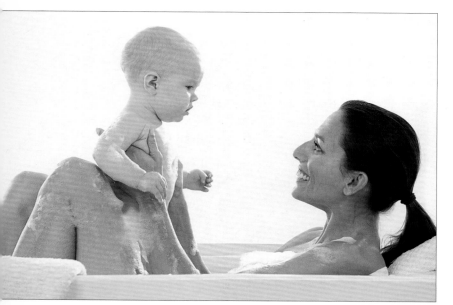

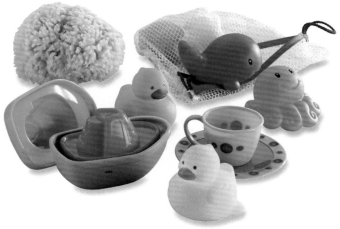

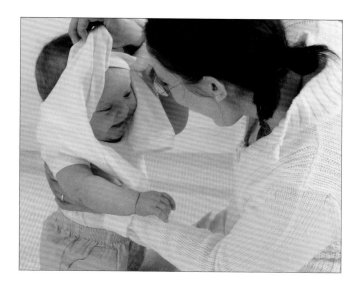

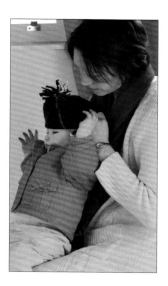

Left: Your baby will enjoy your cry of "Where's baby?" as his or her face disappears inside a top, and your start of surprise when a face is revealed. Play peek-a-boo with baby's hands and feet as you slip them into clothes.

Right: It may take lots of perseverance and patience to convince your baby to wear a hat.

CLOTHING YOUR BABY

Some older babies take an active role in getting dressed, pushing their hand through a sleeve opening or "helping" you pull a jumper off. But if they are not in the mood, dressing can be a challenge. Try to make it as much fun as possible – smile, make eye contact, chat, sing and play games. Clothes that are easy to get on and off make the whole process easier: look for wide necks and sleeves, stretchy fabrics and popper fastenings. If your baby is crawling, choose clothes that keep the knees covered.

A hat is important for warmth in cold weather and to give protection from the sun. But getting a baby to wear one is tricky. If your baby pulls it off as a matter of course, wait until he or she is distracted and then put it back on. Alternatively try saying "No" firmly and replacing it. You may have to do this many times, but once the baby realizes you mean business the hat may stay in place – for a while at least. It will help if the baby has a coat with a hood that you can pull over the hat, or if you choose a hat with straps that fasten under the chin.

Babies don't need shoes until they are walking. Keep the feet bare whenever you are in the warm. If your baby is wearing socks, make sure they are the non-slip variety in the right size: the tiny bones in a baby's feet are very soft, and tight socks can cause damage. Outdoors, a baby's feet may need some extra protection: soft pram shoes are best. Once your child learns to walk, buy proper shoes with lightweight, flexible soles from a specialist shop with trained fitters.

SAFETY IN THE BATH
- The water should be warm but not hot. Always check the temperature before putting the baby in the bath.
- Keep the room warm; babies lose body heat very quickly when they are wet.
- Keep the bath shallow – no more than waist-deep when your baby is sitting down.
- Never leave a baby alone in the bath, or under the care of another child.
- Don't let your baby pull himself or herself up in the bath unless you are holding on. It's best to discourage standing in the bath altogether.
- Wrap a wet facecloth around the hot tap as soon as your baby is old enough to reach for it.
- Put a non-slip mat in the bottom of the bath.

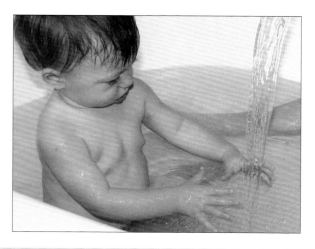

SAFETY IN THE SUN
- Keep your baby out of the sun as much as possible.
- When using a buggy, attach a parasol or, better still, a UV-filter sunshade.
- Dress your baby in lightweight fabric with a tight weave to protect the skin.
- Make your baby wear a wide-brimmed hat.
- Use a sunscreen of factor 20 or above, and re-apply frequently. Choose a natural sun cream specially formulated for children.
- Take precautions on warm cloudy days as well as on sunny ones.

When to wean

By the age of six months, your baby will almost certainly be ready to start eating solid food. The iron stored at birth will have begun to run out, and the baby may need more calories than he or she can get from milk alone. At this age, most babies are interested in new experiences and are more likely to take to eating than if you wait until much later in the first year. Ideally you will start giving solids at six months, but some parents start earlier, and so long as the baby is not at risk of developing allergies and you give only recommended foods, this shouldn't be a problem. However it is important not to start giving your baby food any earlier than four months, because a young baby's intestines are immature. Starting solids early or giving certain foods may encourage long-term digestive problems or allergies.

Young babies also find it quite difficult to eat – which suggests that they are not ready for the experience. They can't sit up properly, so swallowing is difficult, and they tend to poke their tongue out when they sense something alien in their mouths. This tongue-thrust reflex protects them from choking. It disappears between four and six

If your baby shows an interest in food, a bouncy chair is a convenient place to have his or her first meals.

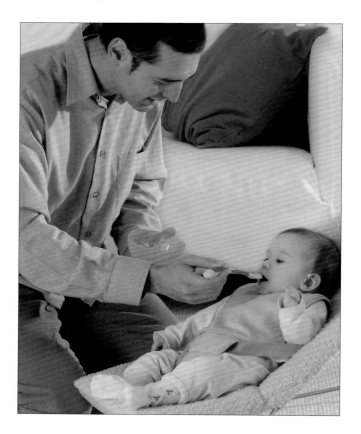

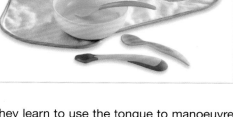

ESSENTIAL EQUIPMENT
You don't need a lot of special equipment when introducing solid food to your baby, but the following are useful.

Baby chair. It is much easier to feed with a spoon when you are facing your baby. If he or she can sit up well, use a highchair. If not, a bouncy chair set at the most upright level makes a good substitute for the first weeks.

Spoons. Shallow weaning spoons are easy to get into a baby's mouth and make it easy for him or her to lick the food off. Plastic spoons are easy to clean and sterilize, and they won't hurt your baby when he or she starts waving them around.

Bibs. Feeding is a messy business so you will need three or more bibs. Cloth ones are the most comfortable, and Velcro fasteners are much easier to use than ties.

Bowls. You can use ordinary bowls, but it is easier to serve tiny amounts in a small, shallow bowl, which also allows the baby to see the food. A bowl with a sucker on the base is good for when a baby starts to feed himself or herself, because it stays steady.

months, when they learn to use the tongue to manoeuvre food to the back of the mouth and swallow it. An older baby can also let you know that he or she wants more food by leaning towards the spoon with an open mouth or has had enough by turning away with a mouth firmly shut.

IS MY BABY READY FOR SOLIDS?
Wait until your baby is showing signs of being interested in food before you think about introducing solids. These are some of the typical signs to look for.
- Your baby still seems hungry after a feed.
- Your baby wants feeding more often.
- Your baby watches you with interest when you eat.
- Your baby begins waking up more frequently in the night after a period of sleeping through.
- Your baby is putting things in his or her mouth.
- Your baby can hold his or her head up well.

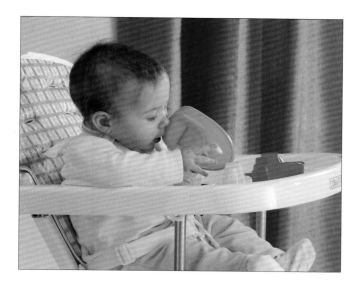

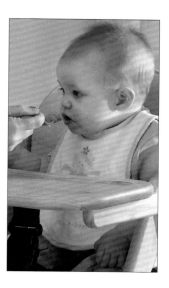

Left: Before you use the highchair for feeding, get your baby used to it. Put some toys on the table for them to play with. If they start putting a toy in their mouth, give them something they can eat.

Right: Starting your baby on solids is quite an event. At first it can feel like hard work, but you – and the baby – will soon get the hang of it.

Talk to your health visitor if you are not sure whether to start solids or not. A premature baby won't be ready to start on solids until at least four to six months from his or her expected, rather than actual, birth date.

WHICH HIGHCHAIR?

The most natural option for a highchair is one that is made from wood from a sustainable source. Make sure the design is simple and that it doesn't have any awkward crevices that will be difficult to clean.

A chair with an adjustable seat or footrest will be more comfortable for the baby, but will probably take up more space than one that folds up. The chair should have a fixed five-point harness for absolute safety. You will need some cushioning to protect the baby's head from banging on the back of the chair.

Some highchairs are designed to be drawn up to the table so that the baby can join in family meals from the beginning. This is a great idea in theory, but you may prefer to choose one with a tray to contain the mess. A highchair with a detachable tray can be used either way.

ALLERGIES

If a baby's father, mother or any siblings suffer from allergies or allergy-related conditions such as asthma, eczema or hay fever (allergic rhinitis), the baby may inherit the allergy. The best way to protect him or her is to breastfeed exclusively for six months, and to continue breastfeeding for the rest of the first year.

Introduce solids very slowly and do not give any foods that you or your partner are allergic to until your baby is at least a year old. Dairy foods, wheat, citrus fruits, eggs, fish, shellfish and nuts are the most common food allergens, so they should be introduced with caution. Sesame seeds and peanuts, and any foods containing them (such as peanut butter, groundnut oil and sesame oil) should not be given until your child is at least three; you may wish to exclude all nuts from your child's diet.

Even if there is no family history of allergy, it is still important to take weaning slowly. Introduce one new food at a time and be on the lookout for any allergic reactions. These usually occur within minutes of eating and can include the following: facial rash (especially around the mouth), sneezing, runny nose, coughing, wheezing. Very occasionally, a baby may develop breathing difficulties or swelling of the lips: this needs urgent medical attention and you need to call an ambulance.

If a baby is intolerant of a certain food – meaning it is difficult to digest – he or she may experience bloating or passing wind, diarrhoea or vomiting within a few hours or sometimes over a couple of days after eating it. If your baby seems to have a reaction of this kind to a certain food, try introducing it again a few weeks later to see if the reaction recurs. If it does, you probably need to eliminate the food from your baby's diet. Children often grow out of allergies and intolerances, so you may be able to re-introduce the offending food later, but get individual advice on this from a health professional.

When a baby is ready for weaning, he or she should take food from a spoon or your finger with just a little encouragement.

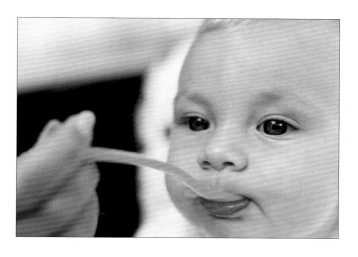

First foods: 4–6 months

Your aim when introducing solids is to get your baby used to different tastes and textures, not to replace milk. Start with just one "meal" a day, offering just a teaspoonful of food to start with. If your baby seems eager for more, you can offer a couple of teaspoonfuls the next time and gradually build up to a couple of tablespoons or so. Don't worry if your baby seems to eat more one day and then less the next; this is quite normal.

A good time to introduce solid food is mid-morning, ideally between milk feeds. That way, your baby won't be so hungry that he or she will be wanting milk, nor so full that he or she won't be interested in trying something new. Once the baby is used to the idea, you can combine solid food with the lunchtime feed. Give milk before the solids, so that you don't cut down on milk feeds too quickly. Or try giving a little milk first, then the solids, then the rest of the milk.

If your baby rejects the food repeatedly, he or she probably isn't ready for solids yet and you should wait a week or two before trying again. Don't try to force the baby to eat more than he or she wants – babies have a good sense of when to stop and it is important to be led by what your baby wants.

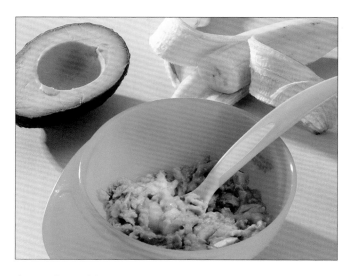

Avocado and banana, mashed together, are healthy raw foods that you can feed to young babies.

INTRODUCING NEW TASTES

Give baby rice for at least a week or two before introducing another new food. Take the weaning process very slowly, introducing new foods one a time. Leave about a week between the first three or four new foods

Starting solids

A good first food is baby rice, which is gluten-free and unlikely to cause any reaction. Commercial baby rice comes in dried flakes and usually has added nutrients such as iron. Mix it with your baby's usual milk (expressed breastmilk or formula) so that this first "meal" has a familiar taste. It should have a soupy consistency.

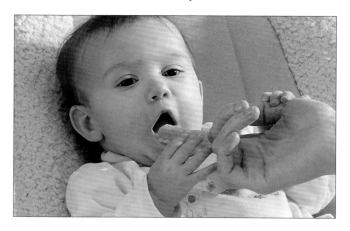

1 Put a little of the milky baby rice on the tip of your finger so that your baby can suck it off. If he or she doesn't seem interested, try dabbing a little on his or her lips or tongue. You may find that the rice is poked straight back out until your baby gets the hang of moving it to the back of the mouth for swallowing.

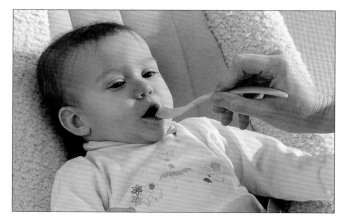

2 If your baby takes well to sucking food off your finger, offer a little rice on a shallow spoon. Give a few more spoonfuls if the baby shows interest by leaning forwards, opening his or her mouth when you offer the food, or grabbing your finger or the spoon. If the baby turns away or pushes your hand away, he or she has had enough.

and wait three to five days before introducing subsequent ones. This will allow your baby's digestive system to get used to each new food, and will also make it easier for you to pinpoint the problem food if your baby develops an allergic reaction.

The following fruits and vegetables make excellent first foods because they are bland and can be mashed or puréed to a smooth consistency. Add a little milk or milky baby rice so that the consistency is fairly runny. To make food more interesting, combine different purées that you have already introduced – try carrot and apple, parsnip and sweet potato, papaya and banana.

Root vegetables. These have a naturally sweet taste and are easy to digest. Try carrots, sweet potato, butternut squash, yams, parsnips and swede (rutabaga). Peel and cut into pieces (remove the seeds in squash), steam until very soft and then purée or mash. Your baby may also like puréed potato.

The best way to cook fruits and vegetables for babies is to steam them – it preserves more nutrients than any other cooking method.

Pears and apples. These fruits are gentle on the stomach and most babies love them. Peel, core and cut into pieces. Steam or cook in a little water until very soft, then purée or mash. An older baby can eat mashed, uncooked pear if it is very ripe.

Bananas, papayas and avocados. These are very digestible fruits that don't need cooking. Simply mash and mix with a little milk to give a suitably runny texture.

COOKING FOR A BABY

The best cooking method is steaming, which preserves most nutrients. Boiling and baking (without oil) are also healthy, but don't boil foods for too long. Avoid frying and roasting, which makes food more difficult to digest. Microwaving not only destroys some of the nutrients in food, but also heats it unevenly, so it is best avoided.

To save time, you can cook and purée a batch of vegetables or fruit, take what you need for one meal, cool the rest and freeze straight away in ice-cube trays. When the cubes are frozen, transfer them to a freezer bag. Don't forget to date and label the bag. Cooked frozen foods cannot be refrozen once defrosted, and if your baby does not eat much of a meal you must throw the rest away, however wasteful that seems. It is fine to defrost frozen food cubes in a saucepan, but make sure that you heat the food through thoroughly, then cool before feeding.

THREE MEALS A DAY

A few weeks after you start giving your baby solids mid-morning, you can introduce breakfast, too. Most babies are very hungry when they wake up, so give a milk feed first and then a teaspoon or two of solids. After another few weeks, start giving the baby some solids in the early evening, too. You can gradually increase the amount at each meal to suit his or her appetite – follow your baby's lead and give what he or she seems to want. Older babies will also need healthy snacks between meals, such as fruit, rice cakes and oatcakes.

The best way to cook fruits and vegetables for babies is to steam them – it preserves more nutrients than any other cooking method.

Preparing a batch of tiny meals in advance takes the stress out of feeding.

Baby rice is quick and easy to prepare, and most babies like it.

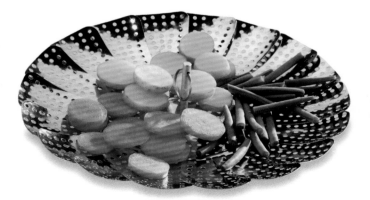

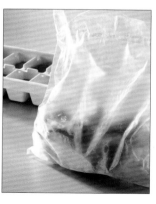

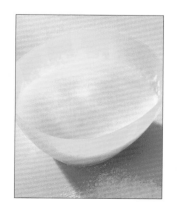

Second foods: 6–8 months

Once you have introduced the idea of eating solid food, the next step is to extend your baby's palate. Don't assume that your baby won't like strong flavours such as, say, courgette (zucchini) or natural yoghurt; he or she may well surprise you. It will help if you introduce each new food in a relaxed and confident way – if your expression says "Beware", then your child will. Often a baby will be more willing to accept a new food that has a distinctive flavour – spinach, say – if it is mixed with the carrot or parsnip that he or she already knows and loves. Start by adding a tiny amount and then gradually increase the ratio of spinach to carrot as the baby gets used to it.

NEW FOODS TO TRY
The following foods are good ones to introduce after the first, rather bland, foods. Remember to introduce them one at a time, and to leave three to five days between each new food.

FOODS THAT NEED TO WAIT
Some foods are more likely to cause an allergic reaction than others, so they should not be among the first foods that you introduce to your baby.

After six months, you can give:
• Cow's milk dairy products – yoghurts, butter, cheese and fromage frais, but don't give unpasteurized cheeses to a young child.

After eight months, you can give:
• Foods containing gluten – wheat, rye, barley or oats
• Egg yolk (make sure it is well cooked)
• Nuts and seeds that have been ground (excluding peanuts and sesame seeds)
• Fish (but children should not have shark, marlin or swordfish because they contain levels of mercury that could affect their developing nervous systems)
• Citrus fruits and juices.

After twelve months, you can give:
• Honey (avoid for the first year because it may contain a bacterium that causes infant botulism)
• Peanuts (crushed) and sesame seeds (avoid until three years if there is a family history of nut allergy)
• Nuts that have been chopped (whole nuts should not be given to a child under five years because of the risk of choking).

CAUTION
Never leave your baby alone when eating: stay nearby in case he or she chokes on a piece of food.

Vegetables. Try purées of steamed courgette, spinach or green beans, broccoli and cauliflower, as well as puréed boiled frozen peas. Home-cooked beetroot (beet) is a good food to combine with mashed potato.

Fruits. Lightly cooked mangoes, peaches and nectarines make good purées, or try mashed ripe melon (cantaloupe is one of the sweetest) from about seven months. Dried fruits such as apricots, dates or prunes can be cooked in water and then puréed, but give them sparingly as they are very sweet. Some babies are allergic to kiwi fruit and strawberries, so wait until at least nine months before introducing these fruits and watch for any reaction.

Grains. Introduce millet or oats (which can be made into a smooth porridge) before wheat-based cereals, which are more likely to cause a reaction. Once your baby is taking textured food, couscous, quinoa and barley are good grain foods and you can also introduce tiny pasta shapes (buy the ones intended for soup).

Dairy products. Give plain unsweetened yoghurt, plain

Babies have a natural instinct to do things for themselves, and most really enjoy feeding themselves with finger foods. Rice cakes are ideal to start off with because they disintegrate when sucked.

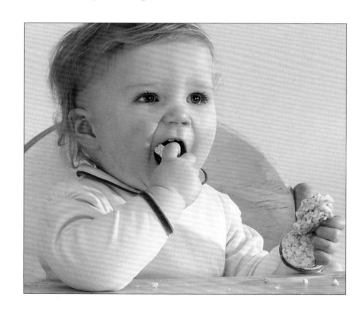

FINGER FOODS

Here are some good first finger foods to try:

- Rice cakes – plain rather than sweet or salted
- Sticks of hard cheese, such as Cheddar or Edam
- Chunks of melon – wash the rind well
- Slices of toast
- Slices of polenta
- Slices of banana and pear.

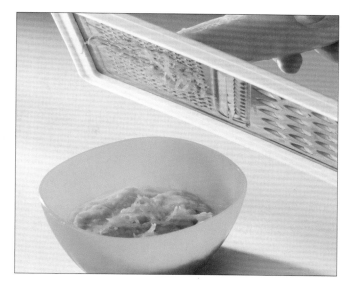

Adding grated food to purées is a good way of getting your baby used to a new texture.

fromage frais, cream cheese, cottage cheese, Cheddar and other hard cheeses. Always use full-fat dairy products – growing babies need lots of calories so you don't want them to fill up on low-fat foods.

Lentils and beans. Try a purée of red lentils – you can add a sliver each of garlic and ginger to the cooking water to add flavour (remove the ginger before puréeing). From about nine months you can try butterbeans, haricots, split peas and soya.

Chicken and meat. Chicken and turkey usually go down well. They can be puréed or mashed with root or green vegetables or dairy products. Once your baby is happy with white meat try lean red meat such as lamb.

Fish. Introduce white fish from about eight months: poach it in milk, flake it and check very carefully for bones before feeding to your baby. Once your baby is happily eating these foods, you can try introducing oily fish such as salmon.

EXTRA FLAVOURS

You can make your baby's food more tasty by adding flavourings such as sautéed onion or leek, garlic and ginger, and finely chopped parsley and other soft-leaved herbs. It is also a good idea to introduce mild spices from about eight months – try sprinkling a little cinnamon on porridge, or adding cumin or paprika to savoury dishes.

Don't add any salt to food for a baby less than a year old, and avoid processed foods such as baked beans, which contain added salt. Similarly, don't sweeten food with sugar or give sugary "treats". There can be a lot of

sugar in fruity yoghurts and fromage frais, baby rusks and processed foods, and all are best avoided.

TEXTURE, TOO

At first your baby can manage only smooth and runny purées. But if you go on giving these for a long time, he or she may reject lumpier food. So it is a good idea to start mashing rather than puréeing food from about seven months, and to gradually increase the lumpiness of the food you serve. Once your baby is eating lumpier food, try stirring in some finely grated or chopped foods to introduce different textures. You can also give your baby finger foods from about seven months.

Don't limit your baby to bland foods. Babies are much more receptive to new flavours than older children, so it is a good idea to expose them to flavours such as ginger, cumin, garlic and fresh herbs.

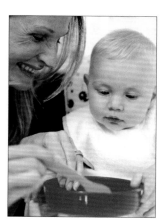

Introduce your baby to different textures and tastes. Try a whole banana, oatcakes, a few raisins or dried apricots, a handful of whole butter (lima) beans, chunks of hard cheese, thin slices of apple or pear and tiny sandwich squares spread with cream cheese.

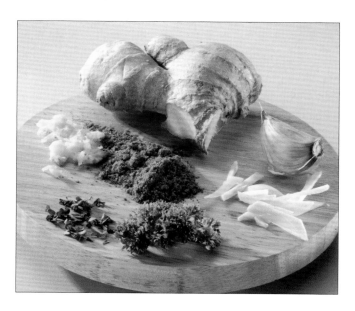

Healthy eating for babies

As your baby's appetite for solid food increases over the first year, he or she will start to take less milk. Once solids become a more substantial part of the diet, you need to start providing a good mix of different foods to ensure that your baby is getting all the right nutrients. A balanced daily diet for a nine- to twelve-month-old baby would include the following.

One or two servings of protein foods. Protein is made up of amino acids, which are needed for the growth and repair of all the body's cells and tissues. Lean meat, chicken and turkey, fish, eggs, cheese, yoghurt and tofu (soya bean curd) are complete sources of protein. Pulses and beans are healthy protein foods but contain only some of the essential amino acids. Your baby also needs to eat some grain foods (rice, oats, bread or pasta) or nuts and seeds over the course of the day to get a good balance of amino acids.

Three or four servings of starchy foods. Carbohydrates are the body's main fuel. The best sources are starchy foods such as oats, rice, bread, barley, rye and potatoes; lentils, pulses, fruits and vegetables also contain carbohydrates. It is best not to feed babies high-fibre foods as this will fill their tiny stomachs without providing the necessary nutrients. Refined grains such as white rice and ordinary pasta are much easier to digest.

Four or five servings of fruits and vegetables. These contain the vitamins and minerals that are essential to good health, and they are the best source of fibre for babies and young children. The best way to make sure that your baby is getting enough is to offer as wide a range as possible.

Grains and starchy vegetables give your baby the carbohydrates he or she needs for energy.

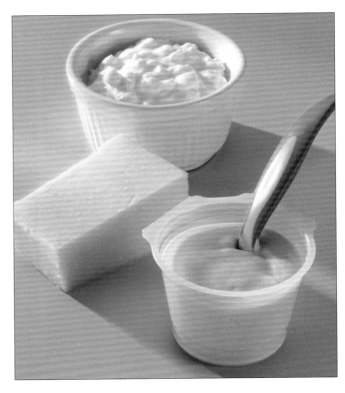

Cheese, yoghurt and other dairy foods are a good source of calcium, but be sure to give full-fat versions.

Calcium. Babies get calcium from their milk, which is still their most important food. If your baby is not drinking quite enough milk, other good dietary sources include dairy products (cheese, yoghurt, fromage frais), almonds, brazil nuts, green leafy vegetables and tofu.

Some healthy fats. Fats are a concentrated source of calories, which growing babies need – both breastmilk and formula have high fat contents. Always give your baby full-fat versions of any milk, cheese, yoghurt or other dairy products you offer. Include healthy

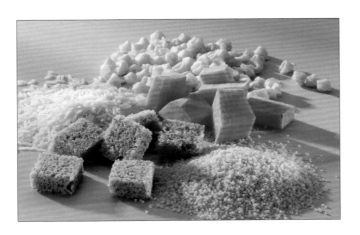

GOING ORGANIC

Buying organic food is an easy way to reduce the chemicals your baby is exposed to: organic fruits and vegetables are produced with fewer pesticides and fertilizers, and the animals used for organic meat are not routinely given antibiotics. Organic farming methods may also produce some food with higher levels of nutrients: one study found that organic milk had higher levels of essential fatty acids, vitamin E and antioxidants, which help fight infection.

PACKED WITH VITAMINS

Vitamin	Needed for	Good sources
Vitamin A	Growth, healthy skin, good eyesight	Green leafy vegetables, carrots, squash, sweet potatoes, apricots, mangoes, liver, oily fish, egg yolks, butter, margarine and cheese
Vitamin B group	Growth, healthy nervous and immune systems, healthy skin, nails and hair, good digestion	Green leafy vegetables, broccoli, oats, lean meat and liver, tofu, fish, fortified breakfast cereals, bananas, avocados, milk and yoghurt
Vitamin C	Strong gums, teeth, bones and skin, healthy immune system, helps with iron absorption	Citrus and berry fruits, mangoes, papaya, nectarines, blackcurrants, potatoes, green leafy vegetables, peppers, tomatoes
Vitamin D	Strong bones and teeth	Salmon, sardines, tuna, milk, fortified margarine, eggs, fortified breakfast cereals
Vitamin E	Maintaining the body's cell structure	Vegetable oils, nuts, seeds, avocado

unsaturated fats in the baby's diet, from vegetable oils, avocados, nuts and seeds, and oily fish. Foods such as processed cakes and crisps contain unhealthy trans-fats and have no nutritional value so they should be avoided altogether.

Some iron-rich foods. Iron is important both for physical and for mental growth, but babies can easily become anaemic (iron-deficient). Use a formula milk with extra iron if you are bottle-feeding. Good dietary sources of iron include red meat and liver, oily fish, pulses, green leafy vegetables, dried fruits such as apricots, and fortified breakfast cereals. Iron from animal sources is easily absorbed by the body. Iron from plant-based sources is absorbed more easily if they are accompanied by a food that is rich in vitamin C (red (bell) peppers, tomatoes and all citrus fruits are particularly good).

Protein foods such as meat, fish, lentils and eggs are an important part of a baby's diet.

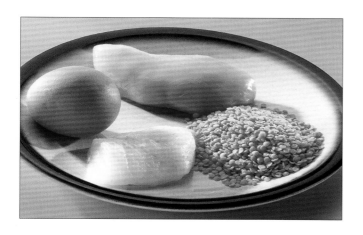

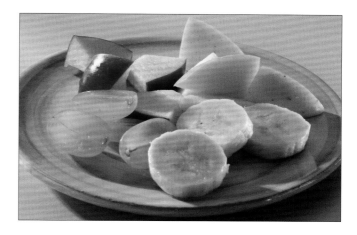

Try to get your baby to try different kinds of fresh fruits, to provide a good range of vitamins.

VEGETARIAN BABIES

A vegetarian diet is perfectly healthy for babies so long as they get enough protein: offer two servings a day. An easy way to increase the protein content of a vegetarian meal is to add cheese, chopped egg yolk or a smooth cashew or almond nut butter (from about eight months). You'll also need to ensure that a vegetarian baby gets sufficient iron, especially if still being breastfed (formula has added iron), and vitamin B12, found in dairy products, breakfast cereals and yeast extract (suitable after one year).

A vegan diet is very restrictive, so it is harder to make sure your baby is getting all the necessary nutrients. You'll have to plan meals carefully in order to provide the baby with enough protein, vitamin B12 and vitamin D, and you may need to give vitamin supplements. It is worth getting advice from a paediatric dietician or doctor before starting to wean your baby if you intend to follow a vegan diet.

Milk and the older baby

Babies need to continue drinking plenty of milk, even after solids are introduced. They need about 600ml/1 pint a day up to the age of twelve months. Give your baby milk first thing in the morning and at bedtime, and at other times if necessary.

Breastmilk is the best milk for your baby for the first year. If you are breastfeeding, it is impossible to tell how much milk your baby is getting. But if you are giving four or more full feeds a day, your baby is almost certainly getting enough.

Bottle-fed babies over the age of six months can continue to drink infant formula or can switch to a follow-on milk if the infant formula doesn't seem to be satisfying them. Cow's milk and goat's milk are not suitable as a main drink until your baby is at least twelve months old, because they don't have enough iron and other nutrients.

OTHER DRINKS

Other than milk, the best drink to give is water. There's no need to give other drinks, which fill your baby up without providing vital calories. It is a good idea to get your child used to drinking water from an early age. Give him or her sips from a cup at mealtimes.

Babies over the age of six months can drink water straight from the tap, but you may want to filter it first to remove impurities. Don't give bottled mineral water – some have high levels of salt and are unsuitable for babies, and the water may have been sitting in the bottle for months.

A spouted cup is useful when you are out and about, and there is a wide range on the market – you may need to experiment to find one your baby likes to use. Remember it is still important to sterilize your baby's cups, bottles and teats.

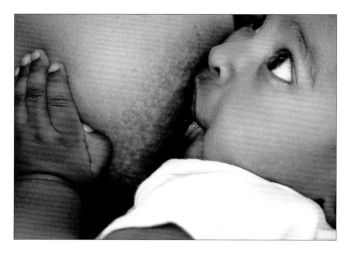

Mother's milk is still the best nutrition a baby can have – it has a high fat content to give energy and plenty of calcium for growing bones.

Fruit juice, even if it is well diluted, is too acidic for young babies. Even after six months, it is best not to give your baby fruit juice to drink because it contains sugars, which can cause tooth decay. Sometimes parents are advised to give babies diluted juice at mealtimes to help

Weaning your baby off a bottle and on to a cup can be a long process. Try cuddling your baby in the same way you would when they were taking a bottle, and maintaining the close association milk has with you.

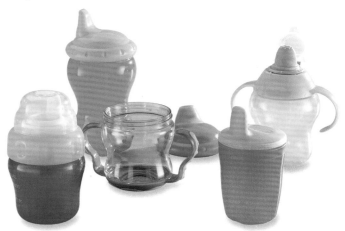

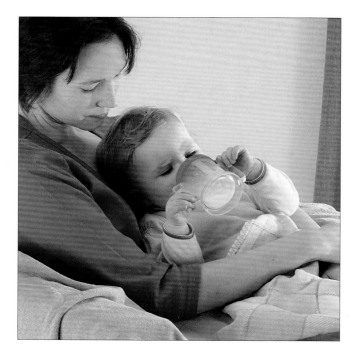

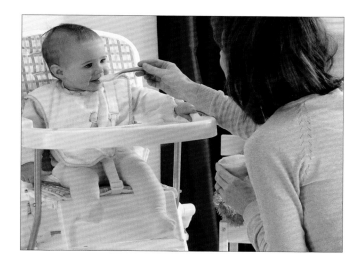

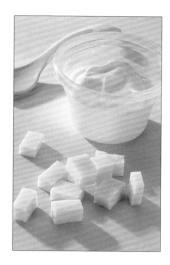

Left: There's no need to give your baby sweet fruity yoghurts. Try him or her on plain bio-active yoghurt, which is better for the teeth and can help the digestion.

Right: Dairy foods, such as milk, cheese and yoghurt, are a good way of ensuring that babies get enough calcium in their diet.

them absorb the iron in food. But fruit or vegetables rich in vitamin C will do the job just as well. If you do decide to give juice at mealtimes, dilute it with water – ten parts water to one part juice – to help protect your baby's emerging teeth, and to stop them getting full on liquid. Other drinks, such as squashes, teas or fizzy drinks, should never be given to a baby.

MOVING TO A CUP

It's a good idea to start getting your baby used to a cup from six or seven months. With a bottle, liquid tends to collect in the mouth and over a prolonged period this can lead to tooth decay, particularly if the baby tends to comfort suck. Frequent sucking on a teat can also interfere with the correct development of a baby's teeth.

The best kind of cup to use is an open one; you can get slanted "Doidy" cups, which are easier for a baby to drink from than the usual baby cup with a spout. You are bound to have accidents when using an open cup, so you may want to restrict it to times when your baby is sitting on your lap or in a highchair and use a beaker with a spout (a sippy cup) for water at other times.

It can take a long time to get a bottle-fed baby used to drinking from a cup. Take your time – and don't be surprised if it takes six months or more to completely wean the baby from a bottle. The bedtime bottle is usually the last one to go, but don't worry, just enjoy the warmth and closeness it brings. Here are some ways to help.

- Let the baby play with an empty cup.
- Introduce a cup at mealtimes first, and help your baby to hold it.
- When you think your baby is ready, give one milk feed from a cup. Choose a feed when the baby doesn't drink as much – usually the mid-afternoon one.
- Keep your baby cuddled on your lap while he or she is drinking the milk – some babies are reluctant to give up the bottle because they associate it with being held.
- Once your baby is taking the cup at one feed, substitute it for the bottle at other feeds, one at a time.

WEANING FROM THE BREAST

The decision to wean your baby from the breast is a complicated and emotive one. Babies benefit from having breastmilk as their main drink throughout the first year, but many nursing women decide that they want to stop or reduce breastfeeds earlier for a variety of good reasons.

- Don't stop breastfeeding abruptly, since this can be traumatic for your baby and uncomfortable for you.
- Accept that weaning takes time. Leave at least a week or two between each dropping of a feed.
- Substitute a bottle or cup of milk for each feed you drop so that your baby doesn't go short of milk.
- If the baby is reluctant, try giving expressed breastmilk until he or she gets used to the idea of taking milk from a source other than the breast.
- If your baby won't take a bottle or cup from you, then try getting his or her father to give it. Stay out of the room so that you don't distract the baby.
- Give your baby lots of cuddles. It is important that he or she doesn't feel rejected and continues to get the closeness you both enjoy when you breastfeed.
- Make the bedtime feed the last one you drop. You may decide that you are happy to continue with this, and a morning feed, say, for a few months longer if your baby is drinking formula at other times.
- Wear a well-fitting bra. Express a little milk to prevent engorgement if necessary.

SUPPLEMENTS FOR BREASTFED BABIES
While breastmilk is generally healthier than formula milk, formula does have iron and vitamins added to it. Breast-fed babies may not get enough vitamin A, C and D from milk alone, so vitamin drops are generally advised. However, once they start eating solids, babies can get these vitamins from other foods; vitamin D is also made by the body when the skin is exposed to sunlight.

Helping your baby enjoy food

Eating is one of life's great joys. It's common for parents to worry about how much and what their baby is eating, but such anxiety can introduce an element of tension into mealtimes that is counterproductive. Having a relaxed, positive attitude towards your baby's food will go a long way to helping him or her enjoy it.

MAKING FOOD FUN

Let your baby eat with his or her fingers. Food will go all over the place, but it will show that eating is fun and that the baby can feed himself or herself rather than having to rely on you to spoon food into his or her mouth. Once old enough, your baby will love to pick up peas or other small morsels and pop them into his or her mouth. Serve easy finger foods alongside mashed or minced food – try steamed strips of vegetables, thin strips of chicken, strips of rolled-up pancakes, butter (lima) beans, small pasta shapes and squares of toast.

Give your baby a spoon as soon as he or she wants to hold one. Let the baby try to use it, while you use a second spoon to get food into his or her mouth, and accept the fact that babies make a mess at mealtimes. Don't hover around wiping your baby's face or hands after

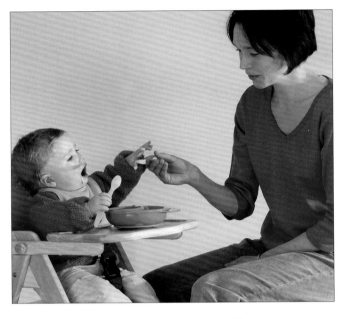

Your baby may assert a fierce sense of independence at mealtimes. Feeding will probably work best at this stage if you both have a spoon.

every mouthful – you'll be sending out the message that food is dirty or bad. Use a bib and put newspaper or a plastic sheet under the highchair to contain the mess. Wait until mealtime is over to clean the baby up.

RELAXED MEALTIMES

Always sit with your baby when he or she eats: mealtimes should be sociable events, and you need to stay close by in case of choking. Include the baby in family meals from as young an age as possible. Offer suitable bits and pieces off your plate, feed the baby a minced or mashed version of what you are eating or provide some finger foods to play with.

Always be positive about your baby's food. Be careful if you are offering something that you personally don't like – your baby may pick up on your distaste and refuse it. And get into good habits yourself. Your child is more likely to eat fruit at breakfast, say, if he or she sees you doing the same.

Let your baby decide how much to eat. His or her appetite will vary from day to day, and from meal to meal. Don't force food into the baby's mouth or spend ages trying to encourage him or her to eat one last spoonful. Your baby will quickly realize that it's possible to get your focused attention by refusing food, and mealtimes could become a battleground.

Setting a good example

Eating food from the same plate as your baby is a good way of encouraging him or her to eat.

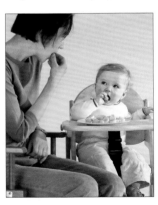

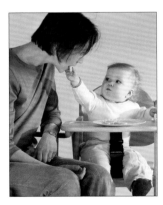

1 If your baby seems uncertain about trying a new food, try popping a bit in your own mouth. Look as though you are enjoying it, and your baby will love to copy you.

2 The next stage will be them wanting to feed you. Accept their offering, however sucked and squishy it might be. They will automatically pick up this positive attitude.

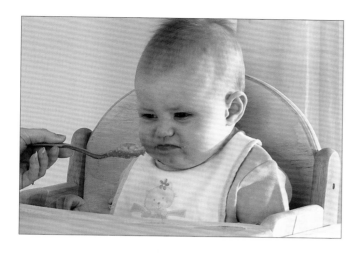

If your baby refuses food, don't keep pushing him or her to accept it – it's more important that the baby sees food as pleasurable than that he or she eats up that last bit of carrot.

EXCITING FLAVOURS

Give homemade food most or all of the time. Most commercial baby foods have a similar taste and they are all processed to the same smoothness. So a baby fed mostly from jars won't experience the distinct flavours and different textures of homemade foods. If you limit your baby to just a few dishes, he or she may be less willing to accept new foods later on, so provide lots of variety. Now is the time to get the baby enjoying as many of the wonderful flavours of food as possible.

REFUSING SOLIDS

Some babies do not take to solids well. If your baby doesn't seem interested when you first offer them, he or she may not be ready for food. Trying waiting at least a week or two before offering it again.

Even babies who take well to solid food will refuse it from time to time, especially if they are ill or teething. The best way to handle this is to stay calm. Continue to offer meals, but leave it up to your baby whether or not he or she eats. Most babies will start eating again when they feel ready, though it can take a few weeks before their appetite returns fully. Similarly, babies will often eat only a few foods – fruit and toast, say – or suddenly refuse foods that they have previously enjoyed. Again, this is normal. Keep offering other foods alongside the ones your baby is eating; let the baby see you eating them. It may also help if you give the baby meals with the rest of the family. Eventually curiousity about new foods will grow again.

WHEN BABIES DON'T EAT

A few babies don't take to eating until much later in the first year. So long as your baby is gaining weight and is healthy, starting solids later is unlikely to be a problem. Talk to a health professional if you are worried. If your

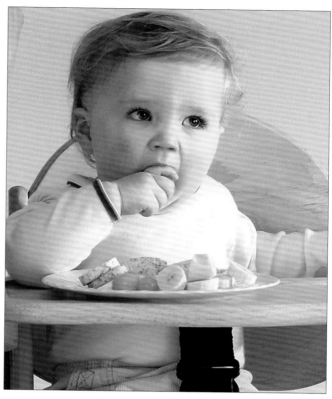

Giving your child a selection of fruit such as grapes and sliced banana after a meal is just as nice – and a lot healthier – than a sugary pudding.

baby is older than eight months and still showing no interest, try cutting down on milk feeds – babies don't need more than 600ml/1 pint per day.

It is worth bearing in mind that a baby who is prone to allergies may be better off feeding only on breastmilk for most of the first year. Nutritionally, babies can get almost everything they need from breastmilk, with the possible exception of iron. Breastmilk contains small amounts of iron, but it is more easily absorbed than that in infant formula, so a breastfed baby may be getting enough.

Your baby will enjoy mealtimes more if he or she is allowed to touch, squash and smear food around. This helps babies to get familiar with food and appreciate it.

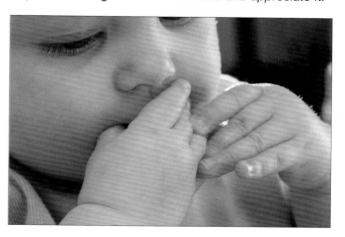

What childcare?

Knowing that your baby is happy and well cared for will make it easier for you to leave him or her if you go back to work. It's important for both of you that you choose the right childcare and that you feel confident about whatever arrangement you make.

DECIDING WHEN TO GO BACK TO WORK

Some mothers are keen to return to work after their maternity leave, while others prefer to take as long a period off work as they can manage. If you are feeling happy with the original arrangements you made about returning, the next step is to decide on the right carer or nursery, but if not you could consider extending your maternity leave. Don't stick with the decision to return to work on a certain date because it seems easier than re-negotiating. Have the courage to follow your instincts about what is right for you and your baby, even if that means admitting you have made a mistake.

Be open and honest with the baby's father (if you are together) about how you are feeling, and listen to how he feels too: he may be unable or unwilling to take on the burden of being the sole breadwinner, he may prefer it if you stay at home to care for your baby or he may want to give up work to do this himself. Often parents have more options than might be immediately apparent; for example, one of you might be able to afford to stay at home if you forego holidays, meals out and so on. It is important that you decide together what is right for your family.

If you want to go back to work but are worried about leaving your baby for long working days, you could consider reducing the number of hours you work. Many women decide to work part-time after they have a baby, and a growing number of fathers are doing the same.

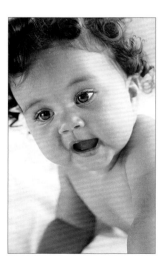

Your baby will prefer to be at home and looked after by you than anyone else. Delaying going back to full-time work for at least the first year is a good option if you can manage it.

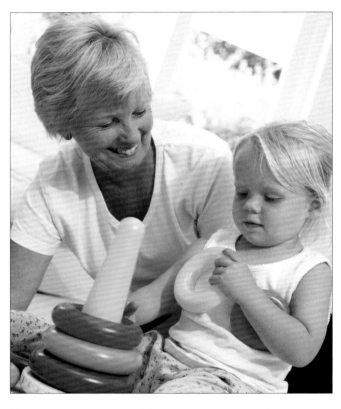

Your parents may be able to help you look after your baby. This form of childcare can work very well, but make sure everyone agrees on who does what.

WHAT'S BEST?

A long-term study led by the respected childcare expert Penelope Leach, which began in 1998, looked at the emotional and social development of 1200 children in Britain, aged three months to four years. It rated childcare options for babies under 18 months old in the following order of preference:

1 Full-time care by parent
2 Nanny in child's own home
3 Childminder (home day care)
4 Grandparent or other informal carer
5 Nursery (commercial day care).

It is important to keep this and other research in perspective. Remember that any study of day care looks at a wide range of children; what is right for your child may be very different. And of course everything depends on the individual carers: for example, a fantastic nursery with attentive, loving staff is better than a lazy and uncaring childminder.

If this is not possible, see if you can change your hours to fit in with your childcare arrangements. It may be that you and your partner can work at different times, to increase the length of time your baby spends at home.

CHILDCARE OPTIONS

These are the main childcare options.

Nanny. A nanny looks after your baby in your own home, so the baby stays in familiar surroundings and has the full attention of a carer. This is the most flexible option, because the nanny can fit around your hours and follow your routine. Most nannies have studied first aid and childcare, but this is not compulsory so it is important to check qualifications. Nannies may live in or out, and it is possible to share one with another family.

A nanny needs a living wage so this is a costly childcare option. If she (most nannies are women) works in your home, you will be her employer. This means that you will need to draw up a contract detailing the job description, hours, sick and holiday pay and so on. You will also need to take out public liability insurance in case of accidents and will have to pay the nanny's tax and insurance contributions.

Childminder (home day care). There are male and female childminders, but most tend to be mothers with children of their own. They usually work in their own homes, caring for a fixed number of children. Hours can be flexible, but some childminders work only in the school holidays or on particular days.

If both parents work flexible or part-time hours, you will be able to reduce the time your child spends in care.

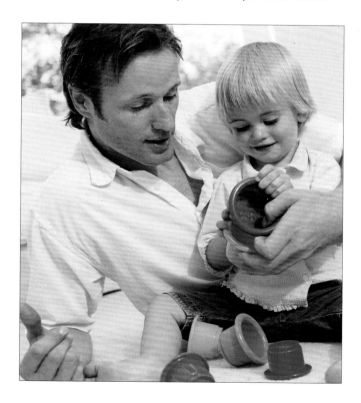

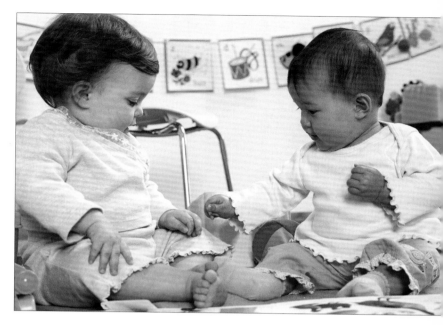

A nursery (day care centre) that takes babies should have a special room where the babies can be cared for away from toddlers and older children.

The legal requirements vary from country to country. In the UK, for example, childminders have to be registered with the local authority and are allowed to look after no more than six children (of whom no more than three may be under five years old). They are also required to complete a basic training course, including first aid. Always ask to see a childminder's registration, insurance and first aid certificates, and sign a written contract covering hours, pay, sick and holiday pay.

Grandparents. Many parents see a grandparent as the ideal carer for their baby. The arrangement is usually unpaid, and can work very well if the grandparent is willing to follow your routine and respect your views on eating and sleeping. However, anyone who cares for your baby must be fit and agile, and aware of health and safety issues. If a grandparent is looking after your baby in his or her own home, make sure it is safe.

Day nursery (commercial day care). Nurseries (day care centres) are often favoured by working parents because they offer reliable and professional care. However, babies cannot go if they are ill, and hours are usually restricted. Some employers offer a workplace crèche, which means that your baby is near you while you are at work. Children are usually looked after in groups, and babies are separated from toddlers and young children.

The main disadvantage of this kind of care is that your baby is likely to be looked after by a series of different people in a day, though many nurseries assign each child to a key worker to provide a sense of continuity. Choose a registered nursery, and ask about staff turnover: if staff tend to come and go, your baby won't get a chance to develop a relationship with the carers.

Arranging your childcare

Start looking for childcare a few months before you need it. This gives you time to evaluate the options properly; you don't want to have to make a decision about where to leave your baby when you are under pressure and in a hurry. Looking for good childcare can feel daunting, and it will help if you work out exactly what you need beforehand. For example, if you work long and unsociable hours, say, then you will need a nanny or childminder who will do the same. If your child is disabled or has special needs, you will need a nursery or carer who is able and willing to care for him or her sensitively.

Spread your search wide. Ask as many people as possible whether they can recommend someone. In particular, the following can be useful.

Your local authority. They should have a list of registered childminders and nurseries in your area.

Other parents. Those with older children may have a trusted childminder they are no longer using.

Nursery workers. If you are looking for home-based care, it is worth asking the staff at your local nursery. Trained staff may be available to look after your baby part-time, or they may know of an experienced childcarer who is looking for a new charge.

Young babies generally do better with a single carer than in a nursery. But if a nursery is well staffed and the carers are warm and loving, it can be a good option.

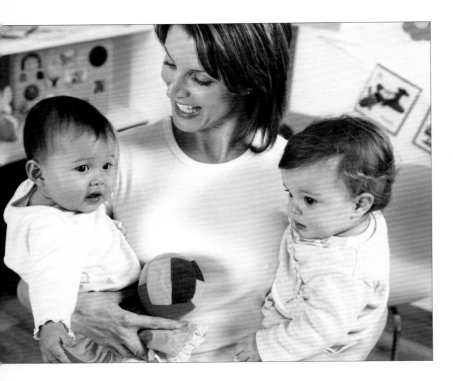

CHECKLIST: CHOOSING A NURSERY

A good nursery should be spacious, clean and light, with some safe outdoor space. It is important that there is be a good ratio of staff to children: for the under-twos this means no more than three children to every member of staff.

- Ask for a tour of the nursery during a normal day. Observe whether the children look happy and well cared for.
- Look at the areas for eating and sleeping – will your child be comfortable?
- Check that your baby will be cared for in a separate area, away from older children.
- Find out if your child will remain on the premises all the time. If not, ask where else they will go and how such outings are organized.
- Chat to as many members of staff as possible: do they seem loving, kind, friendly and interested in the children?
- Take your baby with you and observe how staff interact with him or her.
- Go back at least once; take your partner or another close person with you for a second opinion.

Health professionals. Your healthcare providers are in contact with parents and babies every day, so they may be able to recommend a good childminder or nursery.

Parents' groups. The co-ordinator of your local playgroup or breastfeeding group may have some useful contacts.

Childcare training college. Ask the principal if there is anyone he or she can recommend.

CHOOSING A CHILDMINDER OR NANNY

It is important to meet any potential carer at least twice. Take your child with you: the way the carer interacts with the baby is a good indication of whether she is suitable for the task of looking after him or her.

Ask the carer why she looks after children as a job, and what she enjoys about it. Discuss the practicalities of the daily routine: when and what your child will eat, when and where he or she will sleep, and what he or she will do during the day, including any trips he or she may be taken on. You will have more say about this if you are using a nanny, but a good childminder should be able to facilitate your wishes to a large extent. Don't forget to ask to see any relevant certificates: childminder's registration, first-

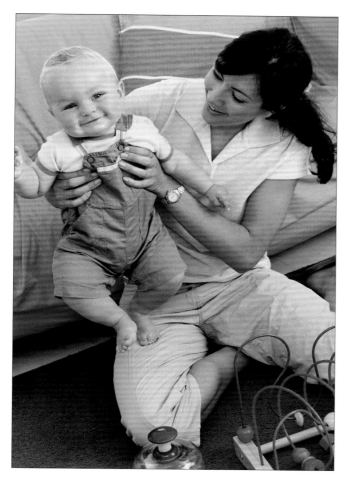

Say a proper goodbye to your baby when you leave him or her with a carer; don't just sneak off and disappear when the baby isn't looking.

aid certificate and so on. Check that the carer knows how to fit a car seat properly if your child will be driven around.

Always see a childminder in her own home. Check that all the relevant rooms are clean, tidy and safe, and that your baby will be comfortable there. Check the ages of any other children who will be present, and time at least one of your visits so that you can meet them.

It is vital that you feel good about the person who is going to care for your baby. Ask yourself if you feel that this carer will look after your baby in the way that you want. Are you happy and relaxed about leaving your child in this person's care? If the answer is yes, follow up the carer's references and ask your partner or another close person to meet her for a second opinion. If the answer is no, even if you can't pinpoint the reason, keep looking.

SETTLING IN

Agree a trial period of two to four weeks for any childcare arrangement, so that you can call a halt without penalty if it doesn't work out.

Arrange for your baby to spend some time with a new carer while you are present before leaving them alone together. A nanny can spend a day with you and your baby, following your usual routine. If you are hiring a childminder, start by spending half an hour at her home with your baby. The next time, leave your baby with the childminder for half an hour or so while you wait outside or walk around the block. Then try leaving your baby for a couple of hours. If all goes well, try a half session and then a full one. Nurseries usually operate a similar settling-in scheme.

Always say goodbye to your baby when you leave. Be cheery and use the same form of words each time, such as "See you later". Your baby may not want you to go, but most children quickly adjust once you are out of sight. Ring to check: if your baby continues to cry after you have gone, this arrangement may not be the right one.

IS IT WORKING?

Your baby is the best barometer of whether childcare arrangements are working. Does he or she seem happy and alert when you return, or fretful or withdrawn? Does your baby seem well cared for? For example, is he or she clean, with a recently changed nappy?

Think about the carer's demeanour and attitude. Is she cheerful and relaxed? Is she happy to tell you about your baby's day? Or does she seem irritable and glad to hand your baby back? Does the carer seem to like and understand your baby?

There are bound to be times when your baby is fractious after a day away from you, but if he or she consistently seems unhappy or the carer is unhelpful, you may need to start looking for a new arrangement. If you are unsure, try arriving early one day just to see what is happening when you are not expected.

Your relationship with your baby's carer should be respectful and warm. It is important that you are both punctual and that you keep each other informed of any developments in your baby's life.

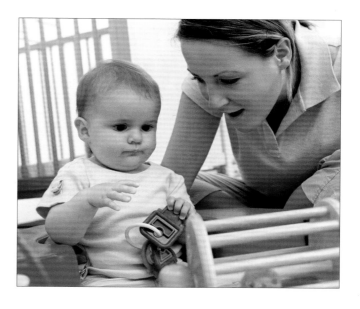

Crying, comfort and sleeping

" Of course, some broken nights are inevitable. They are an inalienable facet of parenthood, well into the toddler years. "

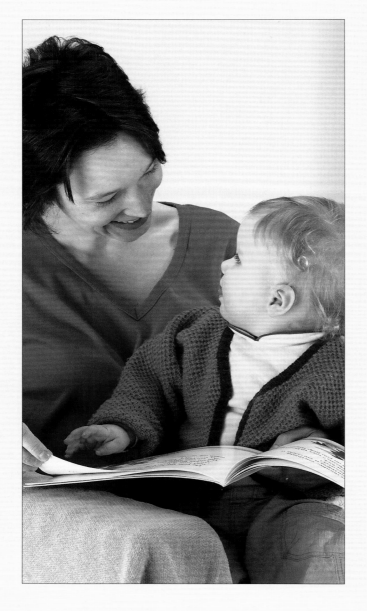

As your baby grows older, you will probably find that he or she cries less frequently. Some of the things that used to be upsetting might now be amusing instead. And while the discomfort of, say, a wet nappy will still trouble a baby, crying will often cease as soon as he or she knows you are attending to the problem. Sometimes your child will just whimper to let you know that something is wrong. In short, your baby has understood that crying is a form of communication, but you still need to respond quickly and compassionately. This can get harder from about eight months, when your baby's intense attachment to you means that he or she may wail in despair if you leave the room. This fear of abandonment, known as separation anxiety, can be very trying for you. When your baby demands to be with you every second, even a simple household task such as boiling the kettle becomes difficult. But the more gently and lovingly you respond to your baby's feelings, the better: he or she needs reassurance to get through this tricky stage.

The bond between parent and child grows stronger in the second six months – and your baby may not want to let you out of his or her sight for a while.

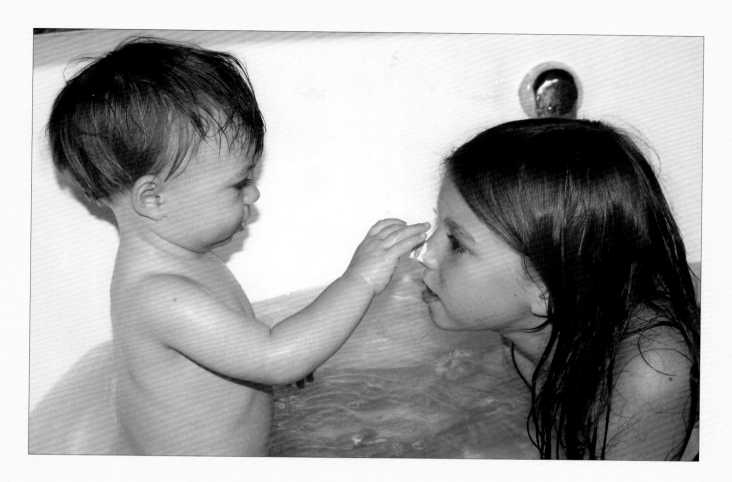

Dealing with nighttime crying is a tougher problem to solve, because you need your baby to spend the nights without your presence. Even babies who have been sleeping well begin to object to going to bed at this age, and no baby likes to wake up in the small hours and find that he or she is alone in the room.

Most babies need guidance to help them sleep well by themselves. This chapter suggests some ways to help your baby to wind down at the end of the day, and how to set clear and consistent rules about bedtime. These techniques will improve a wakeful baby's nights, but to make them work you need to make a clear decision about how you want your baby to sleep, and you must plan to achieve it. Of course, some broken nights are inevitable. They are an inalienable facet of parenthood, well into the toddler years.

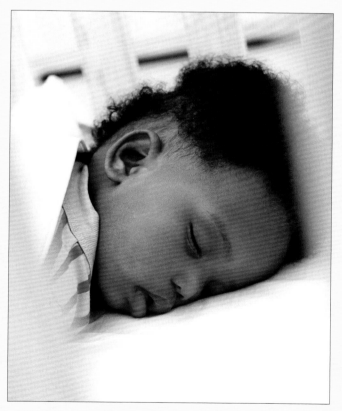

Top: Adopt a bedtime routine that stays the same each evening and gives time for your baby to settle down and relax. This will help him or her to fall happily asleep.

With a little forethought and determination, you and your baby can look forward to a refreshing night's sleep more often than not.

Why your baby cries

Older babies cry for many of the same reasons as younger ones: hunger, fear, teething and so on. Older babies cry when they are tired, but don't realize what they need is to go to sleep: unlike young babies they can, and do, keep themselves awake. Good daytime and nighttime sleep routines will help to avoid this problem.

There are also a few new causes for tears, arising from babies' increasing activity and growing perceptions of their world. As your baby learns to crawl, pull up to standing and cruise around the furniture, there are bound to be a few bumps. Crying is more likely to be caused by the shock than any pain, but he or she needs your reassuring hug fast. Older babies also need more stimulation and may cry from boredom: gone are the days when you could walk around shops with the pram for hours at a time. Your baby may quickly get fed up with being confined, and probably has a new moan or whining cry to signal displeasure.

Older babies may scream with fury when things don't happen the way they want. They hate it when they cannot quite make a toy work or find that they are propelling themselves backwards when they are trying to crawl forwards. This sense of frustration isn't necessarily a bad

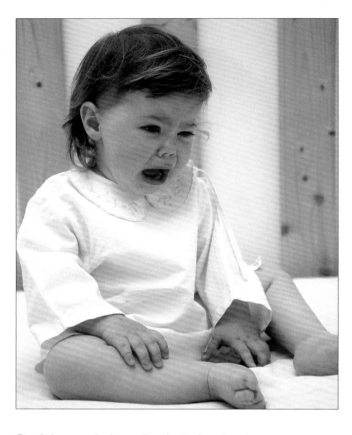

Babies have intense emotions, but unhappiness doesn't last long if they are given comfort or distraction. Older babies are quite capable of crying simply from boredom and lack of stimulation.

Don't leave a baby crying in their cot unless you are following a controlled crying routine. If a baby is crying they are calling for your care and attention, they are not being "naughty".

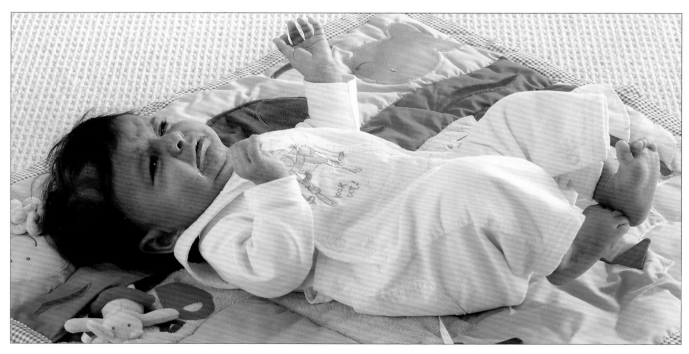

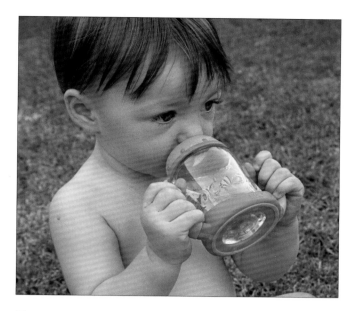

Try not to get into the habit of offering your baby something to eat to stop him or her crying – a few sips of water or an interesting toy will do just as well, and will avoid creating a link between comfort and eating.

thing. It eggs babies on to new achievements, and the screams that accompany their attempts are sometimes a way of expressing the effort they are putting in, but you will obviously want to reduce and minimize any distress.

Help your baby out by showing how to make that troublesome toy work or by removing an obstacle in his or her path. But don't take over – encourage the baby to have another go if the task is within his or her capability. Distraction is the subtlest tool that a parent can deploy. If your baby is getting very frustrated, divert his or her attention by doing something unusual, like making a funny face or a new noise. Remain calm yourself. Cries of frustration are a normal and inevitable part of your baby's development, and patience and reassurance are sometimes all a parent can offer.

THE START OF DISCIPLINE

Lots of people talk about babies being manipulative when they cry. It is true that once a baby learns that you will come running when you hear crying, he or she may do it simply to get your company. But this doesn't make the baby "naughty" or "cunning"– it simply means that he or she wants you to be there. The fact that the crying stops as soon as you arrive shows how delighted your child is to see you.

The next few months, though, are the time to lay the foundations of discipline. As the baby learns to assert himself or herself, you are bound to find that your wishes conflict. For example, your child may scream and resist whenever you try to put him or her in a car seat, or howl in protest when you take that sharp pencil away. Try not to forbid your baby to do things if there is no need. Going

into the car seat is obviously non-negotiable, but perhaps it doesn't matter if the baby pulls all the food containers out of the cupboard: this is only exploring after all, and your baby doesn't know that they are not toys. So choose your battles wisely: it will make life easier for you both.

Be firm. If you have decided that your baby cannot do something – such as playing with your mobile phone – don't suddenly give in.

Be consistent. Don't stop your baby pulling books off a shelf one day and then ignore this same behaviour the very next day.

Be inventive. If your baby is resisting going into the highchair, say, put an exciting object on the tray to encourage him or her to go willingly.

Think prevention. You can avoid a lot of tears by ensuring your baby's environment is safe to explore.

Reinforce words with action. Don't expect your baby to stop doing something because you call "No" from the other side of the room without moving towards them; it is good to say "No" in a firm way but you should also go and gently take the troublesome object away to reinforce the message. Add some easily understood words of explanation as well – for example, "Hot!" as you move the baby away from the oven.

If a child is crying from anger or frustration try to keep calm yourself, and keep giving love and cuddles.

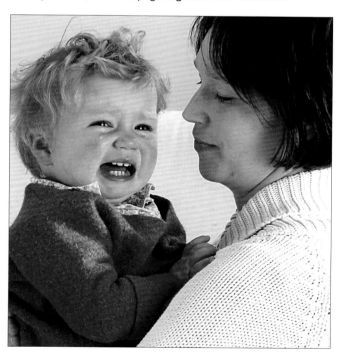

Fear and anxiety

There is a whole category of things that can make your baby cry that are nothing to do with the physical world but are psychological in nature. By now your baby has built up an expectation of how things happen in his or her world. If something out of the ordinary happens – even if it is not a bad thing in itself – the baby may cry because it is unsettling. For example, if you take your child to a swimming pool for the first time, he or she may cry even before you go into the water, because the smell, look and sound of the pool environment are very unfamiliar. Similarly, if a babysitter appears when the baby wakes in the night, instead of you or your partner, he or she may become very distressed – even if the babysitter is somebody your baby loves.

The best way to help your baby through these difficulties is to try to let him or her know whenever something new is about to happen. The babysitter could call to your baby while approaching the room, so that the baby knows someone different is coming in before he or she is picked up and comforted. And, of course, your baby will be much easier to soothe if left in the care of someone he or she knows well. At the swimming pool, cuddle the baby for a while and point out other children playing in the water before you even attempt to get in there too. Babies are very adaptable and usually enjoy new experiences, so long as they are introduced gradually and from a home base of safety.

FEARS

Older babies may develop very specific fears of everyday things. A classic one is the vacuum cleaner. Even if you used the sound of a vacuum cleaner to lull your newborn to sleep, you may find that an older baby develops a real fear of it. This may be so great that the baby whimpers on catching a glimpse and cries at a similar sound – such as the blender, say, or a hedge trimmer being used outside.

Although your baby's fears may seem irrational, don't dismiss them as "silly" or try to force him or her to confront them – you will only increase the fear. Babies need to feel safe in the world and to know that they can trust their carers to look after them. So if your baby is scared of the vacuum cleaner, keep it out of sight and use it only when he or she is sleeping or in another room. If the baby seems to be scared of the dark, get a nightlight or leave the hall light on and the bedroom door open.

As your baby is reassured about being protected from frightening things, his or her confidence will grow. Eventually the baby may start to get curious about the very thing that was scary – he or she may want to look at that vacuum cleaner and even touch it. Don't rush this – let the baby conquer such fears one step at a time, when he or she is ready.

SEPARATION ANXIETY

Young babies think of themselves and their main carers as one: they have no sense of themselves as individuals and are completely unaware that those tiny fists waving in the air belong to them. As they learn to control their movements and make things happen, they gradually become aware that they are independent beings. One clue is the realization that they can make the carer come by crying out, which happens at about four months.

By about seven months, they have worked out that they and their carers are separate entities. This marks a huge leap in understanding, but it also makes babies anxious: for if they are separate, that means they can be left alone. Separation anxiety, as it is known, manifests as

Fathers need not be upset if their baby cries when handed over. Babies naturally feel closest to their mother at first: the uniquely wonderful and complex bond with the father takes longer to develop.

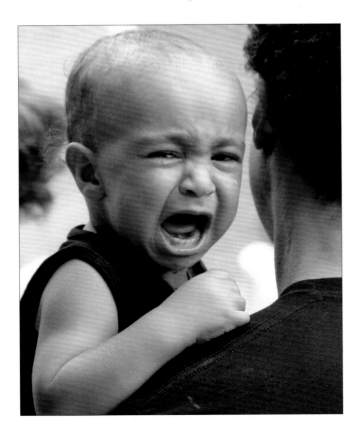

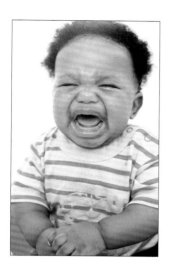
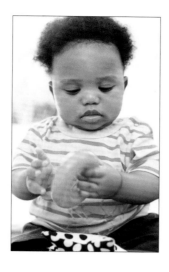

Left: It is amazing how the most heartbreaking tears can be soothed and then forgotten by a live-in-the-moment toddler.

Right: If you are leaving your child, be sure to say a proper goodbye that isn't rushed or stressful. Sneaking off may avoid some tears at the time but it will make him or her feel insecure.

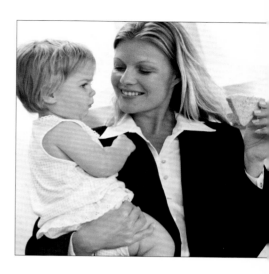

a tendency to cling. It usually starts between eight and twelve months; but it can be later and some babies are not affected at all.

Your baby may start to cry if you try to give him or her to other people, especially if they are not very familiar. The baby may also protest or burst into tears if you leave the room for a moment, even when being cuddled by the grandfather he or she loves. At this stage, your baby cannot understand that you will return – all he or she feels is abandonment.

All the effort you put into your baby's feelings of security and confidence in the early years helps them as they get older and spend more time without you.

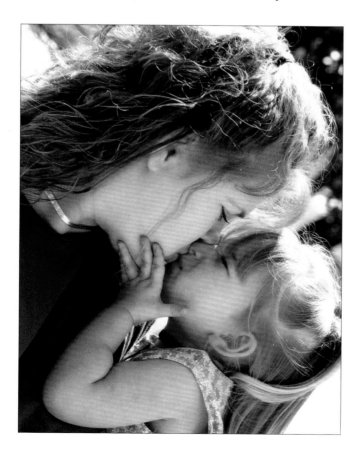

HANDLING SEPARATION ANXIETY

Your baby needs to be secure in his or her attachment to you. Only through love and reassurance do babies gain the confidence to explore the world.

Keep your baby with you as much as possible. It is often easier to take the baby with you into the bathroom, say, than to cause unnecessary distress. If your baby becomes nervous of strangers, which is very common during the second half-year, don't pass him or her over for a cuddle. Ignore anyone who says he or she is spoiled or clingy; your child will go to other people when he or she is good and ready. If possible, however, get your baby used to being with at least one other trusted person beside you and your partner. This means that there is someone else to care for him or her in an emergency, or if you really need a break.

When you are leaving, always say goodbye – sneaking off when your baby's attention is distracted for a moment will undermine his or her trust in you. But keep goodbyes short, cheery and calm – if you show that you are upset or anxious, you will be reaffirming and increasing the baby's sense of unease. It's a good idea to use the same form of words (perhaps with an accompanying gesture) each time. For example, say "One minute" (and hold up one finger) if you are just popping into another room to get something; say "See you later" (and blow a kiss) if you will be away for longer. And if you have said you will be "one minute", don't be gone for ages – always stick to your promises. Your baby doesn't understand the concept of time yet, but will come to realize that "one minute" means a short separation.

Give your full attention to your baby when you get back. Have a loving cuddle straight away if the baby wants one; if he or she is happily absorbed in doing something, watch and perhaps join in until your baby is ready to come to you. Be cheerful but calm so that the baby learns your return is quite normal and not something to make a big fuss about. Gradually your baby will learn that you always come back.

Changing sleep patterns

By now your baby will almost certainly be sleeping a lot more at night than in the day. Babies over six months commonly sleep for ten to twelve hours at night, as well as having daytime naps. But your nights are still unlikely to be the long unbroken stretch you may be craving. Even though your baby may be sleeping for as much as six to eight hours at a time, the longest sleep will probably coincide with your evening and the early part of your night. Most babies wake up at least once a night until they are twelve months old.

It is still important to put older babies on their back to sleep. If you find that your baby rolls over, gently move him or her back again. However, if this happens repeatedly or if the baby wakes up when turned, it is probably better to leave him or her be.

DAYTIME NAPS

Most babies need at least two naps a day – one in the morning and one in the early afternoon – until the end of the first year. Ideally, the afternoon nap should be the long one, as it will help keep your baby going until bedtime.

Some babies drop a nap even before they get to twelve months. You might find that they just enjoy a quiet period at that time for a couple of weeks.

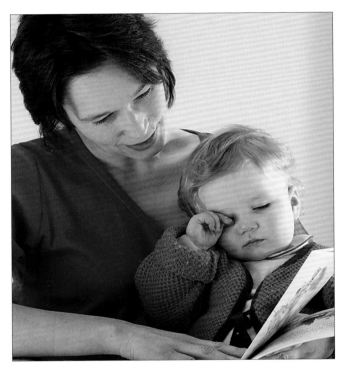

Your baby may be happy to play with some toys in the cot even if he or she doesn't want a nap. If not, schedule in some quiet time – look at a book or do a simple jigsaw – as a break in an action-packed day.

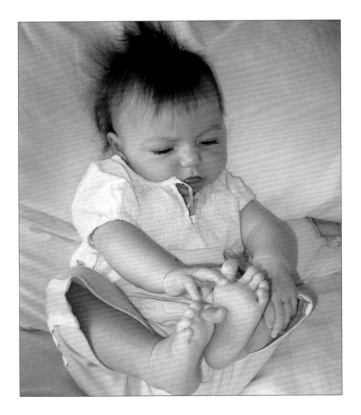

Now that your baby is more aware of what is going on, he or she may resist going to sleep during the day, because who wants to nap when there is all that exploring to do? But rest is important, otherwise the baby will become irritable during the day and, paradoxically, will find it harder to sleep at night.

Do what you can to facilitate naps, whether this means putting the baby down in a darkened room or rocking him or her to sleep in a buggy. If possible, put your baby down soon after lunch, even if there is no sign of tiredness. Without a sleep in the early afternoon, he or she is likely to be exhausted by late afternoon, the worst time for a nap because bedtime is not far away.

Don't worry too much about how long your baby sleeps. Although the average baby naps for about three hours a day, yours may need a lot less sleep than this. Be guided by your baby's humour and habits – if he or she is in a good mood during the day and sleeps well at night, then it doesn't matter if the naps are very short.

Some babies drop a nap before they reach twelve months. Usually the morning nap is the first to go, but some drop their afternoon nap, which means they have a

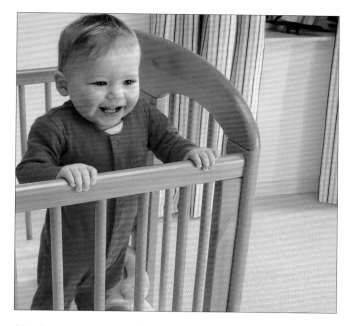

Moving your baby to his or her own room may improve the nights for all of you. The baby may be more inclined to settle him or herself after waking at night.

long time awake before bedtime. One solution might be to give your baby an early lunch – 11 am, say – and to put him or her down for a nap after that.

BABY'S OWN ROOM

Six months is a good age for a baby to move out of your bedroom and into his or her own space. Your baby is now more likely to wake up when you go to bed or if you turn over in the night. But if you don't have a lot of space, are still breastfeeding or feel that your baby benefits from sleeping near you, you may prefer to go on sharing a room for longer.

Avoid changing your baby's sleeping arrangements when in the throes of separation anxiety, during teething

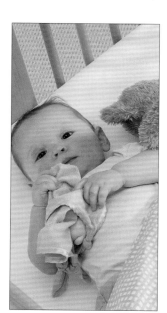

Left: If your baby whimpers in the night, don't pick him or her up too quickly: make sure that the baby really is awake. Try to settle the baby without picking him or her up if you can.

Right: A quiet cuddle before bedtime will help to get your baby into a relaxed state conducive to sleep. Make this the final thing you do, after toothbrushing or a nappy change.

or illness, or if the baby is experiencing change of another kind – for example, a new carer – and make sure that the baby is happy in the new room before you move the cot there. Buy or borrow a few new toys and place some favourite books there to make it fun. Spend as much time as possible in the room during the day for at least a week before moving the baby in. If your baby is easy to settle, you can use the new bedroom for daytime naps – in the buggy or a travel cot if you have one.

Move the cot in the morning. Put a couple of interesting activity toys in it plus one or two old favourites, including your baby's comforter if he or she has one. Give the baby two or three play sessions in the cot during the day. Stay nearby for these; if possible, busy yourself in the room so that the baby plays independently. Take the baby out as soon as he or she starts to get fed up. Follow your usual bedtime routine, and then put your baby to bed at the usual time in the cot. If he or she wakes up, make sure you get there quickly to help him or her settle back to sleep. You could consider putting a spare bed or mattress in the baby's room, so that you can sleep there if the baby becomes distressed rather than taking him or her back to your room.

Don't forget to give your baby plenty of attention and cuddles during the day to help him or her feel secure. Avoid any unusual absences or making any other changes to your baby's routine for a few weeks.

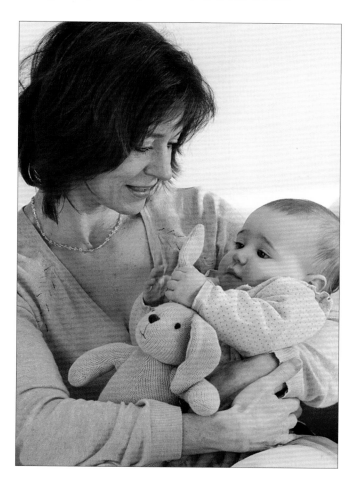

Improving sleep in an older baby

How you deal with broken nights depends very much on whether you think a baby should learn to fit in with your routine or feel that it is your job as a parent to tend to the baby's needs, even when it causes you a lot of inconvenience. Both attitudes have their supporters, but whatever you do, some sleepless nights are inevitable. Here are some simple ways to minimize them.

The baby may be getting hungry. Try to ensure that he or she gets enough food during the day by prioritizing mealtimes and by giving a full breastfeed or a bottle at bedtime. If the baby falls asleep during this feed, give it a little earlier – before a bath or story.

Check that your baby's bedroom is conducive to sleep. Some babies are more sensitive than others and need a carefully controlled environment in order to get through the night. Is it dark and warm enough? If your baby pulls the covers off and then wakes up because it is cold,

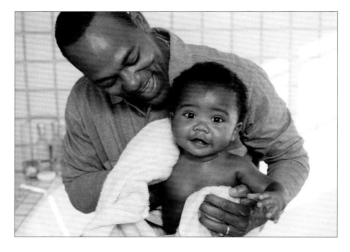

A warm bath is the ideal way for many babies to wind down before bedtime. You can encourage sleepiness by adding a couple of drops of lavender or chamomile essential oils, well diluted in a carrier oil or in milk.

consider using a baby sleeping bag instead of blankets. Your baby may need quiet to sleep, but some find it easier to drop off if there is some noise – try leaving the door open so that the baby can hear the household sounds, or leave a ticking clock, a soothing musical mobile or a radio turned down low. A nightlight can also help some babies to sleep better.

Have a consistent bedtime routine that allows your baby to wind down properly – say, a warm bath, a story or song on your lap and then a feed. If you can, get your baby into bed while sleepy but still awake, to learn to drop off on his or her own (this is hard if you are breastfeeding and have a baby who falls asleep at the breast). Introduce a comforter if your baby doesn't already use one. This can be particularly useful if you are trying to move your baby into a cot from your family bed. And if you are breastfeeding and want to stop night feeds, get your partner or a supportive helper to attend to the baby during the night for a while.

LIGHT MORNINGS
Early-morning waking is very common, especially in summer, and it is hard to handle. Generally speaking it doesn't work to start putting your baby to bed later – he or she will almost certainly wake up at the same time. The most helpful thing that you can do is to ensure your baby's room is really dark – put up blackout blinds or curtain lining to eliminate the first chinks of light. It is also a good idea to treat all feeds before, say, 6 am as quiet night feeds. You can also try putting a couple of toys in the baby's cot so that he or she discovers them on awakening. You may find that he or she will then play happily in the cot for 20 minutes or so while you enjoy a few precious minutes' extra sleep.

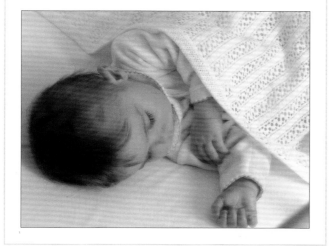

ADOPTING A COMFORTER
You can encourage your baby to adopt a comforter if you think it will make settling at night easier. Over time your baby will associate it with love and sleep, but remember that once this association is made, the comforter will be extremely important to your child – you won't be able to go away for a night without it.

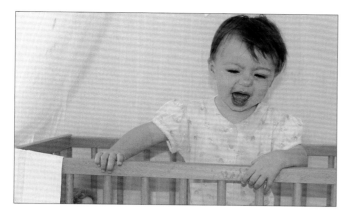

Children do tend to wake up earlier than their parents, and protest vigorously if they don't get a response.

Make sure that you are allowing your baby the opportunity to settle him or herself. It's easy to get into the habit of picking up your baby as soon as he or she makes a sound, especially if the baby is sharing your room. But babies often whimper, cry out or cough in their sleep without actually waking up properly. Wait for a few moments and listen – your baby may continue sleeping if you do not disturb him or her unnecessarily.

CHECKLIST: WHY IS MY BABY WAKING UP?

Here are some of the reasons why an unbroken night's sleep might be eluding you and your baby.

Hunger. If your baby wakes up and won't settle, he or she may need a feed. Keep the room dark as you feed and put the baby back to bed straight away.

Comfort feeding. Lots of breastfed babies wake up several times a night to nurse. Sometimes this is hunger but it can also be because they enjoy having their relaxed mother to themselves.

Anxiety. Babies may become more restless if they are unsettled by a major change – starting at nursery, for example. If your baby is experiencing separation anxiety, he or she may start to resist going to bed.

Developmental leaps. Your baby may be more wakeful at night when acquiring a new skill.

External disturbances. An older baby may be disturbed by noises or by your movements. This doesn't mean your home has to be kept silent – normal household noises can be comforting.

Physical needs. Teething pain – and any accompanying fever – can make for very disturbed nights. Your baby may also wake if too hot or cold, with a soiled or very full nappy, or if he or she is ill. If you think your baby's wakefulness may be due to illness, see your doctor.

Habit. Babies who are used to being nursed to sleep, for example, may find it hard to drop off on their own when they wake up at night.

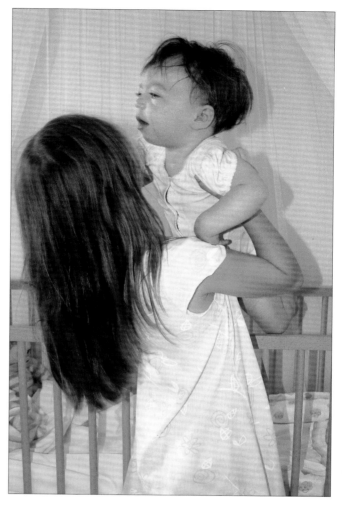

A responsible older sibling may be willing to amuse the baby for a short period so that you can get more sleep.

If your baby doesn't seem to like being in the cot, let him or her have a few play sessions there during the day while you potter about in the room. However, take most of the toys out of the cot at bedtime: one stuffed animal or a comforter is enough.

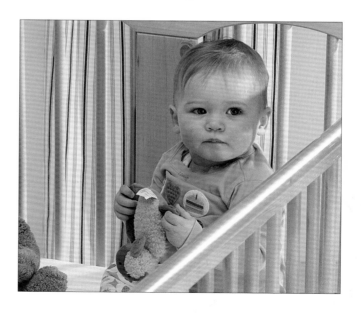

Sleep training

All babies wake up from time to time throughout the night. But if your baby is used to being fed or stroked to sleep at bedtime, he or she will need the same help to drop off during the night. The point of sleep training is to teach a baby to get back to sleep on his or her own.

If your baby is continuing to wake up several times a night, you may decide that now is the time to take action. Unless there is a medical reason for the crying – and it is important to check this with your doctor before embarking on sleep training – you should be able to teach your baby to sleep better using one of the methods described below. Set aside at least a week to do it, and don't choose a time when any major change is going on in your child's life, when your partner will be away or you will be going out in the evening.

Don't forget that your baby's sleep, or lack of it, is only really a problem if it is affecting his or her mood and ability to function, or making daily life difficult for you. If you are both happy, it doesn't matter if your child continues to wake up at night – some mothers are happy to give night feeds for the first year and beyond.

If you can, continue with the method throughout the night. But it is also fine to do the sleep plan until a certain time – 1 am, say – and then to revert to your usual methods if you find that easier. Stick with your sleep plan for at least a week if you can, to instil the idea that once your baby goes into the cot, he or she stays there. It is important that you and your partner agree your approach to sleep training if you are both going to be involved.

Sleep training aims to teach a baby to get to sleep without your help, so that he or she doesn't need to disturb you during the night unless something is wrong.

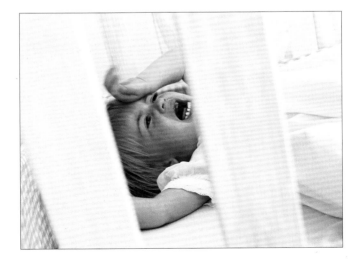

Make a decision about what you want, and work out what steps you are going to take to get there. Be clear about who is going to do what – it is difficult to make sensible decisions when you are faced with a crying child at 3am.

CONTROLLED CRYING

This is the sleep-training method recommended by many health professionals. It doesn't involve leaving your baby to scream unattended for a long time; instead you keep checking so that your baby knows you are there. This can make the baby furious – if you are coming in, why aren't you picking him or her up? – and the process can take longer than if you simply leave the child to scream it out. But it won't leave your baby feeling abandoned and it will mean you can check that nothing else is wrong – such as wind, or a lost dummy (pacifier) or comforter.

Controlled crying is stressful for everyone concerned, so try gentler methods first. If you do decide to do it, be certain that it is the right choice for both parent(s) and child. Be clear with your partner about who is going to do what before you begin. Stick to the method for at least four days – crying often peaks on the third. Remember that you can adapt the method to suit yourself. For example, you may decide that ten minutes is your limit for crying or that you will stroke your baby when you go in.

1 Follow a bedtime routine and put the baby to bed when sleepy and relaxed. Kiss goodnight and leave the room.

2 If the baby cries, wait one minute then return. You can shush, but don't linger or pick up. Gradually increase the time that you leave the baby to cry – to two minutes, then three, then five, then eight, ten and finally 15. Don't leave the baby crying any longer than 15 minutes at a time.

3 Be resolute – if you give in, your baby will hold out for longer the next time you try the method. Continue checking every 15 minutes until your baby falls asleep.

4 If your baby wakes up later in the night, go through the same process of checking and leaving for increasing periods of time, up to 15 minutes. Never just leave your baby crying without checking.

> **CAUTION**
> Any form of sleep training is stressful. Be clear about what you want to achieve and stay calm. It works best if one person tackles each night, but it is a good idea to have your partner or a supportive helper on hand to take over if you become overwhelmed.

Settling a reluctant baby

Some babies do not want to go to bed on their own because it means being away from you. They may be in the habit of falling asleep while breastfeeding, or coming into bed with you to get to sleep. Unless you want to sleep with your baby and go to bed very early every night, this is something you do need to tackle. Here is a gentle way to settle a reluctant baby. It involves gradually reducing the amount of soothing you do. Once you are down to the bare minimum, you should find that your baby finds it easier to drop off on his or her own.

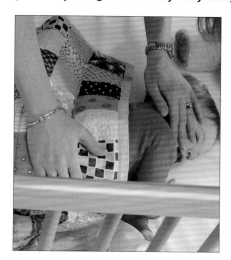

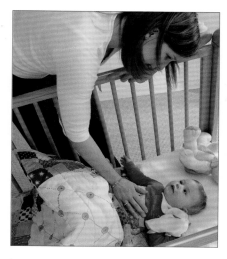

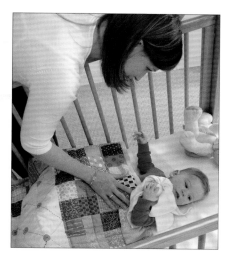

1 Go through your usual bedtime routine. Cuddle or feed until your baby is sleepy, and then put him or her in the cot. Stay in contact – leave one hand underneath the baby's back and stroke his or her head or tummy with the other. Soothe the baby verbally at the same time – try shushing, repeating a key phrase such as "Sleepy time", or singing the same song.

2 If your baby gets very distressed, you may want to pick him or her up. Once comforted, put the baby back in the cot straight away – you may have to do this many times before he or she becomes calmer. If your baby is standing up, lie him or her down. Often a baby will scramble up again immediately. Just keep lying them down again until he or she gets the message and gives in.

3 Once your baby is lying down, keep reassuring them. Combine physical comfort with verbal soothing, reducing the volume as your baby calms down. Stay calm yourself – do some deep breathing if you need to. You should find that the baby's protests gradually become less vocal and insistent, but it can take a lot of patient perseverance before this happens.

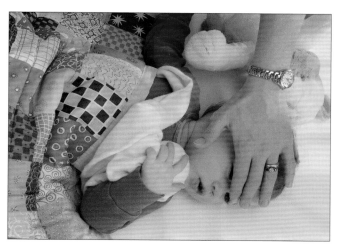

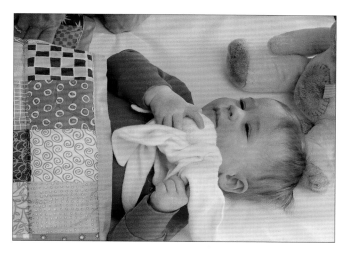

4 Once the baby is calm and sleepy, try stroking your hand from the forehead downwards. As your hand passes over the baby's eyes, they automatically shut and this can help lull him or her into sleep. Continue the verbal soothing, becoming quieter and quieter as the baby drifts off. Slowly remove your hand as you continue to shush or sing. Stand by the cot for a few minutes before retreating.

5 After a few days, your baby should be quietened more easily. Once he or she starts to go into the cot calmly, try simply sitting beside the cot and comforting him or her from a distance – but still go and offer physical comfort if he or she cries. Eventually, when you judge the time is right, you may be able to leave the room and let the baby drift off alone.

Development and play

" This new ability to get around will make your baby more physically independent, but emotionally his or her attachment to you will grow. *"*

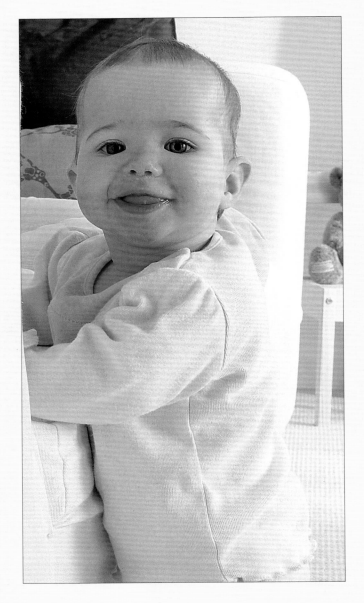

The second half-year of your baby's life is a most eventful time. In the space of a few short months he or she will learn to sit up, and then to get about – by crawling, bottom-shuffling or simply wriggling across the floor. No longer does your baby have to wait to be moved or given interesting things to examine – now he or she can just go and get them.

At some point during these months, your baby will discover how to pull up to a standing position, and will figure out how to edge around a room by holding on to the furniture. This new ability to get around will make your baby more physically independent, but emotionally his or her attachment to you will grow, and a strong bond will also develop with other important people in the baby's life.

Excitingly, your baby will also have some new ways to interact with you. Older babies understand the word "no", although they may not always obey it, and they know their own names and turn round when you call them. By the end of the first year, many

Cruising gives your baby a degree of independence, which he or she will exercise to the full. Standing and moving about will become a favourite activity.

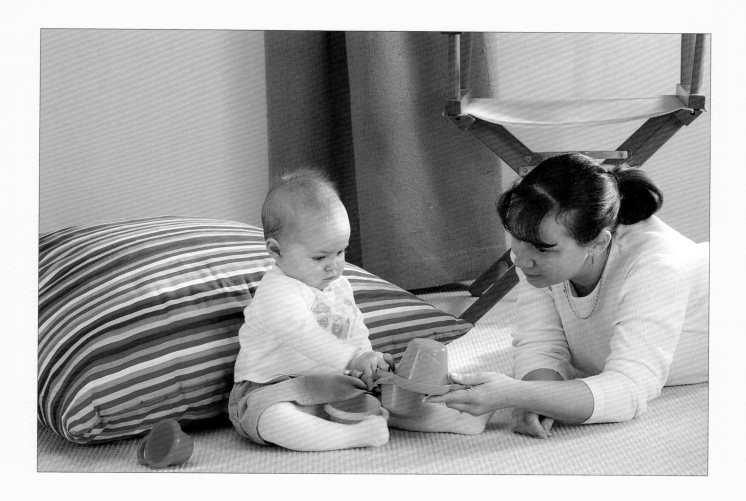

babies can use a few hand signals to communicate: they may wave goodbye, point at something they want and clap hands. Most babies love showing off these new skills, especially when they meet with approval and delight in those around them.

All these new developments mean that outings become more fun. Your increasingly curious and sociable baby will really enjoy music classes now he or she can see what is going on, and will love to shake a percussion instrument or clap with the music. Baby gyms provide your baby with the opportunity for a bit of rough and tumble.

At a developmental review (well-child visit), during this time you will be asked about your baby's eating and sleeping and new achievements. This is a good opportunity to raise any concerns you may have.

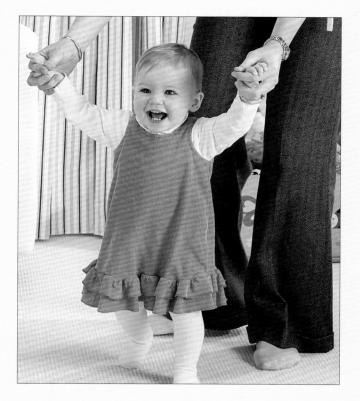

Top: The time when your baby sits up but cannot yet move about is probably the easiest stage of parenthood. He or she will be contented to sit and explore toys.

Babies who are beginning to stand will love being walked round. Some babies start walking independently, though most won't do this until well after one year.

Sitting and crawling

Babies love to sit, but it usually takes six months before they can stay upright by themselves. Before then, you can help your baby practise by sitting him or her in a circle of cushions or rolled-up blankets; the baby will rock from side to side as he or she tries to balance.

Sitting is great fun for babies because it gives a much more comprehensive view of what is going on. It also allows them to stretch further to grab interesting objects, and of course their hands are now free for exploring any item within reach. Expect your sitting baby to topple over a lot. Even after mastering the skill, it takes time to learn exactly how far he or she can reach out without tipping over. Until then, continue to use cushions or rolled-up blankets to give a soft landing. Stay close by: if your baby falls head-down into a pile of cushions in an awkward position, he or she could get stuck.

Most babies are at least nine months old before they can move from a lying-down position to sitting up, without help. Before this they will use any means available to haul themselves up, whether this is your hands, a tablecloth or the sides of a buggy. Be vigilant about strapping your baby into the buggy and highchair, so that he or she can't fall out. If you are still sitting your baby on a sofa or bed, it is definitely time to stop: he or she could easily tip on to the floor.

Babies who are just learning to sit haven't yet worked out how far they can lean forwards without falling over. They need a helping hand to explore safely.

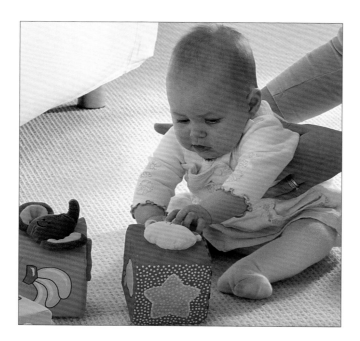

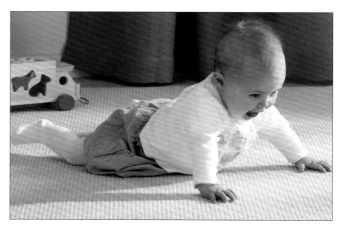

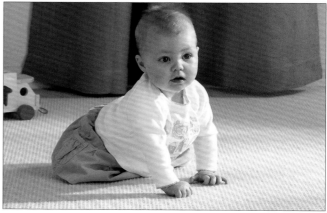

Because motor control develops from the head down, babies' arms are much stronger than their legs at first. So they may use their arms to pull themselves along, commando-style, before they start to crawl properly.

CRAWLING

Not all babies crawl. Some get about by shuffling on their bottoms, using one hand to push themselves forward. Others travel on their hands and feet with their bottoms

CHECKLIST: SAFETY FOR MOBILE BABIES
- Dress your baby in clothes that cover the knees to protect them from hard surfaces or carpet.
- Check wooden floors for splinters, gaps and any protruding nails.
- Put up stair gates.
- Check your child proofing.
- Remember that babies can learn a new skill quite suddenly. If your baby is getting ready to crawl, take precautions straight away

MOBILITY

Babies vary so much in when and how they start to get mobile that crawling isn't included as one of the developmental milestones. It doesn't matter if your baby doesn't crawl, just so long as he or she finds some way of moving around. But if your baby isn't mobile by the age of one, or doesn't seem to use all his or her arms and legs when moving, you should consult a health professional. Remember that premature babies often do things later than other babies born at the same time.

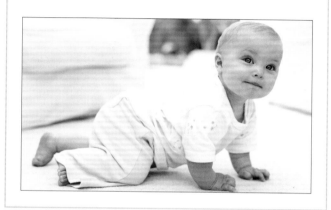

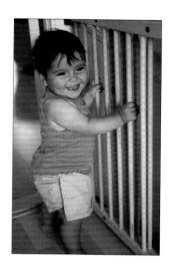

Once your baby becomes mobile, you will need to make sure that your home is safe and be on the lookout for hazards when you are out. Keep one step ahead of your baby's development, since he or she may progress quite suddenly.

high in the air – the "bear-walk". And some cut out this middle stage altogether, going straight from sitting to cruising and walking. Babies who do crawl usually start between eight and ten months, but they start to practise well before this. Often they start by pushing themselves up on their hands and knees when they are lying on their stomachs. It can take them many weeks to figure out how to move forwards from this position: they tend to rock backwards and forwards without going anywhere.

When they do start to move, it is often backwards. This is because their arms are stronger than their legs, but they soon learn how to push with their knees to move forwards. And once they work out how to use opposite arms and legs together, they can go much faster.

You can't help a baby to crawl, but you can provide the opportunities to practise and a safe space to play in, and put the baby down on his or her front often. Placing an interesting toy just out of reach can encourage a baby to try to move forwards. Once crawling starts, it is fun to make a mini obstacle course using cushions, which your baby then has to go around or climb over in order to get to you or to a favourite toy. This can help build confidence and improve balance and coordination, but do help out if your baby gets stuck or frustrated.

CHILDPROOFING YOUR HOME

It is a good idea to crawl around your living spaces to look for hazards such as trailing cords, sharp corners and uncovered plug sockets. A mobile baby will investigate

anything on the floor, so check for dropped coins and stray objects under sofas and so on. Put up stair gates, but once your baby is confidently mobile, let him or her practise crawling up stairs while you follow. You can also let your baby come down the stairs feet-first on his or her tummy, so long as you are there in case of a fall. Consider investing in a playpen or travel cot so that you can keep your baby safe if you need to cook, say, when he or she is awake. But don't use it for long periods.

You can buy childproofing safety packs from DIY stores and pharmacies. They include plug guards to prevent your baby poking things in a socket, and corner protectors to cover sharp corners of coffee tables.

Loop up trailing wires of appliances and secure with an elastic band.

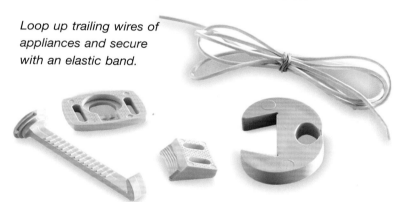

Fit catches to cupboard doors so that your toddler can't open them.

Cushions fitted to doors will stop them slamming on little fingers.

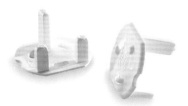

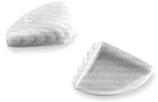

Unused electrical sockets can be made safe with these plugs.

The corners of eye-level tables can be cushioned with covers.

Standing and cruising

Babies long to stand on their own two feet in every sense. Moving independently is a great step towards other kinds of independence: they can entertain themselves, reach toys, and set off to find the people that have moved out of view. Babies seem to sense these possibilities for extending their experience: you need only look at the delight on a child's face after negotiating the route from sofa to table leg, from table leg to chair to see this. But learning to walk, like learning to sit, doesn't happen suddenly, it will develop in stages.

From the time they are a few months old, babies love to stand when being held on a lap. They quickly discover that they can bounce up and down if they bend and straighten their knees, and this will probably be one of their first games. At about seven months, they may start to alternate their feet as if they were walking. But most babies haven't yet developed the strength to take their own weight, and they feel insecure if they are "walked" along the ground before they are ready.

Early walkers may take their first steps at eight or nine months, but most babies don't walk unassisted until they are between 12 and 15 months old. A few are older than 18 months when they start.

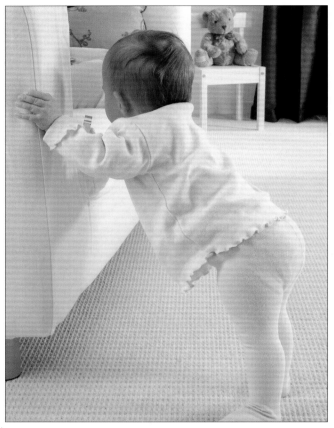

Once your baby starts to cruise, you will probably be astonished by some of the clever ways he or she finds to navigate a room. He or she will use this new skill whenever and wherever possible, so look out for unsafe items on furniture that they will be able to reach.

Most babies have developed enough strength in their legs to stand properly by the time they are about eight or nine months old. But apart from a few early developers, they can't usually maintain the necessary balance to stand independently or to walk. However, they quickly learn to pull themselves up with the help of a chair or the bars of their cots and playpens. They will also enjoy "walking" with your help.

This is a tricky stage for both parent and baby – your baby will repeatedly pull himself or herself up and stand holding on to something at every opportunity. However, the baby hasn't yet worked out how to sit down again. So he or she will shout for you to help – and then promptly stand up again – or will fall on his or her bottom and be shocked by the impact. Be patient: it will take only a few weeks for the baby to figure out how to get back down to the safety of the floor.

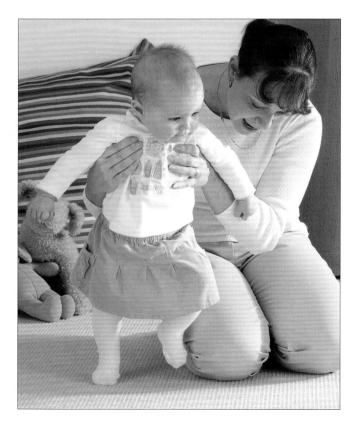

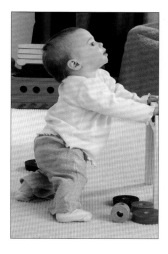
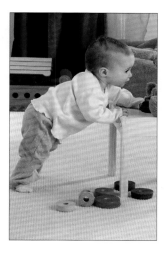
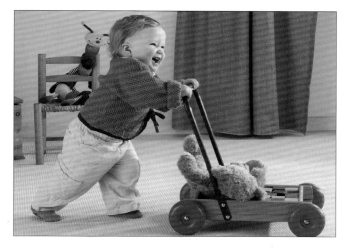

Babies start pulling themselves up from about eight months. But they won't work out how to get down for another month or two.

A toddle truck is the perfect toy for a cruising baby. Look for one that has a stable base and won't tip over. Wooden trucks are often sturdier than plastic ones.

CRUISING

Once your baby can pull up, he or she will soon start to "cruise" – that is, walk while holding on to something. Cruising is likely to become your baby's favourite activity, and he or she will spend many happy minutes walking from one end of the cot to the other, or shuffling along the edge of the sofa.

As he or she gains in confidence, your baby may surprise you with ingenious ways of getting around a room: leaning with the flat of a hand on a wall, stretching up to grab the edge of a table or even pushing a chair along like a walking aid. The baby may navigate to the corner of the refrigerator, say, and then pause to consider how to get to the next piece of furniture. He or she will eventually take the odd unsupported step – like a leap into the unknown – without being aware of it. Your baby is ready to walk, but doesn't quite know it yet.

Don't get shoes until your baby is walking (and even then put them on only when he or she is outside). It is

It's best for babies to learn to walk in bare feet, since this helps with balance and coordination. So hold off putting your baby in shoes indoors.

much better for babies to learn to walk barefoot, which allows them to feel the ground and make the tiny adjustments they need to balance. If socks are necessary to keep a baby's feet warm, make sure they are the right size and the non-slip variety.

STANDING AND CRUISING SAFELY

You can't help a baby to stand or cruise; all you can do is provide a safe environment in which to practise. When ready, your baby will pull himself or herself up by any means possible: it is up to you to ensure it is a safe one.

Move flimsy pieces of furniture out of your living space or put them somewhere out of reach. Your baby can easily pull a light table over, which will not only hurt but will damage his or her confidence.

Remember that once your baby can stand up, he or she will be able to reach for things overhead. So, don't put coffee cups or anything else that can be pulled over on the edge of a table, and take any breakables off low shelves. Abolish tablecloths.

If you haven't been using a baby sleeping bag, don't start now. If your baby isn't used to one, he or she will try to stand up in it and fall over.

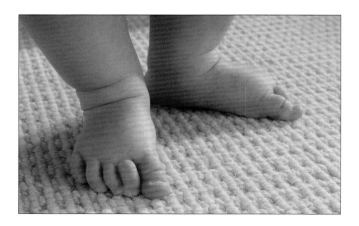

CAUTION
Never put your baby in a baby walker. These toys are dangerous: in 1991, almost 28,000 American children were admitted to hospital following accidents with baby walkers. They are not even a good development aid because they tend to reduce a baby's interest in getting around under his or her own steam. They may also even affect the proper development of the leg muscles if used a lot. Reputable baby stores no longer sell them.

Aqua baby

Swimming is a wonderful activity for you and your baby to enjoy. Water provides a whole new environment for babies to explore and in which to enjoy their bodies. In water they don't need strength or balance: they can experience what it is like to move freely. Swimming can help with muscle development and coordination, and it may also improve sleeping and eating patterns.

If you want your baby to be able to dive underwater and swim at an early age, it is worth joining a specialist swimming class. Most baby swimming classes are held in private or hydrotherapy pools, which are heated to a higher temperature than ordinary swimming baths. Swimming teachers recommend starting classes early, because young babies have no fear of water and have a natural dive reflex that enables them to hold their breath underwater. Babies are most likely to enjoy swimming if they go for the first time before the age of nine months. It's fine to take a baby who is older, but be prepared to proceed very slowly and gently since he or she is now more likely to be frightened of the water. Visit the pool when it is quiet or during a parent-and-baby session. Your baby may feel nervous if the pool is crowded and noisy.

GETTING STARTED

Remember that the point is to get your baby comfortable in the water. Hold the baby close to you at first, and gradually lower yourself into the water until the baby is immersed up to the shoulders. Don't rush this first stage.

Babies love playing games in the water, so it's a good idea to make swimming a group activity with a few parent-and-baby friends. Try making a circle with your babies, and then swooshing them out of the water and into the middle of the ring.

CHECKLIST: POOL KIT
- Swimming nappy (usually optional)
- Baby swimming pants (usually compulsory)
- A hooded towel
- A couple of pool toys (such as a ball)
- Milk and a snack for afterwards
- Your usual nappy bag
- Swimming costume and towel for yourself
- Toy or book for while you are dressing

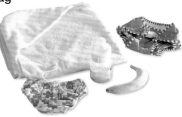

If your baby is nervous, start by bobbing up and down so that only the tips of his or her toes hit the water. Then, as the baby relaxes, go a little further.

When your baby seems happy and confident in the water, slowly move him or her away from you and then back again, holding securely under the baby's arms. Have a big smile on your face, talk to your baby and keep eye contact. If he or she is happy doing this, swish him or her from side to side while you keep them at arm's length. Keep your face on a level with your baby's to help him or her feel safe. If the baby's face goes underwater, give him or her a cuddle and reassurance if necessary.

A good teacher can show you how to get your baby so comfortable underwater that he or she will dive with you. Choose a small class that offers plenty of individual attention. Your baby will be in the water for a while so it must be very warm.

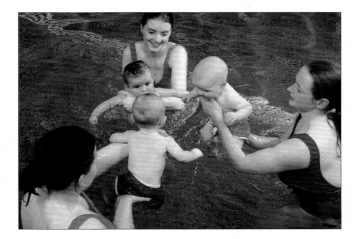

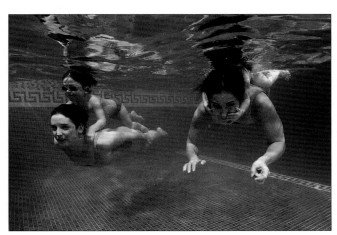

One-arm hold

Once your baby is comfortable in the water, and you are feeling confident too, try this more relaxed hold. It gets babies used to having less support without making them feel insecure. Eventually you can try using a foam woggle instead of your arm.

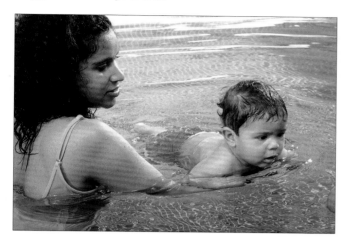

Rest your baby's chest on your forearm, so that his or her arms are in front of it. Place a reassuring hand on the baby's back. At first, keep your baby close to your body. Then slowly extend your arm outwards in an arc-like movement. Gently take your hand off the baby's back. Turn so that your arm traces a circle through the water. Put a ball in front of your baby to keep him or her amused and encourage use of the arms. Keep your arm relaxed.

Next, try turning the baby around to face outwards; keep your hands on either side of his or her ribcage below the armpits. Dip the baby in and out of the water, matching your words to the actions: for example, "Up we go" and "Splaaaash". Hold the baby at arm's length and swish from side to side. Put a ball or interesting bath toy a little distance in front and move the baby forwards as he or she reaches towards it. Young babies naturally kick in the water, but older ones may not. If your baby doesn't

Practising back floating

This is a good exercise to encourage your baby to float on his or her back. Start with the baby in the water in a sitting position, using one hand to support the bottom and the other to support the neck, back of the head and top of the shoulders.

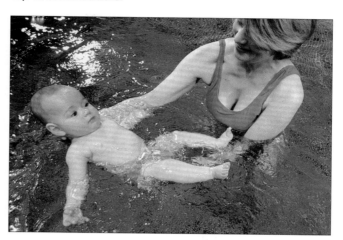

Gently lower the baby backwards into the water, then sit him or her up again. Do this several times in a rhythmic movement – try saying or singing "Baaack, uuuup" as you do so. In time, the baby will be able to spend longer lying on his or her back and you'll be able to remove the hand under the bottom. Once the baby finds his or her buoyancy, you can lessen the support under the neck.

kick spontaneously, wait until you can support him or her one-handed (see below) before trying to help. Then use your other hand to move the baby's leg in a kicking action. Say "Kick-kick-kick" whenever your baby is kicking, and eventually he or she will learn to kick in response to the words. Don't worry about the kicking style – babies have different ways of kicking, and there is no point in trying to refine their technique until they are swimming without assistance.

SWIMMING WITH A BABY: KEY POINTS

- Don't take a baby swimming if he or she is unwell or has a cold.
- If your baby has eczema, the condition may be exacerbated by chlorinated water. Keep a close eye on the baby's skin, and stop if it gets worse.
- If possible, choose a pool that has steps rather than a ladder. If yours has a ladder, get someone to go with you so that you don't have to negotiate the rungs while holding your wet, slippery baby.
- Keep swimming sessions short – start with ten-minute sessions and build up slowly to 30 minutes.
- Always take your baby out of the water as soon as you think he or she is getting tired or chilly. Wrap the baby in a towel (with his or her head covered) as soon as you leave the water.
- Don't give your baby solid food just before swimming (it is fine to give a milk feed).
- Don't use armbands or rubber rings, which stop your baby from discovering his or her natural buoyancy.
- Always respect your baby's feelings. Even babies who have been swimming since they were very young may suddenly develop anxiety about being in the water. Never force a baby to do anything that he or she is unhappy with.

Dexterity, doing and thinking

By the age of six months, babies have already learned to grasp an object, put it in the mouth and to pass it from hand to hand. Now, although they still like to put objects in their mouths, they start to use their hands more: watch your baby stroke and pat an object before picking it up, and then shake, roll or bang it on the ground. Try laying your baby on different surfaces – grass, rough carpet, a soft rug, a silky cushion – so he or she can explore the feel. Offer textured books – the baby will quickly work out which part of the page to stroke – as well as toys with interesting textures and shapes.

Over the next few months, your baby's dexterity will improve dramatically. Babies learn to hold objects in their palms by wrapping their fingers and thumb around them, the thumb working like an extra finger rather than a separate unit. This clumsy hold doesn't allow them to manipulate the object very well. At about seven months, they learn to use the four fingers and the thumb as different units, making it much easier for them to pick up and handle things.

The next stage is to control individual fingers. The first sign that your baby can do this is when he or she starts to point, at about eight months. Some time around nine months, babies learn how to hold an item between index finger and thumb, using the pincer grip that is unique to

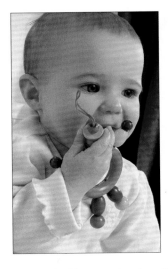
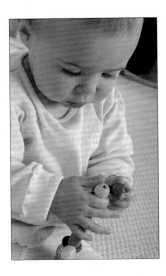

Young babies predominantly use their mouths to explore things. But as they become more dextrous, they start to use their hands a lot more.

humans. This enables them to pick up even very tiny objects and to perform sophisticated movements such as turning the pages of a book. You can help your baby to practise the pincer grip by putting a few cooked peas or grains of rice on the highchair's feeding tray at mealtimes: he or she will enjoy the task of picking them up one by

OBJECT PERMANENCE

Very young babies are unaware that anything they cannot see continues to exist. So if they have dropped a toy, say, they won't look for it because in their mind it is no more. Experts differ on when babies start to understand that objects are permanent, but most put it between four and seven months. At some point around this age you will notice that your baby will pull a cloth aside to find a toy that is partially visible. By nine months, a baby will look for a toy even if it is completely hidden. This leap in understanding means that an older baby will be much harder to distract when you take something away. You can help your baby to learn about object permanence by playing variations of the game "peek-a-boo". Cover your face with your hands and then reappear. Hide a squeaky toy under a cloth and make it sound before the baby can see it. Your baby will also enjoy surprising you by playing peek-a-boo back – covering his or her face and then slowly uncovering it. He or she will love it if you respond with surprise.

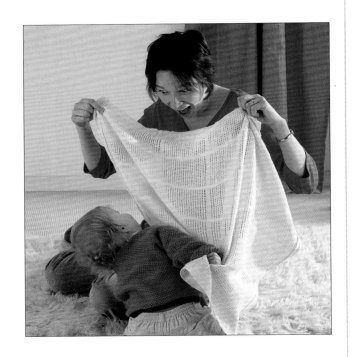

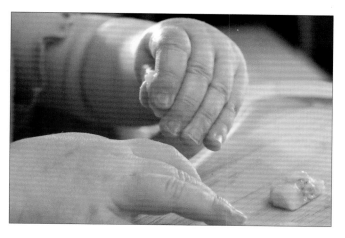

The pincer movement shows that your baby has control over individual digits. A key sign that it is about to happen is when he or she starts to point.

one. Unfortunately this also goes for any other small item, which will also go in the mouth. This means that you have to be vigilant about what is on the floor: a dropped button or pin could be a real danger.

Your baby will be able to hold only one thing at a time at first and will hold on until he or she loses interest and drops it without noticing. If you try to offer a second toy, he or she will automatically drop the first one in reaching for it. But by seven or eight months, a baby is able to hold two things at once, one in each hand.

Your baby will love to hand things to you. Say "thank you" when he or she puts a toy into your hand – this is the very start of learning to share.

DROPPING AND THROWING

Babies have to learn how to let go of things. At first, they simply hold on until you take an object from them, or they drop it accidentally when their attention is caught by something else. But at about the same time as they learn the pincer grip, they discover how to open their fingers and deliberately drop something that they are holding. This quickly becomes a fun activity they will want to practise again and again. Your baby will love it if you give him or her a small toy and then ask for it back – put your hand under it so you can catch it as it drops.

Be prepared for a few weeks of picking things up whenever your baby is in the highchair – it will add to the baby's fun if you exclaim in mock protest every time you have to do this. You could put a metal tray on the floor where the objects fall so that your baby can hear that different items make different sounds when they hit it: try a metal spoon, a soft toy, a wet flannel and a bouncy ball. To stop your baby's new game becoming a real annoyance, restrict toys for the buggy to those that can be attached to it: the baby can then enjoy throwing them over the side and hauling them back in.

Your baby will also enjoy batting a ball back to you after you throw it. This is a good way to practise hand eye coordination. At first he or she will swipe at the ball and probably miss, but will quickly learn to how to hit it back in your direction.

Once your baby has discovered how to drop things, he or she will enjoy your reaction as they repeatedly hurl toys or dishes down from the high chair.

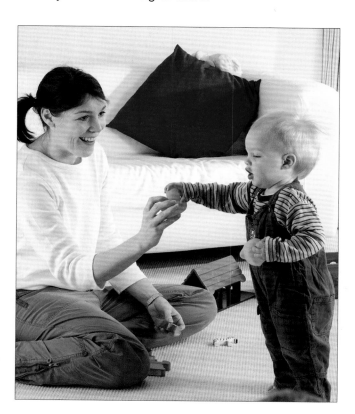

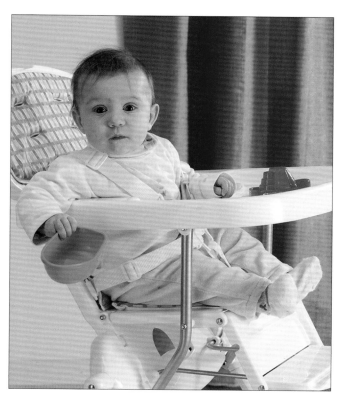

Sociability and language

Now that your baby can sit up and look around, he or she will get a lot more from going out and meeting people. You'll notice that your child starts to become more interested in other babies and children, and may stretch out to touch another baby's hand or face.

Babies love to socialize, and from the age of six months it is important to give them plenty of opportunities to interact with others. This can be as simple as taking your baby with you to the supermarket – it is good to experience positive interactions with strangers, who may smile and play little games while you are in the checkout queue. Your baby will also enjoy classes and parent-and-baby groups, as well as visits to the park to see other children playing.

As the first birthday approaches, you'll notice that your baby becomes more aware of the distinction between familiar people and strangers. For a while, new acquaintances will be scary. One moment the baby may be happy to be cuddled by another adult or to play in front of another baby; the next he or she may be crying for you. This is an aspect of separation anxiety and a normal stage of baby development. Your baby's budding

Your baby won't yet have any understanding of social skills, but you can certainly introduce the concept of being gentle when touching you or another baby. This is the root of empathy, the important notion that you should treat other people kindly.

LANGUAGE SKILLS AT 12 MONTHS

A few babies say their first word by 12 months, but most take longer. Your baby is likely to recognize the following words at one year old.
- His or her own name – the baby may turn towards you when you call it.
- "Hello" and "bye bye" – the baby may start to wave on hearing them.
- "No" – though babies take real delight in ignoring it.
- A few naming words for familiar items – such as "ball", "duck" and "teddy".
- Some basic commands, such as "Give it to mummy."
- Simple questions such as "Where is your nose?" – which the baby may then point to.

awareness of whom he or she belongs to and who belongs to him or her is the beginning of a sense of community, of being part of a family, a friendship group, a nation and a wider world.

LANGUAGE AND THE OLDER BABY

Most babies have started to manifest the rudiments of language by the end of their first year. At this time, you will probably find that your baby babbles more often and in a conversational tone that sounds like real language, as if

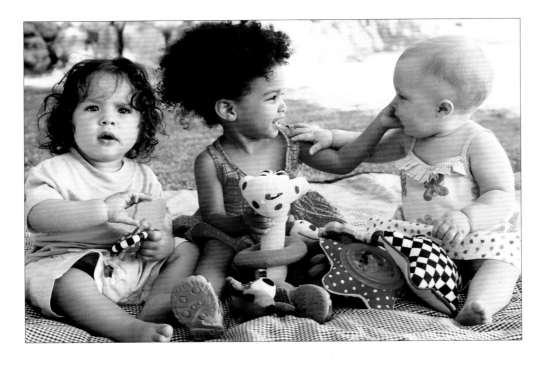

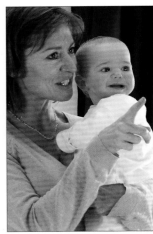

Pointing out things of interest and telling your baby about them is something that most parents do instinctively.

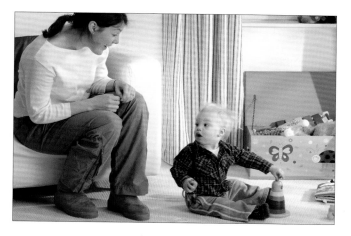

One of the first words that babies learn to recognize is their own name. If they hear it often, they will quickly learn that this particular sound means them.

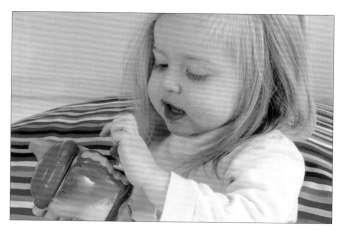

Talking to your child about things that are in front of him of her is the best way to encourage him or her to learn useful everyday words such as "cup".

telling a little story. He or she may even say a few words, though these are unlikely to be perfectly enunciated – for example, "duh" for "duck" or "ook" for "look".

We tend to judge language development by when a baby says the first word, but your child's understanding is racing ahead of his or her ability to articulate. A one-year-old knows a lot more than he or she says, and when a baby chooses to speak the first word is not an indicator of developmental level.

Before your baby speaks, you will see the first green shoots of verbal communication in his or her behaviour. You may notice that the baby listens with greater attention when you talk, and seems to understand words that crop up often. He or she seems to know when you are asking a question – a quizzical expression shows this. And your baby may even know the answer to some frequently asked questions – pointing to a photograph when you say "Where's granny?"; shaking his or her head when you offer another piece of banana (though sometimes this will be for fun, and the baby will take the banana from your hand straight afterwards).

Your baby will also begin to associate certain words with particular situations, which is a stepping-stone towards linking a fixed sound with a definite concept. The baby may, for example, routinely say "Peep-oh" when playing the hiding game or invent words that seem to bear no relation to his or her native language. All this is thrilling for you as a parent. The time when your little baby can tell you what is on his or her mind is just around the corner. Some fascinating and sometimes hilarious conversations lie ahead.

HELPING YOUR BABY TO TALK

Your baby will pick up the meaning of words naturally, but here are some ways you can help.

Talk about things your baby can see. At dinner time, talk about the baby's food, cup, spoon; if you are in the park, talk about the swings, the children and so on.

Use simple sentences that include key labelling words such as "Here is your teddy", "Pass the teddy to daddy", "Where is teddy?" Your baby has to hear a word in context many times to understand what it signifies.

Get down to your baby's level. Make eye contact when you speak, use big hand gestures, exaggerated facial expressions and a sing-song tone to help your baby grasp the gist of what you are saying.

Spend time talking to your baby each day. Find some time when there are no other distractions (such as older children wanting your attention) or background noise (such as the TV or radio).

Be on the lookout for first words and respond to them, even if they are made up. Your baby will be delighted to see that you know what he or she means.

Second children may spend less one to one time with their parents, but they will benefit from having a sibling to talk to, play with and learn from.

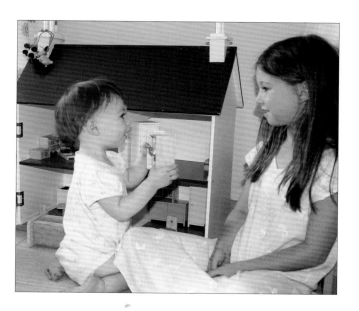

Signing with your baby

There is nothing out of the ordinary about babies using signs to communicate. This is something that they do quite spontaneously and without conscious prompting. From about eight or nine months, your baby may start to clap, wave "Bye-bye", point to things, shake his or her head, lift his or her arms to be picked up and so on. Babies learn to signal before they can speak because hand signals are more visible and easy to copy than the complicated mouth movements that constitute speech.

Teaching your child baby sign language takes this natural process one step further. All it requires is for you to match an action to a word that crops up regularly, and to perform the gesture whenever appropriate.

WHY LEARN BABY SIGNING?
Baby signing can have real benefits for both baby and parent, because it allows a baby to communicate beyond his or her ability to articulate speech. It is fun for both of you – you get to find out more about what your baby is thinking, and the baby enjoys telling you.

Baby signing can facilitate language development, one study found that signing babies recognized more words and had larger vocabularies than non-signing ones. Baby

Signing isn't necessary for language development, which happens quite naturally as a result of interaction, but it can be a fun extra activity to do with your baby.

signing teachers claim that signing babies often learn to speak earlier as well. Baby signing may also help with brain development. Advocates say that signing, because it involves visual awareness as well as language skills, uses more parts of the brain than normal speech, and therefore creates more synapses (conceptual pathways) in the brain.

Another possible benefit is that signing can reduce frustration and possibly tantrums. If your baby can make signs that you both understand, it may be easier to tell you what he or she wants (a sleep, a drink, a favourite toy) rather than having to wait while you work it out.

WHEN CAN YOU START?
You can start signing with your baby any time from about six months, but the baby probably won't start to sign back until between eight and ten months. Toddlers can also benefit from signing, and since they have more advanced motor skills may reward you by signing back much more quickly – an 18-month old could pick up some simple signs within a few days.

HOW DOES IT WORK?
You can use a sign language developed for the deaf – American sign language (ASL) or British sign language (BSL) – to sign with your baby. Some of the signs are too difficult for a baby to reproduce, so you may need to

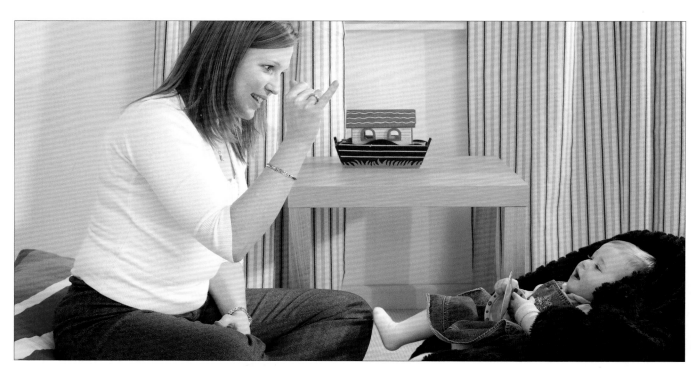

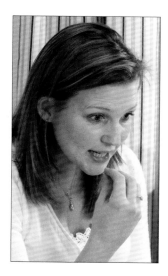

Eat: Bring your fingers together and then move your hand towards your mouth several times.

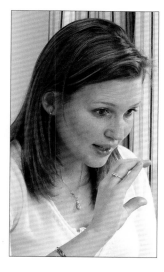

Drink: Hold your fingers and thumb apart to make a C-shape. Bring your fingers up to your face as if drinking from a cup.

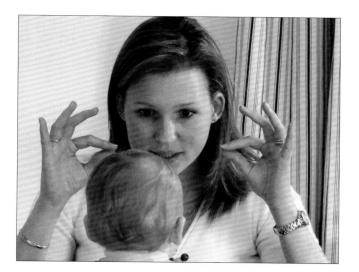

Cat: Pinch the index finger and thumb of each hand together under your nose and then draw them out to the sides, as if preening a cat's whiskers. For "dog" slap your right hand against your leg a couple of times, then click your fingers as if attracting a dog's attention.

teach a simplified version. Alternatively, you can use your own invented signs – such as a few pats on the head for "hat" or your hands cupped together for "ball".

Unless you want your baby to be able to sign to a deaf person, it doesn't really matter what system you use – your baby will adapt to any signs and is unlikely to continue signing once he or she can speak fluently. It can be easier to use an established system like ASL or BSL than to think up a host of new signs yourself, but you'll need to go to classes or buy a signing dictionary.

SIGNING AT HOME

Start with a manageable number of signs – six is enough – and make sure you have your baby's attention before you sign. Get close up, make eye contact and then do the gesture. Make sure that you always say out loud the word for the sign you are using. Remember that the point of the exercise is not to teach your baby perfect sign language,

but to provide a temporarily useful way of communicating until the baby is able to speak well. Try to sign in exactly the same way each time – your baby will learn by repetition. It is important to sign in different contexts – for example, sign "cat" when you see one in the garden, when you come across one in a storybook, and as you draw one. Sign one thing at a time at first – don't sign two words in succession, or your baby may be confused.

Be on the lookout for your baby's first attempts to sign back. It doesn't matter if this sign ends up being different from the "real" one; the baby may refine it as his or her motor skills improve, and you can then perhaps adapt yours. Make sure that you respond to your baby's signs, and give lots of praise. If possible, let other carers know what signs you are teaching, so that they can use them too. And be very, very patient. It may take many weeks for your baby to use a sign that you teach, or for you to recognize it as such.

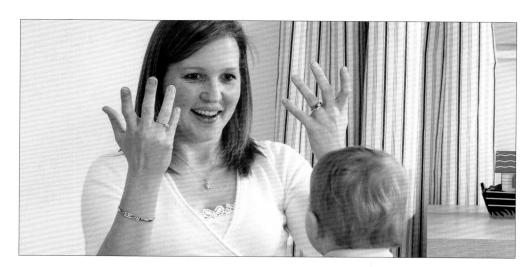

Right: To signal "finished" open your hands, palms facing your chest, then turn them outwards in a flicking movement.

Fun for older babies

New manual dexterity means that your baby can explore toys more thoroughly, and you'll notice that he or she starts to have more interest in what they can do. So the baby may push a toy car along the ground, but place one building brick on top of another.

The best way to encourage your child's learning is to tailor play to abilities. Babies tend to be most interested in skills that they are just about to master or have recently learned. It is up to you to provide activities that are just hard enough to be fun and stimulating: if they are too easy or familiar, the baby will get bored; if they are too difficult, he or she may become upset. You will have to be the judge of when your baby is ready to give them a go.

ROLLING TOYS

A mobile baby will love to chase after toys that roll: a wheeled car or truck, a soft, slow-moving ball or even a toilet roll. Make sure that any rolling toys are too large to fit in the baby's mouth and that they are suitable for this age (don't let your baby play with an older child's car, say, which may have lots of small parts). The baby will also like pulling or pushing toys.

Babies are equally interested in "boy" and "girl" toys, so don't try to limit them. Your little girl may enjoy playing with planes or cars, which she can push along the floor; a little boy may love cuddling a baby doll, which, after all, looks just like him.

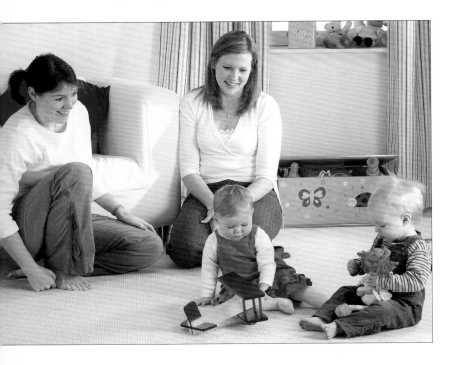

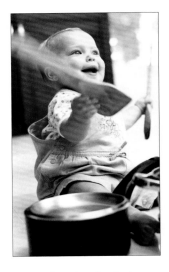

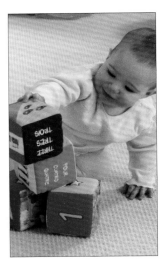

In the hands of a baby, a couple of saucepans and a wooden spoon can be magically transformed into a drum kit.

Babies love to knock down towers of bricks, and will eventually start to try building them up for themselves.

TOYS THAT DO THINGS

As your baby gets more dextrous, he or she will enjoy playing with toys that do something, especially if they offer the thrill of surprise. A truck that takes off when you push a button or a jack-in-the-box that pops up when you turn a dial will be a source of real fascination. Let the baby practise setting the toy off: this will help develop dexterity and strength. Toy telephones (and real ones) that ring or buzz are universally popular.

EMPTYING GAMES

Older babies love to empty things out of containers, drawers, cupboards, bags and boxes. To make a game out of this you can fill a fabric shopping bag or a box with a selection of small objects that the baby can take out one by one. Change some of the items every so often to keep the game interesting. As well as toys, you could include things like a wooden spoon, a baby hairbrush, an old notebook, a set of clean, unwanted keys on a ring, an old purse, a plastic pot or an orange. It is a good idea to let the baby help you put them all back in the right place – showing that "tidying up" can be a fun part of playtime.

DISCOVERING WATER

Water is a source of wonder to all babies: it changes shape, cannot be held and glistens in the light. Your baby will love to play pouring games in the bath. Provide a variety of containers of different sizes, and show how to pour water from one to the other. Natural sponges make great bath toys: fill one up and then show your baby how to squeeze the water out of it.

STACKING TOYS

A set of stacking cups will provide months of amusement. At first your baby will simply enjoy exploring similar objects of different sizes. Then he or she will have endless fun putting one of the small cups inside a larger one. This is one way that he or she starts to work out how things are different, and learn important concepts such as big and small. The baby will love to knock down a tower when you build it, and will want to do it over and over again: it is an early way of showing that he or she can change what is happening, giving an enjoyable sense of power and achievement. Eventually, the baby will have a go at putting one cup on top of another, or threading a set of stacking rings on a pole.

MUSICAL TOYS

Babies love things that make noises. Wooden maracas, a tamourine and various shakers will be popular with babies of this age and older, but you don't have to buy musical toys; you can also make your own. An upturned saucepan make a good drum to bang with a wooden spoon, while a few cotton reels in a well-sealed plastic container make a great shaker.

HELPING YOUR BABY ENJOY PLAY

Keep giving your baby new things to play with: babies need lots of variety and get bored if they play with the same toys all the time. But they don't need lots of expensive playthings – your baby really will be as happy exploring a cereal box and other household items as an expensive toy. Reignite your baby's interest in toys he or she has enjoyed by hiding them away for a while and then letting the baby discover them afresh. Allow your baby to make a mess. Babies scatter toys everywhere, and they

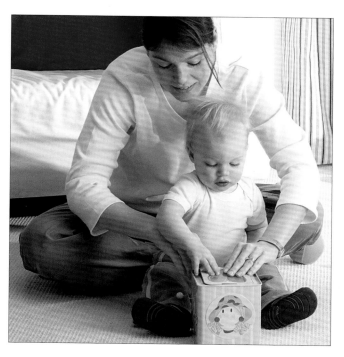

Babies learn by watching other people as well as by exploring things for themselves. So get down on the floor and show your baby how each toy works. He or she may not succeed in copying you, but will have a go – and will remember what to do with that toy next time.

love to empty out a cupboard or a bag of shopping. Be prepared for a less-than-spotless house for a while; you can always tidy up when the baby has gone to bed.

It will help to contain the mess if you restrict emptying games to a special cupboard filled with non-breakable things that can be flung on the floor. Whenever the baby tries to do the same to other cupboards, gently say "No" and lead him or her back to the special cupboard. If you do this consistently, your child will eventually get the message. Be reasonable about what your baby can and cannot do. Move things that you don't want played with, rather than constantly saying "No" every time the baby goes near them.

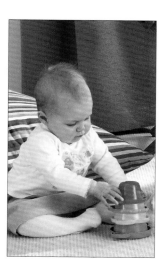

Left: Stacking cups or rings will give good value for months as a baby's manual skills develop.

Right: As your baby explores objects by handling, he or she starts to work out how things relate to each other. A baby will become totally absorbed in the task of putting a small beaker into a larger one.

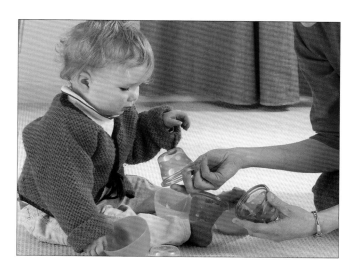

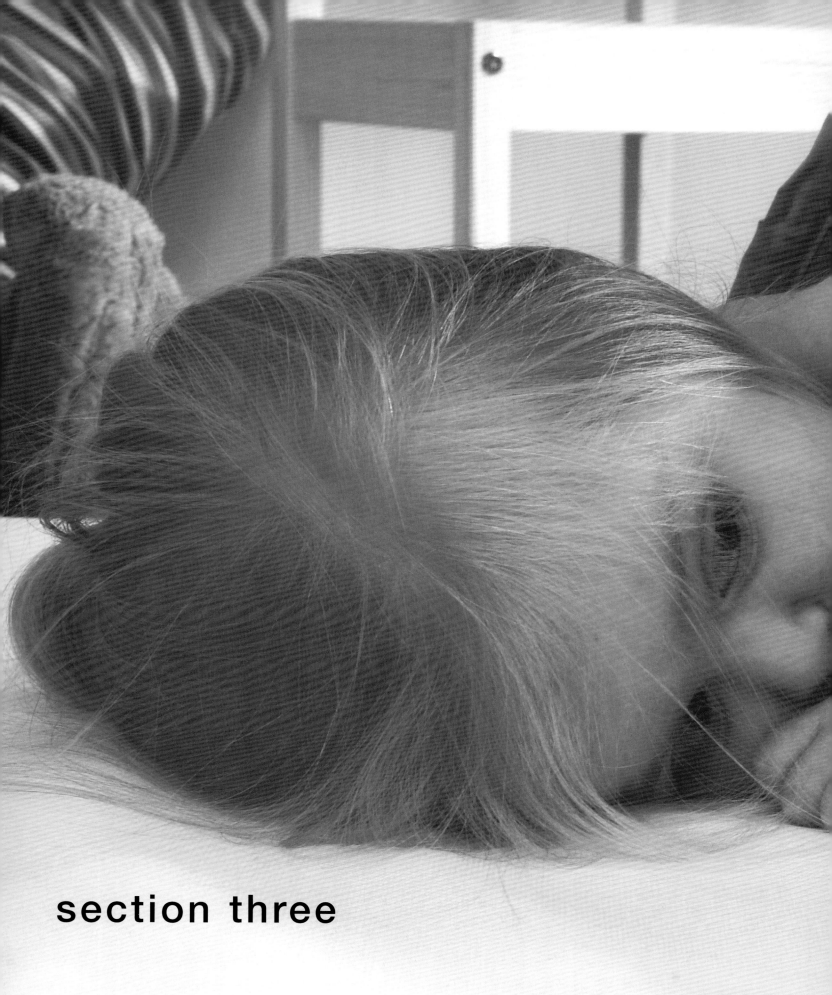

section three

toddlers and older chidren

Toddlers are amazing creatures: they are
curious, strong-willed, unselfconscious, as
changeable as the weather, and always ready to
share love and laughter. You will find that it is a
real education to go for a walk with your child
and to get a privileged glimpse of the world
through his or her eyes. Once your child learns
to talk, you will have some of the most engaging
conversations you will ever have.

General care and feeding

“ It is delightful to watch your little child wash his or her own face with a flannel or to put their wellingtons on the wrong feet. ”

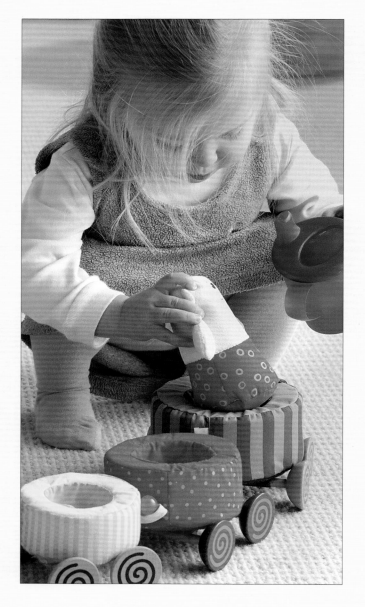

One of the real delights of being a parent to a toddler is seeing how their determination to do things for themselves gradually grows into true independence. But toddlers can have very strong opinions, so simple daily tasks such as getting dressed and washed or eating breakfast can turn into a battleground. Mealtimes are a flashpoint in many families. Your toddler may start to eat more messily, spread his or her dinner everywhere or hurl his bowl on the floor.

It is essential to keep your perspective. After all, it doesn't really matter if your child wants to wear, say, odd socks, or a fairy costume. Don't make a confrontation out of things that don't matter.

The key developmental goal at this age is bladder and bowel control. Toilet training is bound to involve a few accidents, but your child will get there more easily and quickly if he or she is keen to use the potty and if he or she is completely ready for the challenge when you start. In this chapter there's information on the key signs to look out for, as well as advice on

It's good to hand over control of small things to your toddler. Even something as simple as letting a toddler manage his or her own drinks can instil independence.

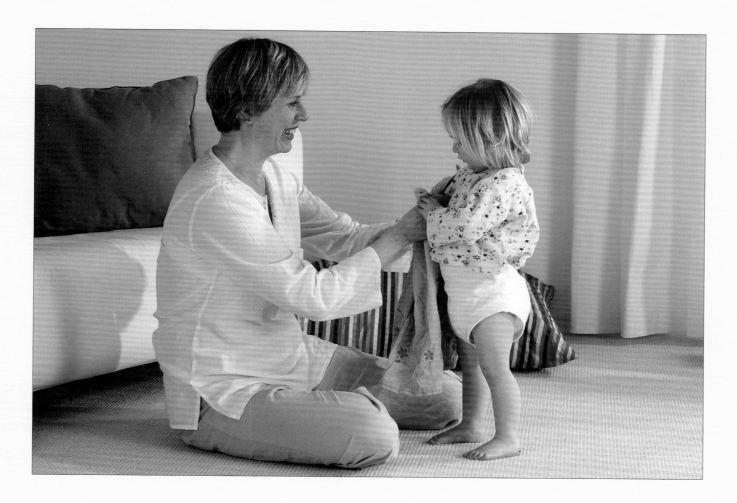

how to introduce the potty and encourage your child to use it. Another common life change in the third year, one over which your toddler has absolutely no control, is the arrival of a younger brother or sister. This is something that has to be carefully managed, but with a little tact and forethought the growth of your family can be as joyful a time for your older child as it is for you.

Always remember that your toddler's growing independence is a positive thing, even if it might make life trying from time to time. It is delightful to watch your little child wash his or her own face with a flannel or to put their wellingtons on the wrong feet, and it gives him or her great pleasure too. So as far as possible, try to nurture your child's natural enjoyment in doing things for themselves.

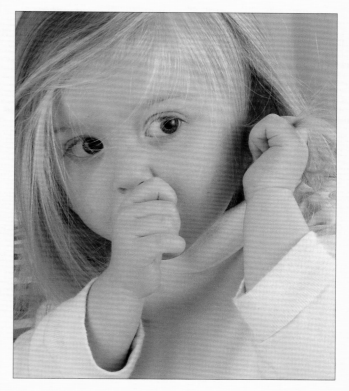

Top: It's fun to see your child gradually working out how to do things for him or herself. Most children want to help get themselves dressed from an early age.

However independent toddlers may seem at times, they are still babies emotionally. Your child may become more needy if a new baby arrives on the scene.

Washing and keeping clean

As your toddler gets older, you begin the process of teaching him or her to become more independent, starting to feed, wash and take care of themselves, or at least becoming aware of what is involved. Your toddler may embrace these new activities with enthusiasm – little children take great delight in doing things for themselves, especially if they perceive a task as a grown-up one. They are also inveterate copiers, and will enjoy performing tasks and jobs with you rather than only under instruction.

CLEAN HANDS

Toddlers inevitably get grubby, and an evening bath is the easiest way to get them clean after a busy day in the sandpit and the garden. In between times, though, it is important that young children wash their hands before meals and after using the potty or helping to take off a used nappy (diaper), so it is a good idea to instil regular handwashing habits early on. Your child will still need your help until about the age of three.

Get a step so that your toddler can reach the washbasin, and teach him or her the difference between the hot and cold taps. Demonstrate how to turn on the cold tap. Teach your child not to touch the hot one – and consider reducing the temperature of your hot-water supply to less than 55°C/130°F to prevent accidental scalding. Begin by lathering your own hands and then gently rub the soap bubbles all over your toddler's. Make it fun by blowing the bubbles into the air, or by having hand-washing races.

A toddler may positively enjoy washing his or her hands just like mummy and daddy. Choose a natural soap without harsh chemicals.

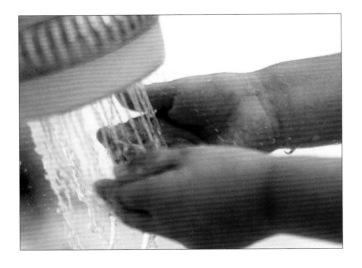

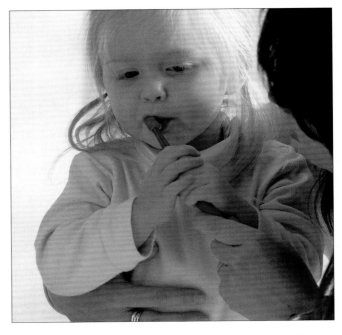

As babies get older, they often enjoy the twice-daily ritual of cleaning their teeth. But they can't brush them properly on their own until they are much older.

GETTING CLEAN

Your toddler's skin is very delicate so it is important to avoid harsh soaps or bath products. A handful of oats gathered in a piece of muslin makes a good alternative to soap, and you can avoid using shampoo altogether if you wish and simply rinse your child's hair with water: the natural oils in the hair will keep it clean. If you want to use products, choose natural ones free from chemicals, and limit hair washing to once or twice a week.

Many toddlers dislike having their hair washed. If you have this problem, you can sponge the hair to get rid of clumps of food. But from time to time, you will have to wash it. If you use shampoo, choose a gentle one that won't sting if it gets in your child's eyes.

NAIL CARE

It's easier to keep fingernails and toenails clean if they are short – long nails can harbour dirt and germs. But most toddlers hate having their nails cut and it is almost impossible to do this safely if your child keeps wrenching his or her hand or foot away. The best solution is to cut the nails when your child is asleep, but you could also try doing it as part of a game such as "This little piggy". Child-sized nail clippers are usually the best way to cut small nails, but some children prefer to have them filed.

TOOTHBRUSHING

If your toddler is reluctant to let you clean his or her teeth, try letting him or her do yours first or brush a favourite toy's "teeth". Tooth cleaning is important, so persevere even if it is difficult. Try doing it after supper rather than just before bedtime if it becomes a flashpoint. Take your toddler with you when you visit the dentist. Children don't need a check-up until they are about two, but it is good to make the dentist's surgery and the "special chair" a familiar environment long before that.

BATH TIME

You don't have to hold your toddler in the bath like a baby, but you do still need to be vigilant. Remember that small children can drown in just a few centimetres of water and in a few moments, so don't ever leave a toddler in the bath unattended or in the care of an older child, however sensible he or she may seem. Encourage your toddler to remain seated in the bath – to prevent slipping – and teach him or her to avoid touching the hot tap (wrap a wet flannel around it as an additional safety precaution).

FEAR OF THE BATH

Most children love baths, but some toddlers become frightened of the water or develop a dislike of the sound and sight of water disappearing down the plug hole. It is as if they fear they will go down with it. Treat these fears seriously – forcing a reluctant child to get in the bath will do more harm than good, and it's not a problem to give your toddler sponge baths for a few weeks. After a while, though, you will want to encourage your child back into the bath. Be sure to go slowly.

Start by getting in the bath together (if possible, have someone else on hand to lift the child in and out). Invest in a few new and exciting bath toys – wind-up toys are particularly good for this – to encourage play in the water. Once your toddler is feeling more relaxed about getting into the bath with you, try putting him or her in alone. But let the child stand up if this is easier (with you holding on as he or she could easily slip). Try scooping water over the child's ankles, then legs, bottom, tummy and back while he or she continues to stand.

Have plenty of toys in the bathwater: empty, cleaned shampoo or bubble-bath bottles, natural sponges, a flannel and plastic pots and beakers are good. Let your toddler bend down to pick a toy up. When you think he or she is ready, put the child in a sitting or kneeling position and then quickly provide a distraction by setting off a moving toy or pouring water from one pot into another. Keep the bath short, let your child hold on to you and have lots of physical contact during the bath, and cuddles afterwards. Don't pull the plug out until your child is out of the water (or out of the room if necessary) if it makes him or her feel scared.

MILK BATH

Here is a fragrant mixture to add to a toddler's bath. Milk is gentle on the skin, and an ideal medium for diluting essential oils. Mix the bath milk just before you need it because it won't keep.

100ml/3½fl oz full-fat milk
3 drops lavender essential oil
3 drops neroli essential oil
5ml/1 tsp blue or red food colouring (optional)

Pour the milk into a bowl or jug and add the essential oils, then the food colouring if you are using it. Stir to mix and pour the mixture into a warm bath.

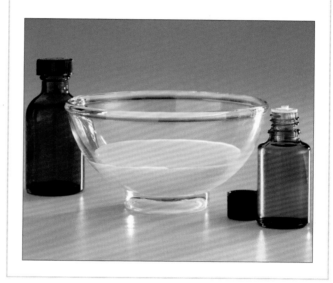

Children usually love baths, and if your child shows some reluctance it is more than likely to be a short-lived phase. He or she will soon be enjoying them again.

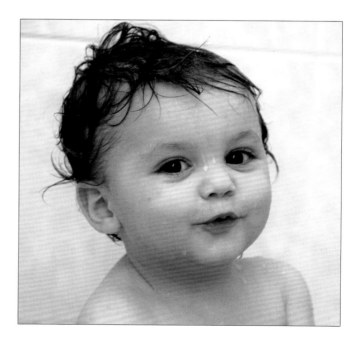

A healthy diet for toddlers

Toddlers have busy lives and small stomachs, so they need to eat little and often. Three meals a day – breakfast, lunch and dinner – is a convenient routine to aim for, but you will also need to offer a mid-morning and mid-afternoon snack to keep your child going between meals. Don't expect your toddler to eat the same amount every day – his or her appetite will vary hugely. It's completely normal for a young child to refuse food on some days and to eat extra helpings on others.

A VARIED DIET
You probably won't be able to get your child to eat perfectly balanced meals every day, but if you offer a wide variety of healthy food, this should add up to a reasonably good mixed diet over a week or so. It is very normal for children to refuse all but a few chosen items from time to time, but so long as your toddler is eating one or more foods from each group, you don't need to worry. Ideally your child will eat a good mixed diet consisting of the following foods each day.

Five or more servings of fruits and vegetables. Try to include as many types as possible.

Four or five helpings of starchy foods such as rice, potatoes, pasta, couscous or quinoa. Don't be tempted to put a young child on a high-fibre diet: wholegrains are bulky and they fill young children up without providing the necessary nutrients.

One or two servings of protein foods such as lean meat, fish, pulses, eggs or nuts. If your child doesn't eat meat or fish, give two servings of other protein a day.

Milk 500ml/17fl oz up to the age of two years; 350ml/ 12fl oz after two, or the equivalent in cheese, fromage frais, yoghurt and so on. Use plain, full-fat dairy products: fruit yoghurts often contain lots of sugar and small children shouldn't eat low-fat dairy products.

Some iron-rich foods the best sources are red meat, chicken or fish, but tofu, beans and lentils, leafy green vegetables, dried fruit, fortified breakfast cereals and bread also contain some iron. Eating vitamin C-rich foods such as brightly coloured fruits and vegetables at the same time helps the body to absorb the iron.

Some healthy fat – olive oil and avocados are good sources. Give oily fish at least once a week.

DRINKS
Drinking lots of water with snacks and at mealtimes will help to keep your toddler's digestion healthy. Juice isn't really necessary, but if you want to give it to increase your child's vitamin intake, make sure that it is well diluted (one part juice to ten parts water for young toddlers, slightly stronger for older ones). Fizzy and sweetened fruit drinks and even fruit juice will coat the teeth in sugary liquid, so, ideally limit drinks to milk and water.

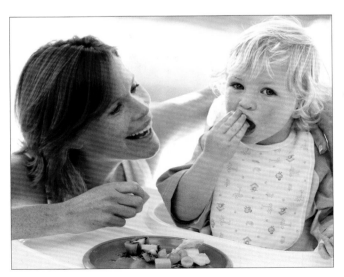

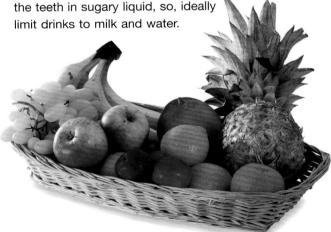

Left and above: It's important to encourage healthy eating habits from an early age. Fortunately most children love fruit – try to give them as wide a variety as possible and keep trying new types.

SWEETS AND CRISPS

It is much easier to ensure that your child eats healthily if you limit the intake of empty calories. All children love crisps and sweets, but they have no nutritional value, and they tend to ruin a child's appetite for more wholesome foods. That is not to say that such foods should be banned altogether (although it is a good idea to hold off introducing them for as long as you can), only that you and your child should see them as occasional treats. Set an example yourself by eating healthy foods: if you enjoy chocolate and biscuits after lunch, then your child will want some too.

If you do give sweets, choose kinds that dissolve quickly in the mouth rather than sticking to the teeth – chocolate instead of chewy sweets, for example. And get your child to eat them in one go: a lot of sweets eaten in a few minutes will actually do less harm to the teeth than eating a few at staggered intervals through the day. If possible, get your child to drink a glass of water afterwards, or to eat a piece of cheese, which helps to neutralize the effect of sugar on teeth.

DAIRY PRODUCTS

Milk is a good source of calcium (which is needed to build strong bones and teeth), vitamin A (for healthy skin, eyes and immune system) and fat (needed for energy), as well as protein. If you have stopped breastfeeding, you can now give full-fat cow's or goat's milk as your baby's main drink, or you can stick to follow-on formula milk if you prefer. Choose organic milk and dairy products whenever possible. Don't give skimmed milk or low-fat dairy products to children under five, because they need plenty of calories. You can start giving semi-skimmed milk to children over two, so long as they are eating and growing well. If your toddler stops drinking milk, give three servings of cheese, yoghurt, fromage frais or milk-based dishes a day. Here are some suggestions.
- Porridge or pancakes made with full-fat milk.
- Homemade fruit milkshakes or yoghurt smoothies.
- Dhal or soup with yoghurt stirred in.
- Quick "rice pudding" made with cooked rice and plain yoghurt (it doesn't need sugar).
- Mini sandwiches made with Cheddar or cream cheese as a mid-morning snack.
- Cooked vegetables with cheese sauce.
- Mashed potatoes made with lots of milk and butter.
- Chunks of Cheddar, hard goat's cheese or edam, served with slices of fruit.
- Greek or plain yoghurt.

NON-DAIRY ALTERNATIVES

There is a lot of debate about the health benefits of eating dairy foods, and it is clear that some children (such as those with milk-allergy-related eczema) are better off

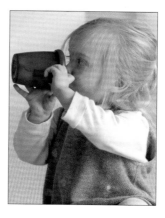

Leave a cup of water close by when your child plays so he or she can help him or herself.

avoiding them altogether. If you want to restrict the amount of dairy products you give your child because of intolerance or for other reasons, here are some good alternative sources of calcium. A paediatric dietician can advise you about planning your child's diet to ensure that it is not deficient.
- Unsweetened rice milk or soya milk with added calcium (don't give sweetened soya milk, which is bad for the teeth). But be aware that some children who are intolerant of dairy products are also intolerant of soya.
- Tofu (made with soya beans) or beans.
- Ground nuts and seeds.
- Canned salmon and sardines (with bones), mashed well.
- Leafy green vegetables: spinach, kale, greens.
- Dried apricots and figs.

Offer your child only healthy food choices for as long as you can. This is much easier if you eat healthily too – your child is much more likely to eat a piece of fruit if he or she sees you eating one.

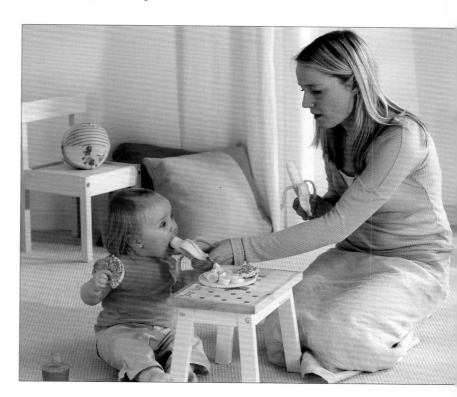

Helping your toddler to enjoy food

Toddlers are often picky eaters and a child's eating habits can cause parents a great deal of stress. But there are many ways you can help to give your child a positive attitude to food. As a general rule, it is best to let your toddler's appetite be your guide. You will naturally find yourself gently coaxing your child to eat vegetables, but it is pointless to try to force a child to eat more than he or she wants. If your toddler is a healthy weight and has plenty of energy, then he or she is almost certainly getting enough. Check with a health professional if you are not sure.

HAPPY EATING

After the age of one your child can eat pretty much everything you eat (with the exception of very salty or spicy foods) provided it is chopped small enough to manage easily. This means you can include your toddler in family mealtimes and make eating a sociable activity. Push the highchair up to the table, and later get a booster seat so that he or she can sit comfortably at the table.

It's best if your child sits down for snacks and there is less chance of choking that way. He or she will love food to be served on a toddler-size table or low stool.

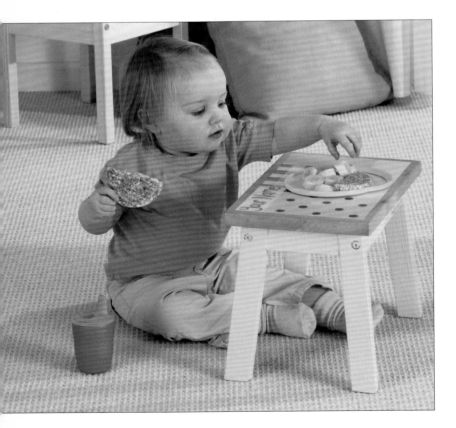

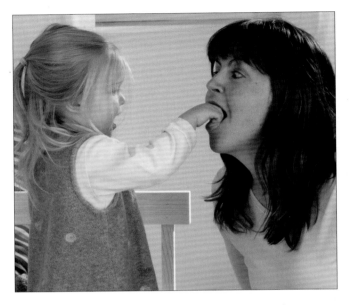

Children like to copy their parents and to try what you eat. Eating together and sharing food is a good way to make food an enjoyable part of life.

If you like to eat a little later than a young child's blood-sugar levels will allow, treat your meal as an extra snacktime for him or her. Don't wait until your child is so tired or hungry that he or she is cranky before eating. Having regular meals and snacktimes will help to regulate his or her energy levels.

Let your child have a spoon and feed himself or herself as soon as he or she seems willing. Having control over how much and what is eaten helps to foster a positive attitude towards food. You can get forks with rounded tines for older toddlers. Your toddler will be more willing to eat an amount that looks manageable than a huge pile of food, so serve small portions. You can always give your child a second helping if he or she wants one.

LIKES AND DISLIKES

Be tolerant about food fads. Most children go through stages when they reject foods they have previously enjoyed, or when they have certain rules about how food must be presented. It is common, for example, for children to dislike "mixed-up" food and to insist that each element of a meal be served in a separate pile that doesn't touch the others. It's often good to humour these fads, but talk to a health professional if you think your child's attitude to food is extreme.

Young children like to copy grown-ups (or older children) and studies show that children whose parents eat lots of fruits and vegetables tend to eat them too. So chop a raw pepper at snacktime and share it with your toddler, or offer some green vegetables off your plate. But children should never be forced to eat foods they dislike or to finish a meal if they are no longer hungry. Remember your own childhood meals. If you were made to eat a food you disliked, or told to sit at the table until you had scraped the plate clean, you may recall how it didn't make you eat any better. Worse still, the child will realize that refusing to eat is a good way of getting your attention and may use this as a way of exercising independence.

Don't assume that your child doesn't like a new food if it's initially rejected. Children may need to be offered a food ten times or more before it becomes familiar enough for them to eat it. So keep serving that portion of red pepper or spinach alongside other foods that your child will eat. It's very tempting to get out, say, bread and cheese if your toddler rejects the meal you have prepared. This doesn't do any harm from time to time, but if you do it often you may be storing up problems for the future.

If your toddler picks at meals, consider whether he or she is having too much milk or snacks at other times. Limit milk to the recommended daily amount, and don't give a snack within an hour of a meal – if a toddler is really hungry, it is better to bring the mealtime forward.

FRUIT AND VEGETABLES

Here are some ways to get your toddler eating plenty of fruits and vegetables.

• Serve fruit at all or most mealtimes. For example, chopped banana or pear in morning porridge; slices of apple after lunch; and peaches and yoghurt after supper.

Make mealtimes calm, happy times. Avoid discussing difficult issues or commenting on your child's eating habits in a negative way.

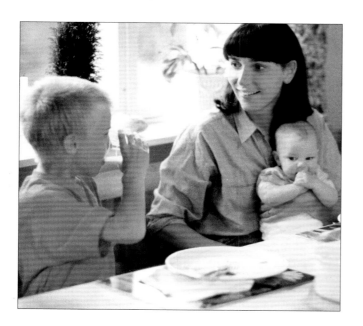

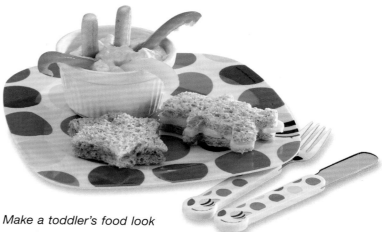

Make a toddler's food look appetising. Offer brightly coloured vegetables with every meal – red and yellow peppers alongside breadsticks with a dip, say. Sometimes you may like to use biscuit cutters to make little sandwiches in the shape of teddies or stars.

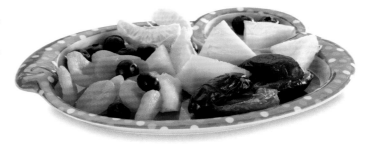

Serving fruit at every snack time will help to up your child's vitamin intake. Encourage them to try exotic fruits as well as the standard apples and bananas.

• Make sure you always have two or three different kinds of fresh fruit in the house. Keep homemade fruit purées in the freezer and serve them alone or stirred into yoghurt or plain fromage frais.

• Give your child raw vegetable sticks as snacks or to keep him or her amused while waiting for a meal – sticks of carrot and cucumber are good served with a dip: hummus or guacamole are good healthy options.

• Include vegetables in every savoury meal. Ideally have one green vegetable and one other vegetable to get a good range of vitamins.

• Keep vegetables in the freezer so you don't run out. If you can't find ready-frozen organic vegetables, make your own: chopped and lightly steamed carrots, green beans, baby sweetcorn and broccoli all freeze well.

• Stir chopped, puréed or grated vegetables into rice, mashed potato, dhal or tomato sauce for pasta. Grated carrot or courgette (zucchini) go well in pancakes.

• Remember that children don't have preconceptions about which foods should be served together. It is fine to use vegetable soup as a pasta sauce or to stir chopped dried fruit into a lamb casserole. And if you are resorting to a tin of (low-salt, low-sugar) baked beans, stir in some peas or spinach to increase the vitamin content.

Preparing for toilet training

Learning to use a potty is an important part of growing up. Teaching your child to do it can be an easy process – provided that you wait until he or she is ready. If you start too early, it will take longer and there will be more accidents along the way. Most children are potty trained somewhere between the ages of two and a half and three years, but some take longer or are ready earlier. Most children master control over the bowel before the bladder, and will be dry during the day long before they can stay dry all night long. Remember, however long the journey, they all get there in the end.

IS MY CHILD READY?

Children start to become aware that they are doing a wee or poo at around 18 months. At this stage, they may clutch themselves and look down at a puddle of wee if they are naked – a sign that they understand they have produced it. It usually takes another year or more before they know in advance that they need to go to the toilet and have the necessary control to wait for a few minutes. When this happens, your child is ready to start potty training, provided there are no other major changes going on – for example, you are about to move house, a new baby is expected or your child is starting nursery. Here are the signs to look out for.

- Your child tells you that he or she is about to do a wee or poo – whether it is communicated in words, by facial expression or by actions.
- Your child remains dry after a nap or for more than two hours at a time.
- Your child makes it clear he or she objects to having a dirty or wet nappy (diaper).
- Your child is able to understand simple instructions, and knows what toilet-based words such as "wee" and "poo" (or whatever words you decide to use) mean.
- Your child is happy to try sitting on the potty and understands what it is for. Some children may ask to use the potty if they see their friends doing it.
- Your child has mastered all the physical skills needed to use a potty successfully – that is, walking well, sitting down and standing up unaided, and pulling his or her underwear on and off.

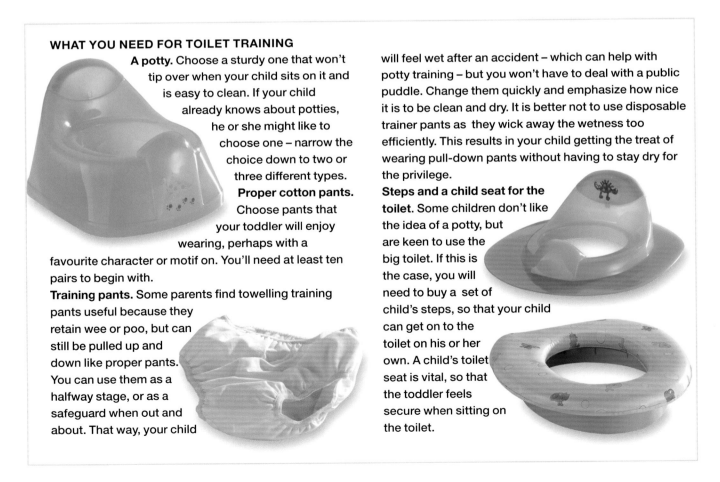

WHAT YOU NEED FOR TOILET TRAINING

A potty. Choose a sturdy one that won't tip over when your child sits on it and is easy to clean. If your child already knows about potties, he or she might like to choose one – narrow the choice down to two or three different types.

Proper cotton pants. Choose pants that your toddler will enjoy wearing, perhaps with a favourite character or motif on. You'll need at least ten pairs to begin with.

Training pants. Some parents find towelling training pants useful because they retain wee or poo, but can still be pulled up and down like proper pants. You can use them as a halfway stage, or as a safeguard when out and about. That way, your child will feel wet after an accident – which can help with potty training – but you won't have to deal with a public puddle. Change them quickly and emphasize how nice it is to be clean and dry. It is better not to use disposable trainer pants as they wick away the wetness too efficiently. This results in your child getting the treat of wearing pull-down pants without having to stay dry for the privilege.

Steps and a child seat for the toilet. Some children don't like the idea of a potty, but are keen to use the big toilet. If this is the case, you will need to buy a set of child's steps, so that your child can get on to the toilet on his or her own. A child's toilet seat is vital, so that the toddler feels secure when sitting on the toilet.

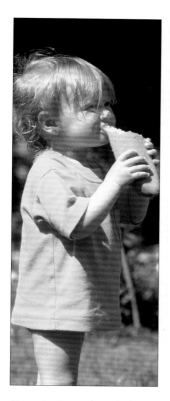

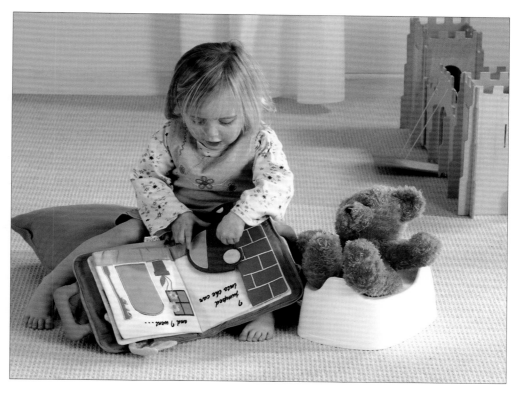

Bare-bottom time helps your toddler to notice how weeing feels. Your child may view the puddle with great interest months before he or she is ready for the potty.

It is very important that children feel relaxed about using the potty. Keep it in the living room before beginning to use it and watch how your child includes it in play.

PREPARING YOUR CHILD

It is important that your toddler feels good about going to the toilet. He or she probably gives some telltale signs that mean a poo or wee is coming: going red in the face, squeezing the legs together, standing on tiptoes, clutching the crotch and so on. Tell your child what is happening in a calm but interested way, and don't look disgusted when you are changing a nasty nappy.

If you feel able to, it is a good idea to let your child see you use the toilet – take the opportunity to explain what you are doing. If you have older children, ask them if your toddler can watch them go to the toilet, too, but don't put them under pressure – they have a right to privacy if they want it. It's particularly helpful if a girl sees mummy use the toilet, and a boy sees what daddy does.

GETTING READY

The first step is to get your child used to having a potty around. Keep it in the bathroom near the toilet, but bring it out to the play area from time to time too.

• Get a colourful book about a child learning to use the potty, so that your child starts to understand what it is for.
• Play at putting teddy or dolly on the potty. Later on, your child may like to have teddy sitting on the travel potty while he or she sits on the real one.
• Put a few toys or books around the potty to encourage the child to sit on it while fully clothed. Don't press or, worse still, force your child to sit on it. It is vital that he or

she feels comfortable at every stage of potty training and that you are relaxed about it.

• Once your child is happily sitting on the potty, put it back in the bathroom and keep it there. He or she may like to sit on it while you use the toilet. You can also try casually suggesting that your child sits on it when naked before a bath – but don't push this.

As your child gets accustomed to the potty as part of their play, you can start to encourage them to sit on it themselves as part of the game.

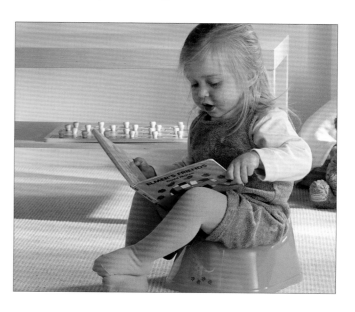

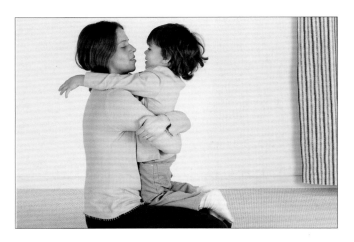

Lots of cuddles can help a child to feel better about accidents or difficulties during potty training.

TOILET TRAINING YOUR CHILD

Once you have embarked on potty training, there are some key things to remember.

Praise. Congratulate your toddler whenever he or she manages to wee or poo in the potty.

Reminders. Your toddler can't wait for long, so keep asking if he or she needs to do a wee.

Make it easy. Keep the potty where your child can find it. If your home has bathrooms on different floors, you may want to put a potty in each one. Dress your child in clothes that are quick to pull off – such as trousers instead of dungarees.

Give privacy. If your toddler wants to turn his or her back or take the potty into a corner, that's fine.

Take it slowly. Wait until your child is dry during the day before you tackle the nights. Back off if the child becomes anxious, and go back to nappies for a few weeks.

Be consistent. Once you've started potty training, keep going unless your child becomes distressed. Don't let the child use nappies one day and the potty the next, or go back to nappies because you are going to stay with friends or going out for the day.

Be patient. Clean up the inevitable accidents without much comment – "Never mind, next time you can do it in the potty" is enough.

BOWEL CONTROL

Children usually learn to control their bowels before their bladder. If your toddler tends to poo at the same time each day (many children go within half an hour of eating a meal), try leaving the nappy (diaper) off just beforehand. Wait until you can tell that the child is about to do a bowel movement, then suggest trying to do a poo in the potty. If your child says no, put a nappy on. If he or she looks interested or doesn't respond, produce the potty quickly. Help with undressing and stay with your child. Remember that he or she may need to concentrate, so don't chat too much. Let the child get up if he or she has tried for a few

USING THE TOILET

It's better for a boy to sit down to pee at first when he starts to use the big toilet, but if he insists on standing up, try putting something he can use for target practice in the bowl: shaving foam, confetti or even coloured ice cubes (if you use blue food colouring his wee will turn the water green – a pleasing "reward"). Make sure the seat won't fall down while he is using the toilet. Show him how to put it up properly and teach him to put it down when he has finished.

minutes and not produced anything and give lots of praise if he or she does poo in the potty.

Clean your child up. You can show older toddlers how to wipe themselves (tell a girl to wipe from front to back), but they still need your help. Wiping is easier with a wet wipe, but choose the flushable variety and don't flush more than two or three wipes at once. Empty the contents of the potty into the toilet and both wash your hands.

Some children love to flush their poo away – especially if they are not usually allowed to touch the toilet at other times. But others find flushing a terrifying prospect. The poo is their own creation, after all, and in their eyes it is something to be proud of. If this is how your child seems to feel, then it is best to flush after he or she leaves the bathroom. Some children are fascinated by their faeces

Some children are fascinated by the process of flushing the toilet and will watch things disappear eagerly. But others find this frightening.

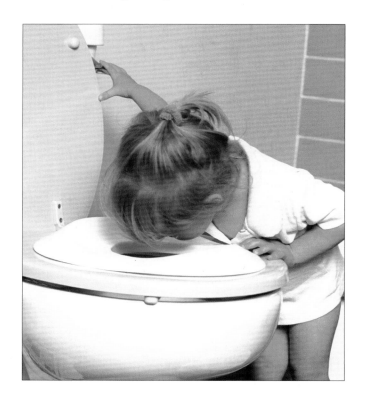

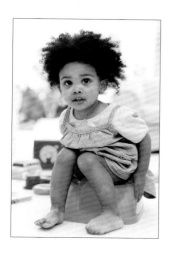

Don't feel that you can't get out and about when you are potty or toilet training. Get in the habit of taking at least one change of clothes with you when you go out, as well as a plastic bag to put the wet ones in.

and want to play with them. It is important not to allow this, of course, but take care not to use words such as "dirty" about the faeces or your child may think that you are referring to him or her.

Make sure your child is eating enough fibre by giving him or her lots of fruit and vegetables during this time – if passing a hard stool causes any pain while on the potty, this may put the child off using it.

BLADDER CONTROL

Urine control can take longer than bowel control, because there isn't much gap between a child recognizing the feeling of a full bladder and the urge to go. It can be a good idea to have a few practice runs before starting potty training for real. Choose a morning or afternoon when you and your child are at home together. Leave the nappy off (perhaps after the first change of the day, or after the afternoon nap) and tell the child that he or she can use the potty for wees as well as poos. Don't make a big deal out of it: be as low-key as you can.

While playing, ask the child from time to time if he or she needs to use the potty – it is also helpful to sit your child on the potty before and after naps, after meals and if he or she hasn't had a wee for a couple of hours. If there is an accident – as there almost certainly will be – be sure not to criticise or tell your child off. If he or she was

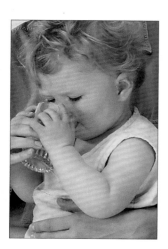

Left: Giving your child plenty of water to drink will give more opportunity to practise bladder-control and potty training. If you are trying to achieve night-time dryness, however, limit their liquid intake after tea time or supper time.

heading for the potty, give your child credit for trying – say, "Well done for trying; next time you'll get to the potty in time." Once you are having more successes than accidents, set aside a few days when there isn't much happening. Take your child to choose some new cotton pants for themselves (or trainer pants if you prefer). If he or she is excited about wearing these special pants, this will help to make potty training fun.

Most parents find it helpful to limit outside activities during potty training, but you can't stay home for days on end with an active toddler. Instead, make outings short, manageable and at child-friendly places; go to the local park or a good friend's house: get your child to use the potty before you go and take a travel potty with you, or use trainer pants.

NIGHT-TIME DRYNESS

Staying dry through the night nearly always takes longer to achieve than day-time dryness. Wait until you notice that your child's nappy has stayed dry for a few nights in a row before you begin (it's a good idea to give praise for waking up dry, even if the child is wearing nappies). Then try washable trainer pants or just go straight to pyjamas. Use a mattress protector on the bed and expect a few accidents. It will help to limit them if you encourage your child to use the potty just before bedtime and restrict drinks after suppertime.

Teach about hygiene at the same time as you potty train and get the child to wash his or her hands properly after using the potty.

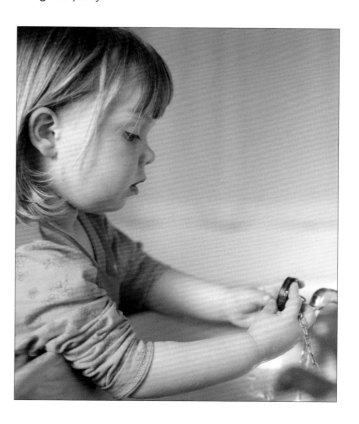

Toilet training problems and special circumstances

The process of toilet training can sometimes create a lot of tension. Parents may feel bad if their child is the last in a group to be toilet trained, or they may be under pressure from family members who insist that their children were trained before the age of two. It is important to know that some children (particularly boys) are not ready for potty training until they are over three. If in doubt, it is better to wait than to force the pace.

If you feel anxious about toilet training, it is worth seeking reassurance and advice on how to proceed. Remember that lots of children have problems with potty training, and an experienced health professional will almost certainly have already encountered any problem that your child has.

SETBACKS

Even children who have been successfully potty trained can start having accidents again, or suddenly refuse to use the potty. This can sometimes be due to a physical problem, such as a urinary infection, so see a doctor to check if this is the case.

If your child is in daycare, take several changes of pants and clothes when you are potty training. Discuss your method with nursery staff to avoid giving conflicting messages or using different terminology.

More often, setbacks are the result of emotional upset, such as the child being unsettled by an event such as a house move. Deal with the mess as calmly as you can and consider whether you need to offer some extra help for a while. Your child may want you to stay with him or her while using the potty, or something may be needed to refocus the child's attention – new pants, for example, or some stickers for the potty, and probably lots of extra loving attention too. If the problem persists for longer than a week or two, you may want to consider going back to nappies for a while and starting potty training afresh in a few weeks. Seek advice from your health visitor.

Children sometimes have a sudden increase in accidents simply because the activity they are involved with is more interesting than going to use the potty. If you think this is what is behind an apparent step backwards, say that it is not right to wait; your child must use the potty when he or she needs to go. Revert to asking often whether the child needs a wee, and put him or her on the potty at regular intervals for a while. But don't get angry.

SOILING

Some children may hold back from doing a bowel movement because they are frightened of doing it in the potty. Eventually they will soil themselves, because they can't hold on forever, and this adds to their distress. Be

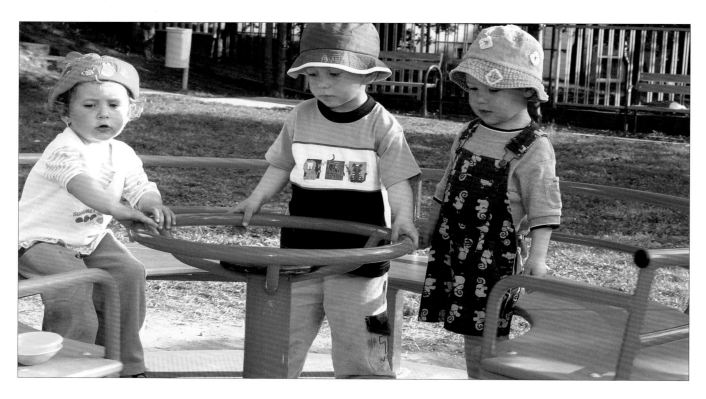

TRAINING TWINS

If you have twins, you may find it easier to train one before the other, or to train them simultaneously. Both methods can work well, so long as the children are ready for potty training when you start, are treated as individuals and their progress is not compared. You will need two potties, and it may be a good idea to get them in different colours and to let each twin personalize their own. However, some twins will want potties that are exactly the same.

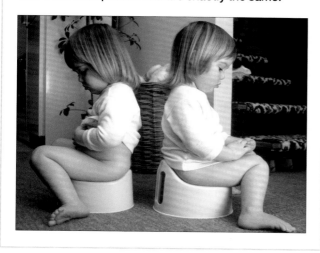

Using a plug-in light in the hallway may encourage your child to use the toilet in the night. It gives a very gentle glow and can provide reassurance as well as enough light to guide the child to the toilet.

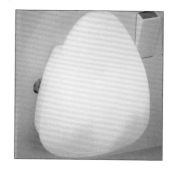

BEDWETTING

Many young children wet the bed occasionally. Most grow out of this by the age of five, but if your child is wetting the bed often, you may want to try the following.

- Consider if you have started night-time training too early – talk to a health professional if you are not sure.
- If your child has been dry but has now started wetting the bed, he or she may be upset about something. It's also possible that a urinary infection or threadworms are to blame, so see a doctor if the cause is unclear.
- Try not to be cross. Remember that your child is not doing this on purpose, and the more calmly you deal with the problem the easier it will be to solve. Shaming or telling off a child will only make things worse. Don't accidentally encourage your child either by, say, bringing him or her into your bed whenever it happens.
- Restrict drinks after 5.00pm – but make sure the child has enough fluid earlier in the day.
- Put a cover on the mattress to minimize the damage, and have fresh sheets and pyjamas on hand so you can clean everything up quickly.
- Wake your child up for a wee when you go to bed. Most children will go back to sleep quite easily.
- Make sure the way to the bathroom is well lit during the night or have a potty in the child's room if he or she is afraid to go to the bathroom in the night.

calmly sympathetic as you clean the child up and explain briefly that this happened because he or she held on. This may be enough to prevent it happening again. Children are more likely to do it if they are unsettled, so give extra attention and cuddles. Again, it can help if you stay with a child who is using the potty, and if you let the child leave the room to play before you flush the faeces away.

Sometimes soiling is the result of constipation, as liquid stools may leak past the hard ones. The child may not even realize that a bowel movement is happening until it is too late. If your child soils regularly and you think constipation may be the cause, seek professional help. Your child may need a laxative, but this should only be given under medical advice. Once the initial problem has been sorted, you'll also need to take steps to prevent your child from becoming constipated again.

CONSTIPATION

If your child is reluctant to do a bowel movement in the potty and is passing hard pellets, adding more fibre to the diet can help. Increase the amount of vegetables and fruits, and get the child eating some prunes and dried fruits. It is also helpful to increase the amount of wholegrain cereals and bread. Avoid bananas for a while and give the child plenty of water to drink. Excess intake of milk can sometimes be a factor in constipation, so keep an eye on how much your child drinks. See a health professional if the problem persists.

If your child won't do a bowel movement in the potty, but is happy to wee in it, try some extra inducement. Fill a special "potty box" with small gifts – crayons, stickers, balloons and little toys – and let the child pick one every time he or she manages to do a poo in the potty.

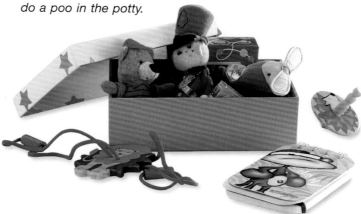

Crying, behaviour and sleeping

“ A good bedtime and sleep routine is one of the key factors that will help your child to behave reasonably. ”

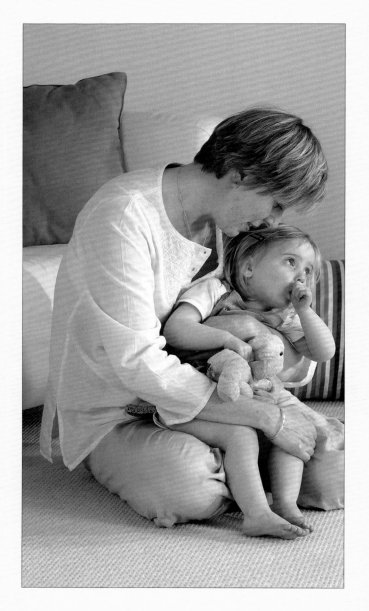

The years between the ages of one and three are probably the most emotionally tumultuous in a child's life. This is a time when your toddler may zig-zag between tearful neediness and fierce insistence on doing things his or her own way. Your child wants to be independent, but lacks the physical skills to manage without help. He or she wants to have you near all the time, but is furious if you try to show the way. This contrariness is what makes hard work of the job of parenting a toddler, but it is also what makes it such an absorbing experience. There are few things more fulfilling than sharing in your child's glee in attainments that bring him or her ever closer to the world of bigger children and adults: walking to the shop, repeating "Woof" whenever a dog appears, wielding a fork or successfully negotiating the stairs.

Your toddler will be testing all kinds of boundaries, so this is the time to start laying down some basic rules. There are simple ways to help your child to behave well when wilfulness spills over into conflict

Tantrums can abate as suddenly and rapidly as they arise, leaving that furious struggling child sobbing, frightened and in need of a loving cuddle.

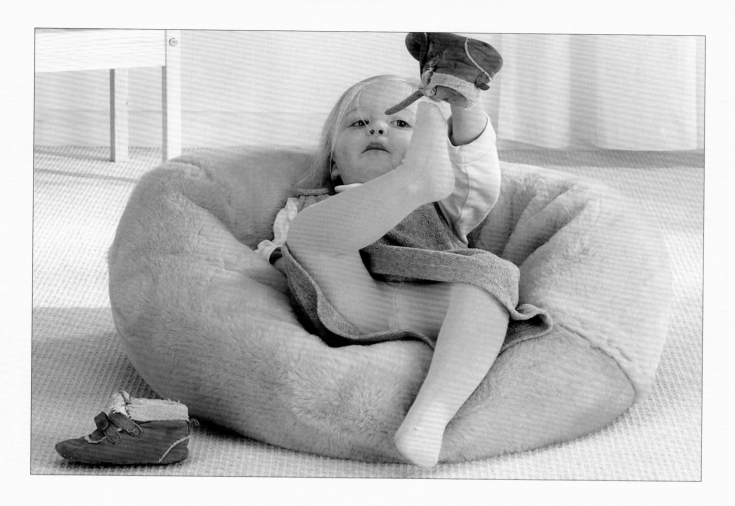

or tantrums. Some children have personalities that are more intense than others, and a very determined, creative or sensitive child is more likely to have tantrums than one who is naturally laid-back or timid. But the way you respond to crying may also play a part in determining how tantrum-prone your child becomes. A good bedtime and sleep routine is one of the key factors that will help your child to behave reasonably. A regular sleep pattern is the foundation of a daily schedule: get this right, and your toddler is more likely to be happy and equable during the day.

In this chapter there are ideas and techniques to help your child manage his or her moods and sleep well at night. Not all the suggestions will work for every child – it is up to you to choose the ones that suit you and your family.

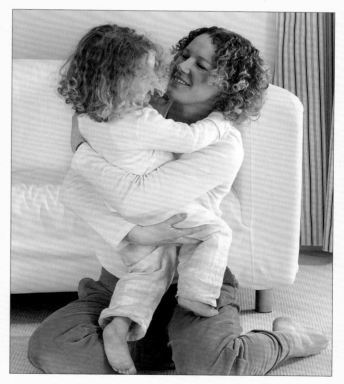

Top: That drive towards independence is ever-present, but toddlers don't understand the easiest way to go about things and need lots of tactful help.

Although parenting a toddler can be hard work, it is fantastically rewarding too. Nothing beats the affection you get from your child.

Why toddlers cry

Toddlers may cry several times a day, and their upset may seem out of all proportion to the cause. But it is important to remember that your toddler simply isn't equipped to deal with difficulties yet. Young children don't have the experience to know that what they are feeling is rage, still less that it will soon pass. Crying is the only way they have of coping with unpleasant emotions. It is also still a key mode of communication, since they can't express their needs or feelings accurately with their limited vocabulary.

FRUSTRATION

There is a huge gap between the things your toddler wants to do and what he or she can manage. Frustration can be positive because it helps to spur a child on to new developmental achievements. But it isn't a comfortable feeling and it can quickly lead to tears of rage. Your toddler will also feel frustrated when prevented from doing something that is enjoyable – a small child doesn't understand, after all, why drawing on walls is bad or why he or she should have to get out of the bath.

FEAR, ANXIETY AND LACK OF ATTENTION

The world can seem a strange and overwhelming place to a young child. Toddlers often develop a fear of, say, the bath, dogs, the dark or certain noises, and will cry when they encounter them. Separation anxiety is normal in toddlers, who want to stay close to their carers and resist being left with other people. Your toddler may no longer cry when you leave a room, but may become distraught if you go out or leave him or her at nursery.

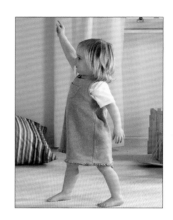

It's important to give growing children lots of ways to release physical energy, it can help to reduce tantrums too. You don't have to go outside for this, try putting on some lively music and having a dance around the house. It will probably improve your mood too.

Most children will cry when they are told off, because they fear the withdrawal of love from you. To an extent, this is a necessary part of socialization, but it is important to reassure children that you still love them even when they are naughty. Young children have an insatiable need for attention. If you are absorbed in another task, chatting on the phone or – worst of all – cuddling a friend's baby, your child may start to cry or behave badly simply because he or she wants you to play.

HOW YOU CAN HELP

Some crying is inevitable, and part of your child's way of expressing themselves, but you can minimize mood swings, and perhaps avoid a tantrum, as follows.

Rest. Your toddler will cry much more readily when tired. Make sure he or she is getting enough sleep and do all you can to help your child relax: a walk in the buggy or some quiet play on your lap can be almost as good as a sleep in restoring a toddler's spirits.

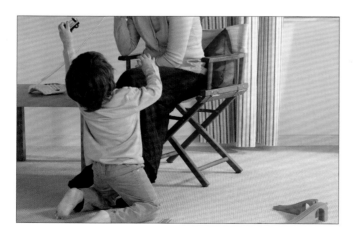

However happily absorbed in a game, your toddler is bound to want your attention the minute he or she notices that you are otherwise occupied.

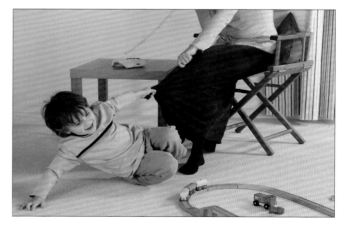

Not getting his or her own way can lead to an increasing sense of frustration and may easily end in an explosive tantrum.

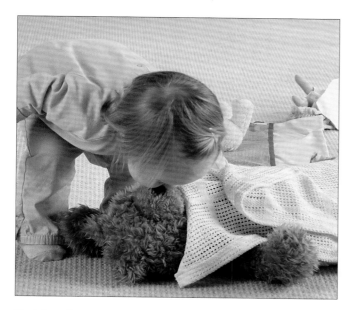

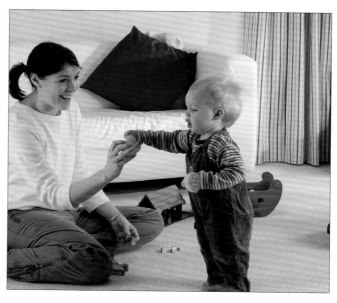

Toddlers have no sense of time and no conception of anyone else's needs. So don't expect them to stop playing just because you need to move on. Give a child time to adjust by saying you will be leaving in a while.

One of the most charming things about toddlers is their desire to be helpful. Your child may wipe the highchair tray or pass you something when you ask for it. This is a good behaviour trait to encourage.

Fuel. Low blood-sugar levels or dehydration make children (and adults) irritable and fretful. So give regular meals and snacks, with plenty of water to drink. Avoid sugary snacks, which give an initial boost but soon lead to a dip in energy and mood.

Physical release. Toddlers have lots of energy that they need to expend. Go on at least one outing a day, more if your child is very active or has regular tantrums. Toddler gym classes are great, but simple outings or indoor activities such as dancing can work just as well.

Sympathy. Be swift to reassure your child if he or she has a bump or is frustrated when playing with a toy. Be sympathetic about any fears – don't dismiss them as "silly" or, worse, try to force your child to confront the thing that is frightening. Your child will almost certainly get over any fear more quickly if you are reassuring.

Independence. Toddlers are determined to do things for themselves, but don't always have the skills necessary to carry it out. Lend a hand where possible, but be tactful – your child will resent being "babied". Offering a few simple choices – does he or she want an apple or a banana, say, or to wear trousers or shorts, can help a child feel that he or she has some small mastery of the daily routine, and will boost self-confidence.

Preparation. Don't demand a sudden change of activity. If your child is involved in a game but it's time to leave, give five minutes' warning, and then a one-minute warning, too, so he or she is prepared for the change.

Distraction. If your toddler starts to get upset, try starting a new game or activity, exclaiming at something you see out of the window, singing a song and pulling faces, or taking the child out for a change of scene.

DELIBERATE CRYING

Toddlers gradually become aware of what crying can achieve and its effect on adults, and realize they can use it to get something that they want – think of young children whining for sweets in the supermarket. At first, this is not so much devious as experimental: your child is naturally going to test all the methods available to see what works and once he or she discovers crying can get results, a toddler is bound to try it on from time to time. It is up to you to differentiate between genuine upset and deliberate whining, so you don't reward bad behaviour.

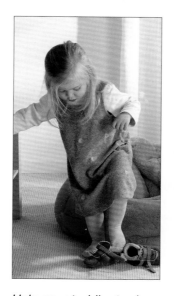

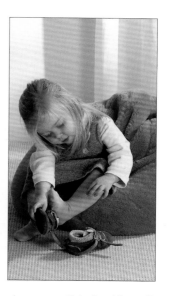

Help your toddler to do as much as possible for himself or herself, even though it is bound to take longer. If a child wants to try putting on his or her own clothes, leave plenty of time to get ready.

Dealing with tantrums

All children have to learn what is and what isn't acceptable behaviour, and this learning process starts early. Toddlers are driven by their own desires and have little sense of other people's feelings, so you can't expect them to know how to behave by themselves. Your child needs clear guidance from you.

Be reasonable. Have as few rules as possible, but put your foot down when it is important.

Be consistent. Make sure you, your partner and any other carers stick to the same basic rules.

Set a good example. If you shout at your child or your partner, your child is likely to copy you.

Encourage your child to ask nicely rather than to whinge or shout for what he or she wants.

REINFORCING GOOD BEHAVIOUR

Acknowledge pleasant behaviour with praise and extra attention and ignore bad behaviour when you can. It is easy to get into the habit of telling a child off for being naughty but ignoring all the good things. If your child gets most attention from you for being "naughty", then that is what he or she will be. So stop your child from doing naughty or dangerous things, but don't tell him or her off unless it is really necessary.

Avoid confrontation when you can. If your child doesn't want to walk up the hill, say, suggest you have a walking race. If he or she wants to play with a sibling's favourite

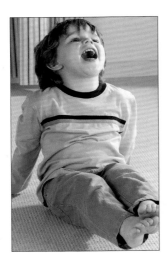
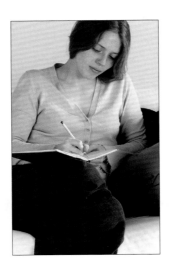

Older children may throw a fake tantrum. This is usually because they have discovered tantrums are a successful tactic.

If your child has lots of tantrums, try keeping a diary to help you pinpoint what the triggers are and then try to avoid them.

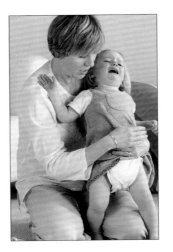
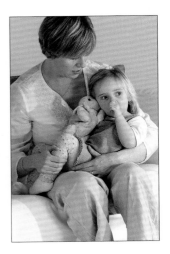

Young children may do best being held during a tantrum; they are then in the best place for a kindly cuddle and calming words once the temper abates.

toy, take it away but give the toddler something as a substitute. If you do need to tell a child off, get down to the child's level and make eye contact. Use a firm, low voice (don't shout) and tell the child the behaviour was unacceptable. Say: "Hitting people is wrong. We do not hit people." Don't say "You are naughty."

TEMPER TANTRUMS

Almost all young children will have temper tantrums from time to time and some intense toddlers have several a day. Tantrums often start at around 18 months, coinciding with a surge in independence. They may continue until

TACTICS FOR DEALING WITH A TANTRUM

When a tantrum starts, do the following.

- Make the environment safe so your child cannot get hurt or hurt other people.
- Some toddlers are helped by being held firmly, but this can make others even angrier.
- Do not engage: do not talk or argue with your child. Either stay nearby but avoid eye contact (read a book) or remove yourself altogether, if it is safe to do so. Deprived of an audience, your child may call a halt to the tantrum more quickly.
- If you are out, pick your child up and go somewhere quieter – your car, a quiet part of the park, a different room in grandma's house.
- Never, under any circumstances, give in.

the age of three or older, when children develop the language skills they need to express themselves. Adults have their own strategies for dealing with anger and fear, some healthy, some not. But all that young children feel is the overwhelming physical sensations that these emotions bring with them – tense body, tingling in the fingers and a head that feels it is about to explode.

A tantrum is usually the result of frustration, or sometimes of fear. It is more likely to happen if a child is also feeling overwhelmed, fatigued, hungry or thirsty. You may be able to prevent tantrums by avoiding key triggers or by diverting your child's attention once you see them building up, but once a tantrum has started there is usually nothing that you can do to stop it: a child in the midst of an explosion of rage is out of control, beyond reason, punishment or reward.

Waiting until the storm blows over is difficult, even for the most laid-back of parents. Most tantrums are awful to watch: children may fling themselves around the room, throw themselves down and drum their heels on the floor, hit out at you and scream. Some children yell so hard and for so long that they make themselves vomit, and others hold their breath until they turn blue in the face or even faint. Rest assured that it is impossible for children to stop themselves breathing for long; the body's natural reflexes step in well before any harm is done.

COPING WITH A TANTRUM

Remember that however hard it is to witness your child in the throes of a tantrum, the experience is worse for the child, who may be genuinely terrified by the maelstrom of emotion that has welled up inside, and who will need your comfort and reassurance as soon as it is over. Calm is the best weapon you have. If you get angry, or show amusement, you will simply add fuel to the fire. And if you

A temper tantrum can erupt in a moment, and is sometimes the only way young children know to release the pent-up rage inside them.

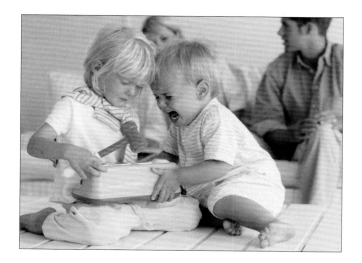

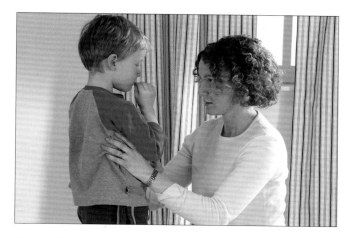

The underlying cause of tantrums is often the child's inarticulacy. As the child grows older, he or she will be able to talk more easily about his or her frustration.

try to draw a screaming toddler into a discussion, you are wasting your time. Your basic aim is to show your child that the tantrums do not frighten you (as they frighten the child), they do not push you into doing what your child wants and they do not stop you loving him or her.

Above all, do not give in. If the tantrum was precipitated by your refusing your child a treat, say, do not suddenly offer it, even if you now think your refusal was unwarranted. If your child learns that tantrums are a good way of getting what he or she wants, there are bound to be more of them. For the same reason, don't "reward" a toddler for a tantrum by producing a treat afterwards.

Don't punish your child, either. When the tantrum stops, be ready to have a cuddle if he or she will allow it, and say that you are glad the tantrum has stopped. Reassure your child that you love him or her but you don't like that behaviour. Then continue with your day as planned; don't cancel arrangements because your child has been naughty.

With an older child, consider talking about the behaviour afterwards. Your child may benefit from discussing the anger, how the tantrum felt and ways he or she could alert you to the onset of this feeling next time. You will help your child to become emotionally literate if you put a name to the uncomfortable sensations of frustration or anger he or she has experienced.

Think about triggers for tantrums and consider ways to avoid them. For example, if the tantrums occur in the supermarket, make sure your child is well rested and has had a snack and a drink before you go shopping. Keep the child occupied: for example, pass him or her the groceries to put in the trolley. And keep the trip as short as possible. If your child has lots of tantrums, give him or her oily fish at least once a week. It may also be worth trying a fish-oil supplement specially formulated for children: a large UK study found that taking fish oils reduced tantrums and difficult behaviour.

Toddlers and sleep

Most young children need 10–12 hours sleep a night, but this won't necessarily be in one long stretch. If your child isn't sleeping through the night, take heart from the fact that you are not alone: around one in three toddlers has difficulty settling at bedtime or wakes frequently through the night.

DAYTIME NAPS

Most toddlers continue with day-time naps until they are at least two and a half. A one year old will probably still need two naps a day: one in the morning and one in the early afternoon. Over the next few months, he or she will probably drop one of these and the second will probably go a year or so later.

Making these transitions can be difficult. Two naps may leave your one year old wide awake at bedtime, but one may leave a child overtired and cranky by the end of the day. When your child drops the last nap, you may want to try having an early supper and then putting him or her to bed at, say, 6.00 instead of 7.00 pm. Be patient at this time, it won't last long. Arrange a quiet interlude at the time when the nap used to be. Your toddler may be happy to lie on the bed for a while, or sit down for a story.

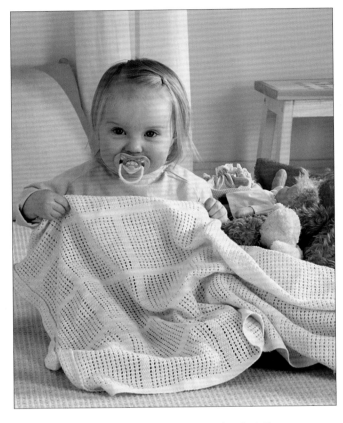

Children become attached to dummies but they can interfere with speech development. Using them at nap times only will make it easier to get rid of them later on.

HOW MUCH SLEEP?
Children vary in how much sleep they need, but this is how long an average toddler will sleep over a 24-hour period:
At one year – 13.5 hours
At two years – 13 hours
At three years – 12 hours

MOVING INTO A BIG BED

A toddler can move from a cot to a proper bed any time between the ages of 18 months and three and a half years. There is no rush – it's better to wait until your child is keen to try a big bed rather than to push him or her into it too soon. If your child has learned to climb out of the cot, but isn't ready for a bed, make sure the mattress is on the lowest level and check that he or she is not using toys as steps. Put a duvet on the floor to provide a soft landing and move any furniture away. Consider keeping the side down so the child can climb out safely. But if your child can easily climb out of the cot, or is too big to sleep comfortably in it, it is probably time to make the move. It is also a good idea to move your child into a bed before you start night-time potty training, since he or she may need to get up in the night.

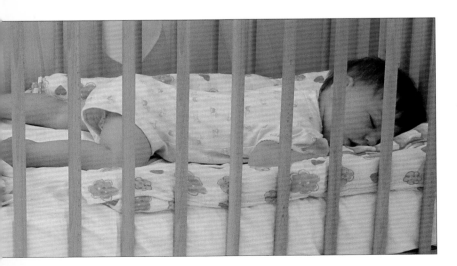

Most toddlers will carry on needing a sleep during the day, to ensure that in 24 hours they are getting around 12 hours sleep in total.

Here are some ways to help your child make the move from the cot happily.

- Don't do it when your child is undergoing any other big change, such as getting used to a new carer.
- If a new baby is due, either make the move to a bed two or three months before the birth, or wait until a few months after it.
- Let your child choose some exciting new bedding for his or her "big bed". It might be easier to pick this from a catalogue rather than going to a store, which could feel intimidating.
- Put the bed where the cot used to be for familiarity.
- Get your child to help you make the bed for the first time, and ask which toys he or she wants to sleep with. Let the child keep his or her cot blanket for comfort.
- Put a guardrail on the bed to stop the child falling out.
- Praise your child for staying in a grown-up bed at night.

LOSING THE DUMMY

Lots of young children like to suck on a dummy (pacifier) for comfort. This can help to get them to sleep, but prolonged use can cause the front teeth to push forwards in some children and it may also interfere with speech development if it is used during the day. Be clear that dummies are for sleep times only. Don't let your child play or talk while sucking on a dummy.

Experts differ on when you should get rid of a dummy – some say by the child's first birthday, others by the age of three. You will have to judge when your child can lose a dummy without causing undue distress. Most children become less interested in their dummies as they grow up,

Moving into a big bed is an important transition that you want your toddler to feel good about. Don't move a child because you are having another baby and need the cot. Borrow or buy a second cot (get a new mattress) rather than oust your toddler too soon.

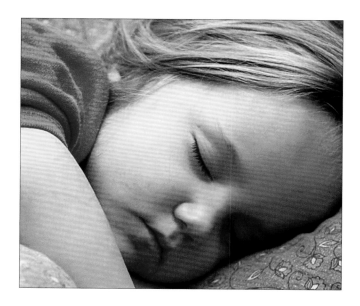

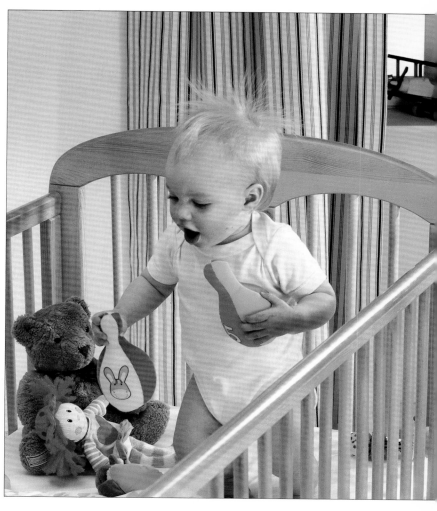

Lots of toddlers wake up at 6.00am or earlier, especially if they sleep through the night. The best solution is probably to go to bed earlier yourself. But your toddler may be happy to play for a while if you leave a different interesting toy in the cot each night.

so your child's dependence on the dummy may be lessening naturally. Try putting him or her down to sleep without it from time to time. If this works, simply offer the dummy less and less frequently.

If your child is old enough, talk about using the dummy. Say that you think he or she is now grown-up enough to stop using it. Ask your child's opinion about this. If the child is clear that he or she still wants it, let the subject drop for a while before bringing it up again. If your child is willing to consider giving up the dummy, suggest that a favourite toy can be used for comfort at night instead. A reward chart – with a sticker every time the child goes to sleep without the dummy – may help. Give lots of praise too. Don't use shame or ridicule to encourage your child to give up a dummy.

Some children benefit from ritual: a dummy fairy may come in the night and take the dummies away, leaving a gift in exchange, or your child could deposit the dummy at the dentist's in exchange for a new toothbrush.

Problems at bedtime

Some children who have slept through the night from a young age start to wake up again or resist going to bed. This is sometimes due to separation anxiety, but often it is simply down to excitement: now that your child can do so much, why would he or she want to go to bed?

BEDTIME ROUTINE

You'll find it much easier to get your child to sleep at night if you have a consistent bedtime routine. This helps a toddler to relax and get ready for sleep. Keep activities after tea gentle and quiet to help your child wind down from the day's events. It is also important to have a set bedtime – somewhere between 6.30 and 7.30 pm works well for most children, but some won't settle until later. If your child is used to a very late bedtime, bring it forwards by ten minutes a day until he or she is going to sleep at a time that works for you both.

Keep your bedtime routine short and simple – it shouldn't take longer than about half an hour. A good routine could be: playtime in the bath, getting into pyjamas, a drink of milk from a cup, toothbrushing, cuddle and storytime, then bed and lights out. Avoid doing anything upsetting at this time: if washing your

Story time is a good part of the bedtime routine, because it gives children focused time with their parent. It often becomes a treasured childhood memory.

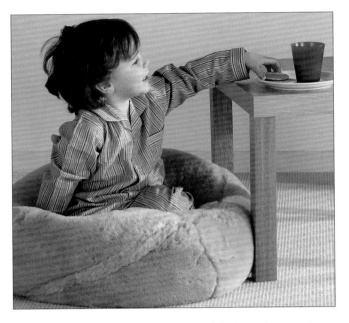

Some children need a simple snack before they go to bed. Avoid giving them anything, such as cheese or chocolate, that may affect their sleep.

child's hair makes him or her scream, do it in the morning. Resist an older toddler's attempts to extend the routine: he or she may ask you to read more stories, say, to delay bedtime. Be firm. Giving some notice of what will happen next – "After your story, it is bedtime" – will help your child to accept the inevitable.

Make sure that your child has any comforters or favourite stuffed animals that he or she needs to help get to sleep. Get a nightlight or leave a light on in the hallway if the child doesn't like to be in the dark. Some children find it comforting if you say goodnight in exactly the same way each night – for example, "Night night, darling, see you in the morning."

GETTING YOUR TODDLER TO DROP OFF ALONE

If you always stayed with your baby until he or she was asleep, your toddler is unlikely to drop off alone now. You may still be happy to stay, but you may find that going to sleep takes longer and longer. If you want your evenings to yourself – or if you have older children who need your attention as well – you will have to make a firm decision to teach your child to go to sleep without you.

Most parents find that they can improve their child's sleep within a week. But you do need to give your child a clear, consistent message about bedtime throughout this time. For this reason, you should start a sleep training

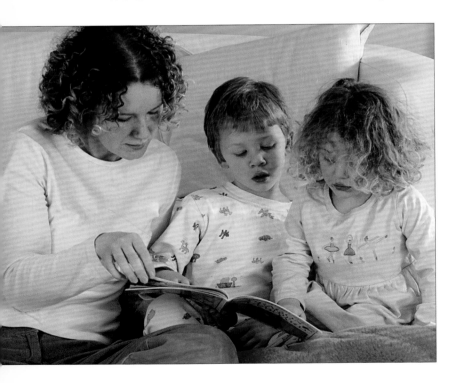

programme in a week when you will be around for every bedtime and when your child is not having to deal with any other disruptions to the normal routine, or other challenges in their life. Younger toddlers can benefit from the routines suggested for older babies, but older ones also respond very well to the kiss method.

THE KISS ROUTINE

This works best if your child is in a bed, so that you can easily bend down to kiss him or her when lying down. It could take a couple of hours and several hundred kisses if your child is very persistent. Kiss your child only when he or she is lying down, and don't be drawn into any discussion or play. Say again that you will be back in a minute to give your child another kiss, and do it as often as seems necessary.

1 Do your usual bedtime routine. Put your child to bed and give him or her a kiss goodnight.

2 Say you will be back in a minute with another kiss.

3 Turn away and then turn back and give your child a kiss straight away.

4 Move away a little further this time, then turn back and give another kiss.

5 Now do something in the room such as putting toys away or folding an item of clothing. Then turn back to your child and give another kiss.

6 Leave the room as if you are going to do something, come straight back and kiss your child again.

7 If your child gets up to follow you, act surprised and lead him or her gently back to bed. Give another kiss and then leave the room again.

8 Continue in this way for as long as it takes for your child to fall asleep. Gradually extend the period you leave between kisses.

9 Do the same on subsequent nights. You should find that it takes less time to get your child to sleep as the week draws on. But don't be surprised if you have a few setbacks: the third and fifth nights are often the worst.

THE MOVING CHAIR METHOD

An alternative method to use is the moving chair method. It can be good if your child cannot bear you to leave the room before he or she is asleep.

After your usual bedtime routine, sit on a chair beside the child's bed and turn the child so that he or she is facing away from you. Switch off the light and tell your child it is "sleepytime" (or whatever phrase you prefer to use) and to close his or her eyes. Then every time he or she tries to chat, simply say "ssshhhh, sleepytime". You will probably have to do this many times, but persevere however long it takes for your child to drop off. Over the next few nights, do exactly the same, but move the chair a little further away from the bed and towards the (open)

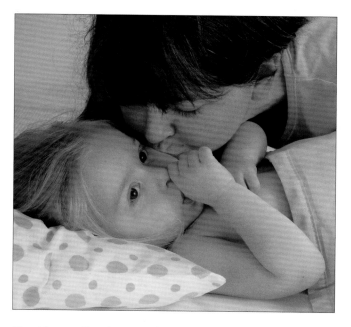

The kiss routine is a gentle way of getting your child to drop off alone, often without even realizing that that is what is happening.

door each night. Eventually you should be sitting outside the door. By this time your child should be able to drop off alone and you can leave the bedroom after you've said goodnight. Go back to sitting outside the door if he or she seems to need that reassurance for a while longer.

Help your child to see his or her bedroom as a pleasant place to be. Encourage the child to play in his or her bedroom and feel happy and relaxed in there. Don't make the bedroom a negative place by using it as a place to send older toddlers as punishment.

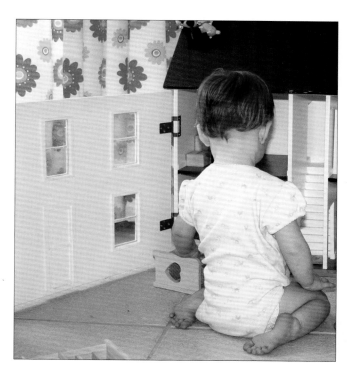

Night waking

It's hard to deal with children waking up during the night. Most of us will do anything to soothe our children so that we can get back to sleep ourselves. If your child is continually waking up and it is affecting your sleep, you probably need to steel yourself to use a sleep training technique to help him or her fall asleep without you.

It's best to start by establishing a bedtime routine first, which may resolve the problem. Give your child as few reasons as possible to get up in the night: leave a glass of water by the bedside if he or she wakes up thirsty, give the child a snack at bedtime and make sure he or she uses the toilet. If your toddler is happy to go to sleep at bedtime, but continues to wake you during the night, try to address any obvious causes first. But if your toddler simply wants your attention at night, you can do the kiss routine, controlled crying or the back-to-your-own-bed method as appropriate. As with any sleep training, you need to make a clear decision that this is what you want to do and to stick with it for a week.

WHY IS MY CHILD WAKING UP?

Night waking can have a straightforward cause and be simple to solve. Before trying any sleep training methods, consider whether your child does any of the following.

Sleeps too much during the day. Try shortening the daytime nap to one and a half hours. Don't let your child nap later than about 2.30 pm.

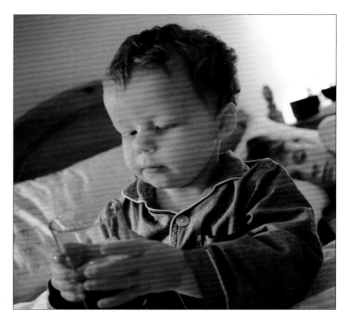

Children have various reasons for calling you in the night. Doing something as simple as leaving a glass of water in their reach can help them settle themselves.

Doesn't sleep enough during the day. Prioritize naptime. If your child won't nap, arrange some quiet time or go out for a restful journey in the buggy.

Is disturbed by outside noises. Consider moving the cot or getting thicker curtains to blot out noise. Leaving a radio set on low in the child's room helps to make outside noises less intrusive.

Is disturbed by you. Don't rush in to soothe your child; wait for a minute or two to see if he or she settles.

Gets too cold or too hot. Modify the bedding as necessary. If your child is waking from the cold when your heating goes off, add another blanket at your bedtime.

Is anxious when alone. Give lots of attention during the day and put your baby in a room with a sibling if you have other children. Consider moving your child's cot into your room, or put another bed in the child's room. When he or she wakes up, soothe your child briefly and then lie down until he or she goes back to sleep. You can then either go back to your own room or stay where you are. You can teach your toddler to sleep alone when the time is right.

Is ill or teething or has nappy (diaper) rash. Accept some broken nights as inevitable, but return to your usual routine as soon as possible.

Has night terrors or nightmares. Comfort your child immediately – don't leave him or her to cry. Put the child back to bed to sleep, but consider leaving a nightlight on.

NIGHT WAKING IN NURSING TODDLERS

Breastfeeding toddlers may continue to wake up at night to feed. If your child wakes often and you are finding it hard to function, the following may help.

- Feed more during the day. Try feeding your child in a quiet, darkened room where there are few distractions.
- Tell an older toddler that you are no longer going to feed at night – sometimes children just need to be given clear parameters.
- Ask your partner to go to your toddler at night. Your toddler is likely to protest at first, and your partner may need to be lovingly persistent in order to settle him or her. This will be easier if your partner first takes over bedtime for a few nights.
- If you are sharing a room, consider moving your child into a different room, or sleep elsewhere yourself for a few nights.

CONTROLLED CRYING FOR NIGHT WAKING

When your child cries in the night, listen to the cries. Go in straight away if you think the child is frightened or in pain. If you are sure he or she is just calling out for you, you can try this method. Remember that you can adapt it: your limit could be five minutes of crying.

1 Wait for a minute or so before you go in. Briefly check that the child's clothing isn't wet or tangled and that his or her comforter hasn't got lost. Soothe the child with a few shushes or by stroking his or her back. Don't pick your child up or linger longer than 30 seconds or so.

2 Let the child cry but go back at increasing intervals to repeat the soothing. Start with two minutes, then three, then five, then eight, then ten, then 15.

3 Keep returning at intervals of 15 minutes until the child falls asleep. If he or she wakes up again, repeat the process over again.

YOUR TODDLER AND YOUR BED

Lots of children get up in the night and come into their parents' bed. This is fine if you are happy with it, and it doesn't affect your sleep, your partner's or your child's. But you will probably find it does disturb you, and that either you or your partner ends up sleeping elsewhere while your child lies horizontally across your pillows.

If you are happy for your child to come in with you:

• Consider setting a limit to give you and your partner some privacy – for example, no toddlers in your bed before 2.00 am.

• Get a large bed that accommodates everyone.

• Put a small mattress next to your bed, and get your child to sleep there. Tell him or her to come in quietly "like a little mouse" so as not to disturb you.

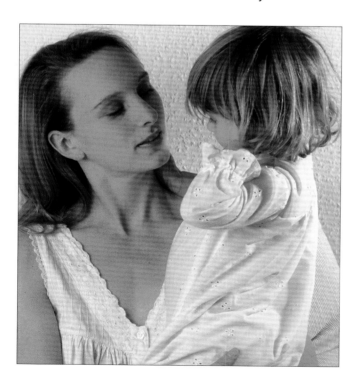

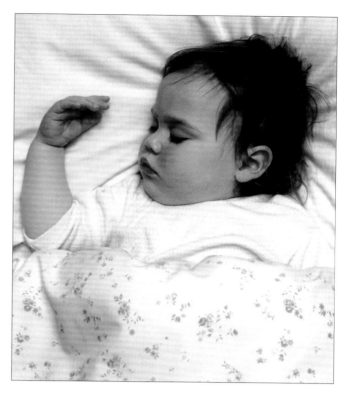

How your child naps during the day can be a cause of poor sleep at night. Think about whether he or she gets too little naptime – or too much.

The back to your own bed method:

1 When your child appears at your bedside, take him or her back to bed. Say it is bedtime, give the child a cuddle and then go back to your own bed.

2 The next time the child appears in your room, do the same thing.

3 If the child continues to appear, then gently lead him or her back to bed in silence. Do this as often as it takes until he or she stays there, even if you have to do it 30 times or more.

4 Don't get annoyed, and don't engage in any chat or explanations. Make sure your partner has the same approach: it is essential to be consistent.

After a nightmare, soothe and reassure your toddler before helping him or her get back to a peaceful sleep in his or her own bed.

NIGHT TERRORS

Some children have night terrors, in which they may scream, thrash about, sit up and look terrified for several minutes. Stay with your child while this is going on, but don't wake him or her. If the terrors tend to happen at the same time each night, try waking your child up 15 minutes beforehand and keeping him or her awake for a few minutes.

Toddler development and play

❝ You will be constantly surprised and delighted by your toddler's skills and attainments and you will bask in the reflected glory. ❞

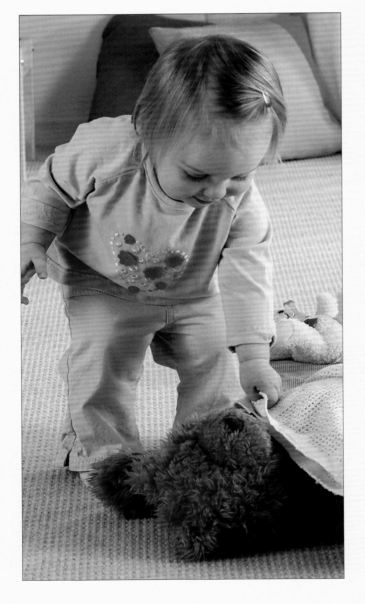

Curiosity is the defining characteristic of young toddlers. From the age of about 16 months, your child will acquire an insatiable appetite for new sights and experiences, novel words and situations, and will want to share this new knowledge with you. He or she may exclaim "Car!" every time one goes past (even if that's every two seconds as you go down the street), or may cry "Woof!" at every four-legged beast in the park, on the television screen or in the pages of a book.

The world is full of interest for toddlers and it is fascinating to watch them explore as their daring and confidence grow. You will be constantly surprised and delighted by your toddler's skills and attainments and you will bask in the reflected glory when your child succeeds in coming all the way down the stairs, sliding on his or her bottom. This is the time of walk and talk. Your child can now get out of the buggy and walk down the street with you and his or her capacity for language will suddenly race ahead at an exponential rate.

A growing emotional maturity may show itself in caring behaviour. Your child may like looking after a teddy or dolly, putting it to bed, "feeding" it and so on.

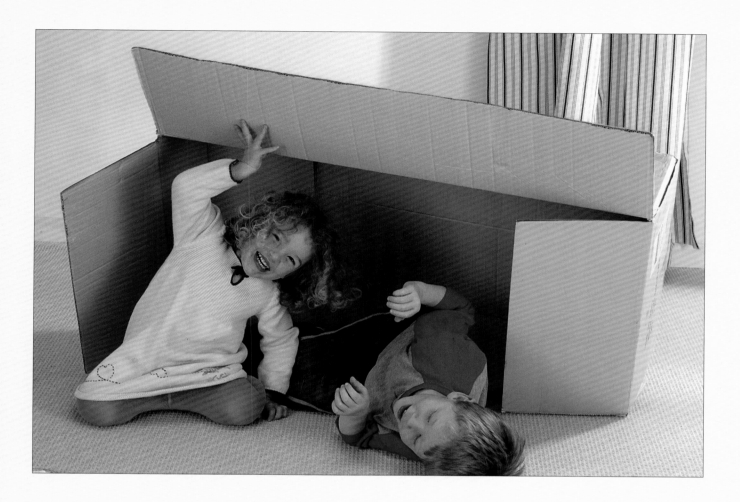

But at the start of their third year, children are in many ways still babies. Toddlers are totally concerned with themselves and do not yet understand about other people and their needs. Yet they already have views of their own about what they should be doing, and will protest loudly if adults try to make them do something they disagree with. This can be frustrating – lots of people dub this time the "terrible twos" – but it is very natural. Your toddler is learning how to be a separate, self-sufficient person. As a parent, you have the tricky job of policing and keeping your child safe, while encouraging this new-found independence and individuality. Your toddler will frustrate and exasperate you at times. But this age is also fun. Your child's emerging personality will make you proud and keep you constantly amused.

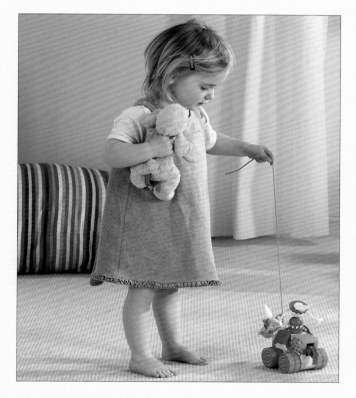

Top: Toddlers enjoy playing alongside other children from the age of about 18 months. An older child will keep your toddler happily engaged for long periods.

A treasured favourite toy may accompany a toddler everywhere for a while, even if he or she is actively playing with another toy.

First steps

Babies officially become toddlers when they learn to walk by themselves. Most children learn to walk when they are between 11 and 14 months, but some children walk as early as nine months and some can wait until 18 months. A child who isn't walking by then is probably just taking his or her time, but it is worth checking with a doctor to be on the safe side.

Your toddler will start walking as an extension of cruising. A gap between two pieces of furniture provides the impetus to take the first step: you can deliberately move them apart when you think he or she is ready to do this. Having been brave enough to take the first independent steps, your child will love to launch himself or herself from a piece of furniture towards you, or, better still, from one person to another – kneel on the floor, hold your arms out and call to him or her as encouragement. It can take several weeks before your baby gains the confidence to go further and walk across a room.

When they first start walking, toddlers rock from one foot to another, keeping their feet wide apart to help them balance. They also hold their arms away from the body for the same reason. As they gradually get steadier on their feet, they walk with the feet closer together. Your toddler will learn to bend and pick something up from the floor without losing his or her balance and will enjoy carrying

Learning walking skills starts early: a baby will enjoy supported standing from a few months old, and, once they learn to step, they will love to walk with your help.

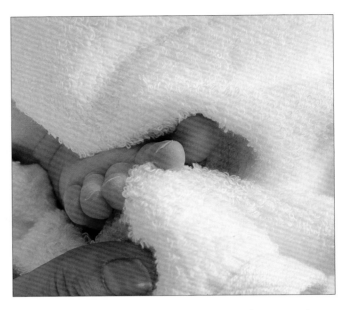

Wash your child's feet every day and dry between the toes – toddlers' feet can sweat a lot. Keep toenails trimmed, or they will press against the shoes and may become ingrowing.

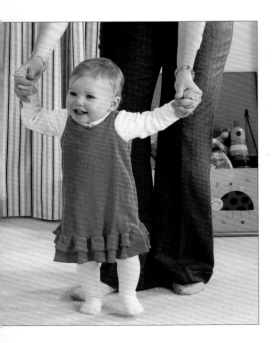
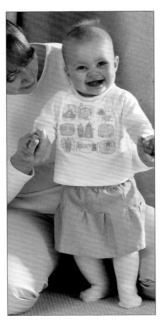

something from one part of the room to another. A sturdy toddle truck will be a favourite toy, but almost anything will be pushed along the ground: a cardboard box, a chair, the buggy. As your child will now be moving more quickly than when crawling, you'll need to watch him or her closely all the time.

Once your child is good at walking, let him or her walk outside. Think of short walks you could do together rather than always using the buggy or car seat. Many parents frown on reins because they think they are restrictive, but they are a good way of giving active toddlers more freedom while keeping them safe.

WHAT SHOES?

Walking barefoot helps to strengthen the muscles in the feet, so don't put your child in shoes until he or she is ready to walk outside. Even then, let your child go barefoot indoors or just put on socks for warmth.

When you shop for shoes, it is very important that you go to a store that measures children's feet properly and offers shoes in different widths as well as lengths. The bones of a young child's foot are very soft so they can easily be damaged if they are constricted by a badly fitting shoe. Never buy shoes off the peg, and don't put your child in second-hand shoes – they will have slightly distorted to the shape of the previous wearer's feet, and

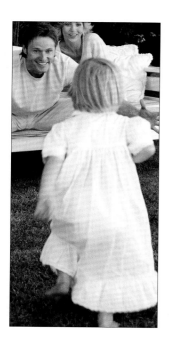

Left: The first steps are short and wobbly. But your baby will be incredibly pleased with himself or herself for managing such an awesome feat, and will be thrilled by your delight in this accomplishment.

Right: Push-along toys can help to give a new walker extra confidence. Later on, your child may pretend it is, say, a vacuum cleaner in imaginative play.

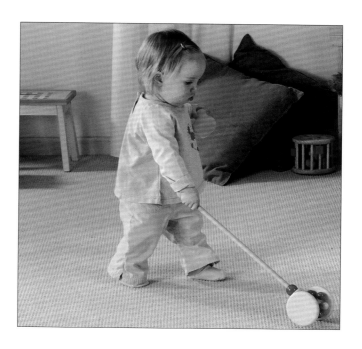

won't give proper support to your child's feet. A properly fitted shoe should have lots of "growing room" in the toe area, and the sole should be flexible, so that it moves with your child's foot. The shoe should fasten securely with a buckle, Velcro or laces. The heel of the shoe should fit securely: it shouldn't come off the heel when your child stands on tiptoes. Choose shoes made of natural materials (such as leather or canvas), which allow the foot to "breathe".

Have your child's feet measured every six to eight weeks, a good shoe shop should do this – and check that your child's shoes are still fitting properly – without putting you under any pressure to buy.

SAFETY CHECK

Your toddler will be able to stretch for things when standing up – which means he or she can get to objects that were previously out of reach. Assess your living space afresh and take steps to make it as safe as possible.

- Don't leave cutlery, cups or glasses near the edges of tables.
- Make sure that carpets and rugs are smooth: a rucked-up rug is a hazard for your uncertain walker.
- If you have a hard floor surface, don't put your child in slippy socks: he or she needs to be barefoot or should wear non-slip socks.
- If older children are playing a game nearby, move a toddler out of their way or he or she is likely to get knocked over.
- Don't allow play with lightweight toy buggies until your toddler's balance has improved to the point where he or she doesn't tip them over.

IS SOMETHING WRONG?

Toddlers walk in a different way to adults – they tend to keep their feet apart, and they "waddle" because they walk with flat feet. Normally these little oddities resolve themselves in time, but do seek medical advice if you are concerned about your child's feet or the way that he or she walks, or if any of the following conditions are severe or affect one leg only.

Pigeon toes (toeing in). Some children walk with their toes turned in. This usually corrects itself in time, but see your doctor if your child turns only one foot in or out, or if there is no improvement by the age of seven or eight.

Dancer toes (toeing out). Other children keep their toes turned outwards when they first start to walk. This usually improves within a year or so.

Flat feet. All children are flat footed when they start to walk; this gives them more stability. The arch of the foot doesn't start to develop until a child is about two, and your child won't walk with a heel-to-toe step for another year after that. If flat feet persist after age three, ask your doctor to refer your child to a podiatrist (foot specialist).

Bow legs. You'll see a gap between your child's ankles and knees until the age of about two. But if the gap is very pronounced or persists, ask a health professional to take a look – very occasionally this is a sign of rickets.

Knock knees. Lots of children hold their knees together when they walk: a gap of up to 6cm/2¾in between the ankles is normal. Knock knees usually go by age six.

SOCKS

Only buy cotton socks for your toddler and make sure that they fit properly. Tight socks can be as damaging as tight shoes.

Your young toddler's development

Six months or so after learning to walk, your toddler will start to run, but he or she will find it hard to stop or slow down to turn corners. "Chasing" a child towards a sofa that he or she can land on safely is great fun and helps to strengthen the leg muscles and improve control. Outdoor games, such as football, will help with balance – your toddler won't be able to kick a ball accurately for a while, but he or she will have a lot of fun trying.

A toddler is hardwired to practise all the movements needed to improve his or her coordination and control. A child who has balance will instinctively squat to pick something up. This builds flexibility in the hips and knees and strengthens the leg muscles. He or she will also practise walking backwards and sideways. Most young children love dancing, which gives an ideal opportunity to practise a whole range of different movements: dance together and incorporate knee bends, swaying, arm movements and different steps into your routine.

The stairs will continue to be a source of fascination. Young toddlers learn to walk up them instead of crawling, but have to bring both feet on to one step at a time, at first holding on to the step above. The next stage is to walk up without holding on, but they can't do this using alternate feet until they are about three. It's good to let

As your child's thinking ability develops, you may notice that he or she pauses before tackling a task to consider how to go about it. Shape sorters teach children about shapes and sizes and give a sense of accomplishment.

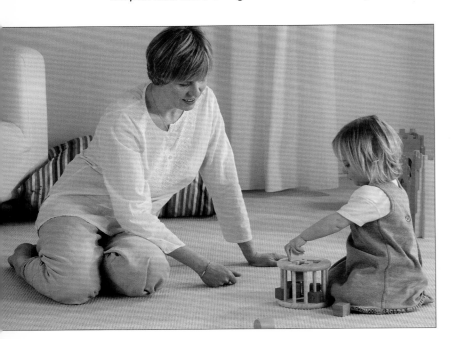

your child practise going up and down stairs, but you'll need to be close behind. A toddler is very likely to pause halfway up and, forgetting where he or she is, may lean backwards with inevitable results. Coming down is harder than going up; teach your child to do it backwards, on his or her tummy. Continue to use stair gates to prevent your child from shimmying up or down unaccompanied.

USING THE HANDS

During the second year, children learn to rotate the wrist, which allows them to be much more controlled in their hand movements. They can build a tower, placing one brick on another: by about 18 months they can manage a tower of three or four bricks, and will be able to add a couple more by the age of two. They can bring a spoon to their mouth without spilling too much food and can learn to drink from an open cup, provided they are given the opportunity.

At the same time, the small motor skills become more refined. Toddlers learn to use just a finger to point rather than involving the whole arm and hand. They can grasp a zipper tag between finger and thumb and pull it open and shut, and can twist knobs on the hi-fi. They learn to use a pencil more deliberately: by the end of the year they can make simple lines and semicircles as well as scribbles.

MENTAL LEAPS

These developing physical skills allow your child to explore the world and to get a better sense of how things work. They go hand in hand with brain development: burgeoning cognitive skills make themselves known in physical achievements, and exploration of the physical world stimulates the child's mind.

Toddlers naturally want to experiment with things, because this is how they learn about them. So they will press buttons on the washing machine, reach for door knobs, and post toast into the VCR. They will test everything – you can almost see them thinking, "What happens if I press this?", or "What does this do?"

INDIVIDUAL DEVELOPMENT
Children progress at different rates, but if you are worried at any time about any area of your child's growth and development, raise it with a health professional. You will be invited to a checkup to review your child's progress at around 18 months.

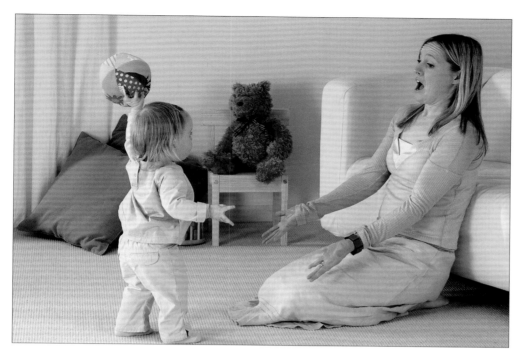

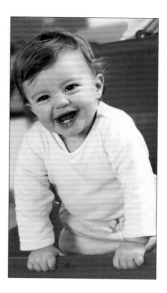

Once they've worked out how to do it, toddlers will love to make you laugh.

At some time in the second year children learn to throw overhand. Give your toddler a foam ball for safe throwing at home.

Memory steadily improves along with motor skills. Your child's new capacity to remember will show itself in play and the ability to anticipate events. If you are getting your coat to go out, your child may follow suit and go and stand by the door. If you were sweeping the floor this morning and have left the broom out, he or she may well grasp it and try to do the same in the afternoon or the next day. This is called deferred imitation.

Memory is, of course, essential for the development of language. There is a huge variation in the amount young toddlers speak, but most are able to name lots of familiar objects and to put two words together – "Mummy phone", "Louis ball", "more milk" – by the end of the second year. You will notice that your toddler's ability to understand you is way ahead of his or her ability to talk – a child will fetch a teddy when you ask for it many months before he or she says the word.

EMOTIONAL DEVELOPMENT

Your baby gradually learns that he or she is an individual, separate from you. Sometimes this feels scary and may make a child anxious and clingy. But a toddler slowly gets more comfortable with the idea. After about 18 months, he or she will be happier to spend longer periods away from you.

A growing sense of self means that a child starts to assert his or her will by refusing to do things that don't appeal – expect to hear the word "no" a lot. It can be quite sad to say goodbye to the compliant and unquestioning baby you have nurtured, but this new

individualism is an essential part of growing up. Your child needs to be allowed to probe the limits of self-reliance, and will do so happily if you provide a loving, stable base to return to. Now, when you go to a parent-and-toddler group, your child will venture farther away from you, returning from time to time for reassurance that you are still there.

Although your toddler's behaviour is bound to test you at times, you'll notice a burgeoning awareness of other people that marks the start of socialization. This starts with you: your child will know when you are sad, for example, and will grasp which aspects of his or her behaviour please or displease you.

During his or her second year, a young child will find it easier to grasp a pencil and make marks.

Children are fascinated by zips, and work out how to manipulate them by about 18 months.

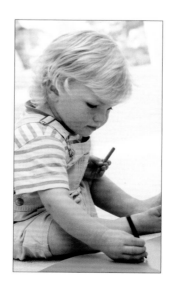

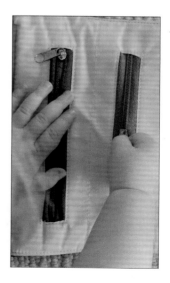

Your older toddler's development

Older toddlers are on the move all the time and they naturally have a lot more physical confidence than younger ones. Their improved sense of equilibrium means that by the age of two and a half they are proficient runners. By the end of the year they can jump off a step. They may also be able to stand on one leg for a few seconds, though they have to concentrate hard. They can kick and throw with much greater accuracy, throwing underarm as well as overarm, and they may be able to catch a ball (though they still miss more often than not).

CLIMBING CONFIDENCE

Older toddlers are much better at climbing, but how high your child climbs will depend on his or her individual sense of adventure. A child who is a natural risk taker may joyfully scramble up a climbing frame or on to a proper chair without considering how he or she is going to get down again. If this is the case, you will need to set limits. If your child is physically timid, he or she may be fearful of climbing. It may help your child to gain confidence if you encourage some practice on manageable pieces of play equipment, such as the first few rungs of the slide ladder, while you stand behind him or her.

If you have stairs in your home, your toddler will by now have had lots of practice at negotiating them. By the age of three, a child may walk up a flight of stairs as adults do, putting alternate feet on the steps. Coming down is trickier, and your child may continue to bring both feet on to each step until around four. If your home is on one level, then you might want to use a friend's home to get your child accustomed to negotiating stairs safely.

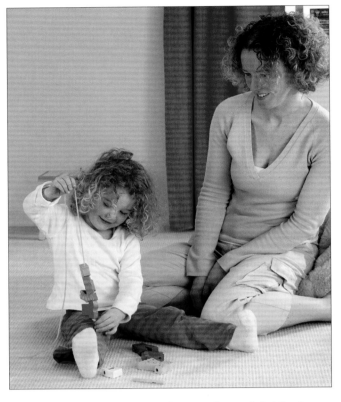

Threading beads on to a string requires a fair bit of manual dexterity. This toy is also great for counting games and learning the names of colours.

USING THE HANDS

At two, children can turn over one page of a book at a time, rather than two or three. They can also thread beads on to a string, provided the holes are large enough. And towers of bricks get higher: they can manage up to eight blocks by the age of two and a half. As children's hand movements continue to become more precise, they are able to tackle more everyday tasks: for example, doing up large buttons or toggles. Get your child to help you with jobs such as setting the table. Tackling everyday tasks will help his or her dexterity and build self-confidence.

Your child will have a lot more control when using a pencil or crayon: he or she won't be able to draw a

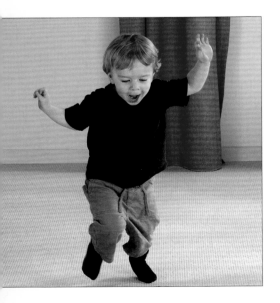

Jumping develops slowly. Most 18-month-olds can't manage to bend their knees and get themselves off the ground at the same time, but they may manage this feat by the age of two. Hopping comes much later.

RIGHT- AND LEFT-HANDEDNESS
Lots of children are ambidextrous until the age of three. But you may notice that your child shows a definite preference for using the right or left hand when eating or playing.

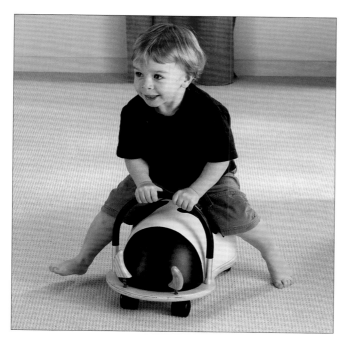

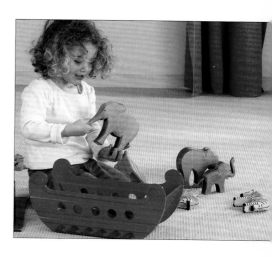

Left: A ride-on toy is good for balance and improves an older toddler's physical confidence.

Right: Your toddler will practise sorting in play: for example, he or she may group toys by colour or size, or put all the animals from a Noah's ark into their pairs.

picture yet, but will do lots of lines, dots and circles. By the end of the year, your child can probably manage a pair of children's safety scissors (supervised by you), though only to cut simple strips rather than complicated outlines at first. Using scissors is a complex manoeuvre, involving forethought, dexterity and concentration. Your toddler will have taken a big step forward when he or she can manipulate a pair of scissors.

MENTAL LEAPS

Your toddler has now garnered enough knowledge about how things work to be able to organize and sort things: he or she may place bricks in a line, say, or put toy animals in one box and toy cars in another. Older toddlers are able to "think" about things that aren't right in front of them, which means they can be much more imaginative in play. Now your child doesn't necessarily need a toy as inspiration – he or she is able to pretend that a cardboard box, say, is a car or a house. In the toddler's make-believe world, ideas are drawn from everything – the daily routine, the people he or she knows, television shows and story

books. Your child's memory has improved to the extent that if you interrupt in the middle of a game, the child will be able to return to it and pick up where he or she left off. Language skills are developing rapidly and he or she will probably be talking in simple sentences by the age of three. You'll also see your toddler playing sorting games with toys, showing the natural urge to classify and categorize that is a very important skill for life: to function in the world, we need to be able to tell what's hot from what's cold, who is friendly and who is not, what is ours and what is someone else's.

EMOTIONAL DEVELOPMENT

During their third year, children develop a much better sense of the world and their place within it. Until now they have seen everything in relation to themselves. Now they start to realize that other people have needs, too. They also become more affectionate.

Toddlers develop a much stronger sense of self from about two years. This goes hand-in-hand with a new possessiveness. Another important part of the sense of self is an awareness of gender. This starts as early as 18 months, and children are sure in the knowledge that they are boys or girls by the age of three. They may start to behave in stereotypical ways at this point, particularly if they feel that this is what is expected of them.

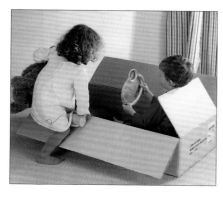

Who needs expensive toys when a large cardboard box can be a car...

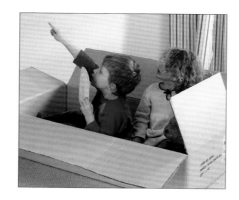

... a spaceship navigating the universe of the living room...

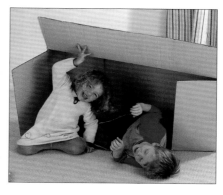

... or a special den in which to hide away from the grown-ups?

An expanding family

Young children love stability and routine, but they inevitably have to deal with change and new challenges from time to time. Probably the biggest upheaval of a child's early life is the arrival of a baby brother or sister, and sensitive handling is necessary to help a toddler accept a new baby.

PREPARING FOR A NEW BABY

Pack away any of your child's baby gear long before the arrival of the new baby. That way, your toddler is less likely to feel that the baby is taking things that belong to him or her when you get them out again. The toddler will also enjoy looking at them all again and helping you decide which toys to put out for the new baby.

Tell your child that you have a baby in your tummy once you start getting large – before other people let it slip. Older children may like to feel the baby kick or to listen to its heartbeat at your antenatal checkups. But ultrasound pictures can look bizarre, so don't show the scan unless you think your child is up to it.

Introducing a second child into your family can have its tricky moments, but your oldest will learn to accept his or her sibling in time.

WEANING A TODDLER

If you are still breastfeeding your toddler when you become pregnant, it is fine to continue. Some mothers decide to feed both their newborn and toddler at the same time (tandem feeding). However, if you decide to wean your toddler before the birth, it is best to start several months beforehand. The most natural way to wean is using the principle of "never offer, never refuse": nurse your toddler if he or she asks, but don't offer a feed. This can work well for some children, but you may also need to do the following as well.

• Give your child a drink and a snack before your usual nursing times.
• Think about when your child likes to nurse. Change your routine so that he or she will naturally ask to nurse less often.
• If your child nurses irregularly, try postponing the feed and then provide a distraction by going out together or playing a game.
• If you usually feed on waking and at bedtime, get the child's dad or someone else to take over at these times.

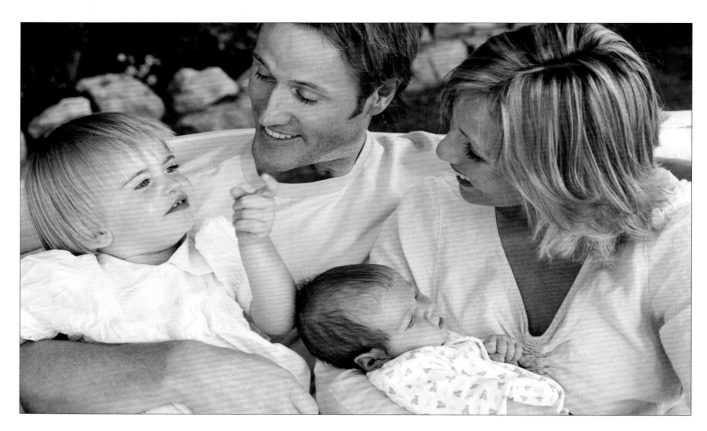

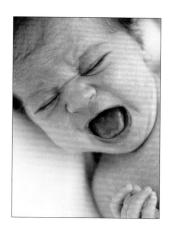

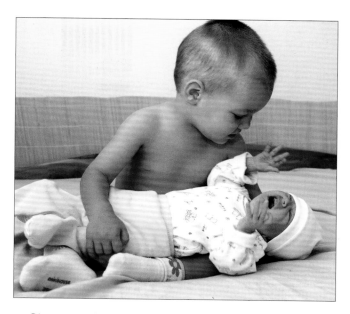

Left: Looking after a new baby and a toddler is hard work, so make sure you get enough rest.

Right: Encourage an older child to play nicely with a new baby and exclaim at how the baby seems to like him or her the most.

Don't make any major changes to your child's routine near the delivery date. Potty training, or moving a toddler to his or her own room or into a proper bed, should happen either a few months before the birth or once the child has got used to the new baby.

Talk to your child about what life will be like when the baby comes. It can help to reminisce about his or her own babyhood: tell stories about how your toddler kept you up all night. Give your child the opportunity to ask questions and voice any concerns, and be honest but reassuring in your answers – for example, agree that things will be different when the new baby comes, but talk about all the things that will stay the same too. If you have friends with small babies, it is a good idea to take your child with you to visit them. If possible, let him or her see other mothers breastfeeding and explain what is happening.

Let your toddler know who will care for him or her while you have the baby. It is much better to get a familiar person to come to your home rather than sending your child to stay with someone. However, if he or she has to go and stay elsewhere, be sure to arrange a couple of practice runs before the birth. If you plan to have the baby at home, you will still need a trusted person to care for your child. Childbirth is intense and messy, even when it is going well: you will need all your energy to focus on your contractions, and your child could be traumatized by witnessing his or her mummy in labour.

INTRODUCING A NEW SIBLING

After the birth, have your arms free for hugs when you see your child for the first time – put the baby in a cot or basket for a while. Tell your toddler how much you've missed him or her. If you are coming home from hospital, get someone else to carry the new baby into your home so that you can give your full attention to your older child. Look at the baby together. Children often find small babies fascinating, and your toddler may enjoy examining the funny squashed-up face or tiny wrinkly fingers with you. Let the toddler stroke the baby gently, and say how much the baby likes it; show your child how the baby will grip his or her finger to say hello.

Give your older child a small gift "from the baby". You can put this at the foot of the baby's cot for your child to discover. You may also like to give a gift from Mummy and Daddy at some point over the next few days – a present can be a tangible reminder of how much you love your child. For an older child, it can be helpful to choose a gift that subtly reaffirms his or her place in the home, such as a new duvet cover or a special cup. Remind grandparents and close friends to say hello to your older child before cooing over the newborn. If they are bringing a gift for the baby, suggest it would be good if they brought something small for the older child as well.

AS TIME GOES ON

Emphasize how lucky the baby is to have your older child as a sibling, rather than how nice it is for the toddler to have a playmate. Try not to go on too much about the "big brother/sister" role – your child doesn't want to be seen as an adjunct to the new baby, and don't expect your child to feel instant love for your new baby. Help him or her enjoy the strangeness of the new baby instead – have a joke about the stinky nappies, the baby's funny little sneezes and yawns. Your child is bound to feel jealous of the new baby from time to time. Acknowledge this feeling and reaffirm how much you love him or her, but be firm that any rough behaviour around the baby is not to be tolerated.

Make the baby's feeding time a special time for your older child too – you can read stories, chat, do a jigsaw or listen to a story tape together while feeding. Let your older child help you care for the baby by fetching nappies or pushing the buggy, and praise him or her for helping.

Stick to your normal routines – bedtime, mealtimes and so on – as much as possible. Spend some time alone with your older child if you can: ideally, go on one outing a week while a grandparent or your partner babysits. Choose something you have always done together.

Helping toddlers play

It is during toddlerhood that children learn to learn: patterns acquired now will stay with them into their school years. But don't feel that you have to hothouse them with endless classes, planned activities and flash cards – too much structured time can be tiring for your child and doesn't leave enough time for imaginative play.

Your child will learn best in a stimulating and loving environment, with plenty of time for unhurried, self-directed play. Play will teach your toddler all he or she needs to know about problem solving, making judgments, being creative, gaining self-confidence, taking risks, developing empathy and – eventually – sharing. Here are some ways to help a toddler enjoy play.

Give your child your undivided attention when you play with him or her. Sit on the floor and do what the child wants. There's no substitute for one-on-one time, and play helps to build a good relationship.

Have fun together. Play is supposed to be enjoyable, and your child will love it if you introduce an element of humour into games.

Follow your child's lead. If your child is playing a game of make-believe, then do what he or she asks you – don't say how things ought to be. If your child needs your help to build a castle, let him or her be the architect and decide which brick goes where. Being in charge of the game helps to boost your child's self-confidence and encourages problem solving.

Don't interfere if your child is playing happily. Wait until he or she needs or asks for your input, and don't interfere or make suggestions.

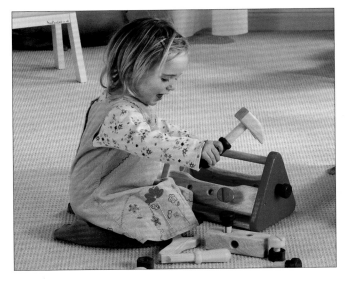

Construction toys are lots of fun, and a kit like this will cover several months of your toddler's development.

BALANCING A CHILD'S PERSONALITY TRAITS

By the time your child is two you may have a clear idea of his or her personality. Your child needs to be loved for who he or she is, but you can still use playtime constructively. If your child can't concentrate for long, for example, help by choosing an activity that he or she enjoys and then praising the child for sticking with it. Look out for the moment when the child gets bored and alter the activity slightly to reignite his or her interest.

Children are often interested in counting at an early age. They may be quick to recognize numbers long before they understand what they are for.

Rough and tumble is good for children, so long as they are enjoying it. It can help to make girls more physically confident and can help boys to manage aggression.

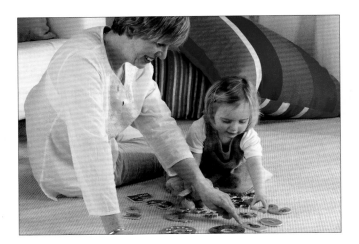

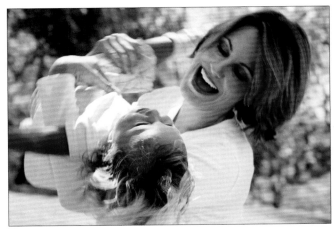

TODDLERS AND TELEVISION

Television has a mesmerizing effect, so it is tempting to allow your child to watch it when you need a break. But watching a lot of television on a regular basis can affect a toddler's ability to concentrate. A study by the American Academy of Pediatrics found that the likelihood of a child developing attention problems at school went up by 10 per cent for every hour of television watched each day – so a child watching three hours a day was 30 per cent more likely to have attention deficit disorder (ADD) by the age of seven. Excessive television at an early age has also been linked to obesity and aggression.

- Don't put a child under two in front of the television. Many children this age won't be interested in watching anyway.
- Limit older toddlers to 30 minutes at a time.
- Choose your child's viewing carefully. Children's programmes often have an educational theme and most children prefer them to adult programmes.
- Be wary of allowing your child to see advertisements. Watch videos instead of commercial programmes.
- Stay with your older toddler while he or she watches a programme and talk about it afterwards.
- Never have the television on in the background while your child is playing.

YOUR CHILD'S TOYS

Toys are more inviting if they are organized than if they are piled in a messy heap. Make tidying up part of play – your child can have just as much fun putting toys back in the box as emptying it. It's a good idea to rotate toys: if you put some away in a cupboard for a while your child will be much more interested in them when they reappear.

Provide some creative play materials, such as play dough or clay, paints, craft materials and dressing-up clothes. Let your child play with natural materials, such as snow, sand, water, mud and grass, as much as possible. Don't feel that you need to invest in electronic

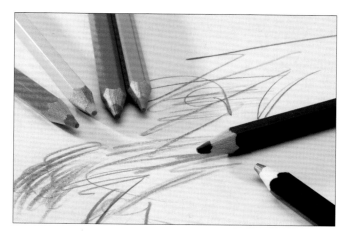

Making marks on paper is something that most children love to do, and it is an important precursor of writing, so keep chunky pencils, crayons and paper at hand.

"educational" toys. High-tech toys are very appealing to young children, but flashing lights and robotic sounds offer less potential for creative play than simple toys and play materials.

Encourage your child to play with a wide range of toys, including those aimed at the opposite gender. Different toys encourage different skills, so limiting your child early on could discourage some aspects of development: for example, playing with dolls can help with social skills, while using construction blocks helps with visual-spatial skills. Look for books that show, say, girls being brave and boys being sensitive to help your child get a broad understanding of how boys and girls behave.

It is important that your child's toys and books should accurately represent his or her world. For example, most dolls are based on Caucasian people, so if you are black or Asian, seek out toys that reflect your skin colour and make sure your child has books that feature people of your ethnic group. Studies show children can become aware of differences in skin colour by the age of two.

If you need to get on with other things, make sure your toddler has something fun to do. But don't expect your child to stay occupied for long periods.

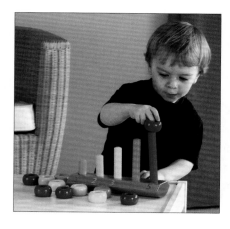
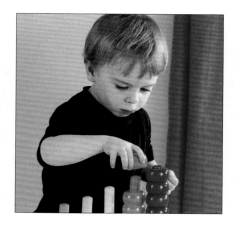
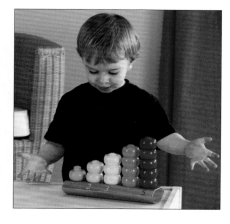

Ideas for play

Give your child a good balance of different forms of play. Toddlers need plenty of running around to let off steam, but they also need quiet activities such as looking at books or playing with bricks to help build concentration. Here are some ideas.

PHYSICAL PLAY

Toddlers have boundless energy, so give them lots of opportunity to expend it. You'll find a toddler easier to manage if he or she gets plenty of physical activity. Spend time outdoors every day if you can. Go to the park, where your child can run, jump and climb. Take your child to the local swimming pool or to a toddler gym (soft room) or go to a dancing class for older toddlers. Take short walks together and point out things that you see, hear or smell – the more children use their senses, the more they learn. On windy days, give an older toddler a length of ribbon and get the child to run so that it streams behind him or her. Some small children take a lively interest in the wildlife that can be found in a garden or park – the woodlice, worms, birds and spiders. You can foster this interest by feeding the ducks or visiting farms and zoos.

If you are stuck indoors with a fidgety toddler, push the furniture out of the way and have a mini-exercise class: touch toes, do star jumps (jumping with legs and arms wide open), run, hop, jump, spin around. Dance to some fast music: your two year old may well have a favourite tune you can dance to. Make a mini-obstacle course: create a tunnel out of a couple of chairs and a blanket, put down large open boxes for your child to crawl through and make a mountain of pillows to climb. For a calming down activity, try doing a few simple yoga poses.

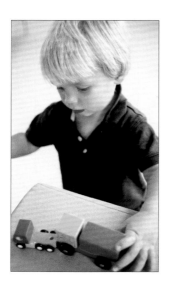

Once children develop the ability to play imaginatively, they can amuse themselves for much longer. A railway set or garage with toy cars will provide fun for many years to come as your child's play adapts to his or her growing abilities.

MAKE YOUR OWN PLAY DOUGH

Toddlers love playing with dough and it's easy to make your own. The dough will last a month or so if you store it in an airtight box in the refrigerator.

250g/8oz water
250g/8oz plain flour
30ml/2 tbsp cream of tartar
a few drops of food colouring
15ml/1 tbsp sunflower or other cooking oil
125g/4oz salt

Put all the ingredients in a small saucepan, place over a medium heat and stir until the mixture forms a smooth dough. Remove from the pan and leave to cool before using.

MESSY PLAY

Making a mess is tremendous fun, teaches your child about textures and encourages free expression. Make it a rule that your child covers up with an apron or similar (an older child's shirt, worn back-to-front, works well) and lay newspaper over the table or floor if you are using paints.
Water. Fill a washing-up bowl with water and let your child play with it, supervised, in the garden. Old yoghurt pots, bottles, straws, a funnel, spoons and a colander are all good to play with. If you have a patio, give your child a paintbrush for "drawing" on the paving, or show him or her how to step in the water and make wet footprints.
Sand. Fill a washing-up bowl with clean sand. Show your child how to make patterns in it. Provide a small jug of water to wet the sand so that your child can build mountains, make "cakes" and so on.
Painting. Younger toddlers can paint with their fingers, pieces of sponge, corks, cotton reels or potato printers. Give your child one colour to start with, and then another so that he or she can see what happens when the two are mixed. Your child may also like to do handprints (which make great cards for relatives). Use non-toxic finger paints or powder paints mixed with water and washing-up liquid (to make them thicker and easier to manage). Two year olds may be able to manage a chunky brush (or chunky non-toxic felt-tip pens).

DRESSING UP

Children enjoy dressing up from about 18 months. Make a collection of items from your own and your friends' or relatives' wardrobes and put them in a special dressing-up box, which you can bring out as a treat or on a rainy afternoon. Hats are good; other favoured items are sunglasses, short strings of beads, bracelets and other jewellery (check for safety), old handbags or briefcases, short nightdresses (for princess outfits), old jackets, gloves, boots, shawls and even odd lengths of glittering or shiny fabric.

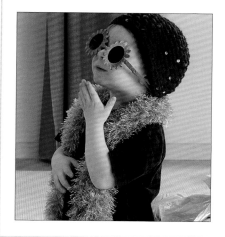 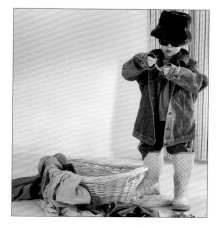 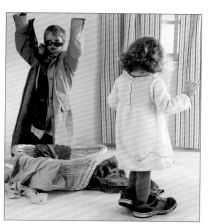

Sticking. You'll need a non-toxic glue pen, plus some small pieces of paper snipped from a magazine, bits of string, wool, ribbon and foil, dried leaves, crumpled tissues, scraps of fabric or cotton wool (cotton balls). Lentils, seeds, dried pasta shapes, loose tea leaves or desiccated coconut can all be shaken on to glued paper.

Model making. This is great fun for older toddlers. You can use all kinds of packaging: cardboard rolls, egg boxes, cereal boxes, corks, yoghurt pots and so on.

IMAGINATIVE PLAY

Toddlers have a natural instinct for copying and love pretend play. It helps them to understand their world and encourages them to use their imaginations.

Domestic play. Pretending to do chores will be a favourite game for several years. Include your child in everyday tasks when you can, such as dusting, watering plants or "cooking". Having a little helper may slow you down, but makes housework more fun. Most household items will be too heavy for your child to play with so you may want to invest in some toy domestic items.

Small world toys. Farmyards, dolls' houses, train sets, garages and so on will give your child hours of fun. Small toddlers will sort the items into groups; older ones may start to role-play with them.

Dolls and soft toys. These will be co-opted into pretend play – and may be assigned the role of a naughty toddler. Don't be surprised if they get shouted at and hit: this is how children act out aggression and difficult feelings.

Nearly fill small plastic bottles with sand and screw the lids on tight to make skittles; arrange them in a corridor and take turns to knock them over with a soft ball.

To make a potato printer, cut a potato in half and use a sharp knife to trace a shape into the cut face – simple shapes work best. Cut round the shape from the side and remove the unwanted pieces. Dip the shape into paint and use as a stamp.

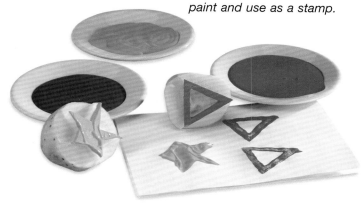

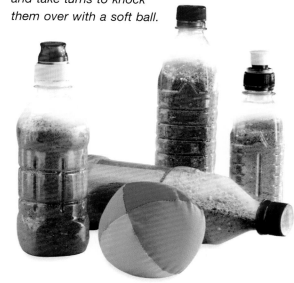

Learning to socialize

Your child's world expands gradually. As a baby, he or she was most interested in you and one or two other important people. Little by little, with your encouragement, your child has learned to interact with people such as relatives, friends, visitors and friendly passers-by. All children need to learn how to get on with other people. It's good to get your child used to being around different grown-ups and other children. This allows a toddler to get used to the idea that not everything revolves around him or her, and encourages the development of empathy, kindness and cooperation.

Most children become more sociable between the ages of 18 months and three years. But they vary greatly in how willing they are to engage with other people. Let your child develop at his or her own pace.

WHEN CHILDREN MAKE FRIENDS

Babies show interest in other children early on, but they don't know how to build relationships with each other. When your baby stretched out a hand to touch another baby's face, he or she was exploring it as much as trying to make friends.

Toddlers often respond to overtures from fun adults or older children. If your toddler has an older sibling or sees another older child regularly, the screams of delighted

Once children work out that it is more fun to play with a friend than alone, they naturally start to exhibit more cooperative and friendly behaviour.

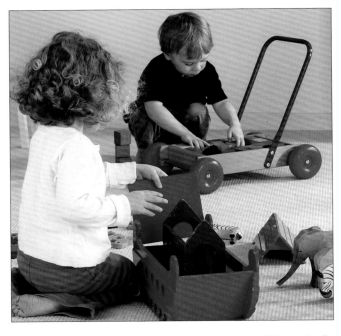

Toddlers enjoy each other's company, even if they don't play together. They may walk side by side, or sit next to each other playing with different toys. The natural instinct to be with people of the same age develops into more collaborative behaviour over time.

anticipation may show just how pleased he or she is to know them. But toddlers don't really engage with children of their own age until they are over two. They start to enjoy each other's company from about 18 months, but at

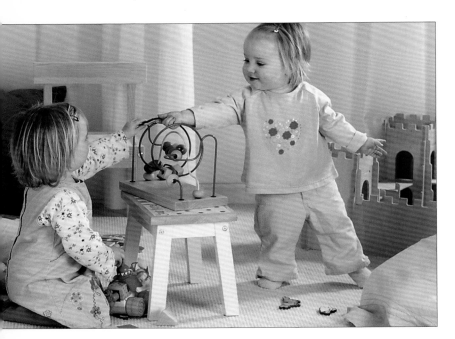

HELPING A SHY TODDLER
Some children are naturally shy and need gentle encouragement to socialize.
- Don't label your child "shy" or talk about your child's shyness in his or her hearing.
- Keep social events manageable – tea at a friend's house, a small music group.
- Give your child lots of cuddles to help him or her feel secure. But don't withdraw from the group into a corner together.
- Hold your child when a visitor arrives. Ask the child to say "hello" or wave and give lots of praise if he or she manages it.
- Look for ways to build your child's confidence: increase activities that he or she enjoys and give lots of attention and praise.

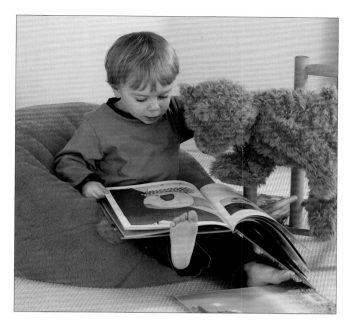

Leave books on a low shelf that your child can reach: you may be surprised at how often he or she chooses a book rather than a more active toy.

three, four or more words together in simple sentences: "Mummy go work now." They may start to use pronouns ("I", "you") as well as connecting words such as "and" and "but". Their pronunciation is clear enough to enable strangers as well as family members to understand them most of the time. They have become, in other words, social beings, able to express themselves and contribute their thoughts to society at large.

DELAYED SPEECH

The pace of language acquisition varies widely. Girls tend to speak earlier and use more words than boys, sociable toddlers talk more than shy ones and younger children in large families tend to acquire language more slowly than only or oldest children. Twins commonly experience delays in their language development: they may develop their own language, or one twin may talk for the other. It is quite possible for an intelligent child to say very little by

TWO LANGUAGES
Bilingual children learn as quickly as monolingual ones, but they may start by speaking a strange amalgam of both languages – picking and choosing words from each. It may seem that they are acquiring English more slowly than their contemporaries at first, but if this happens they will usually catch up by the age of two. Bilingualism never means that a child grows up less proficient in the language of his or her home country, and a native speaker's knowledge of more than one tongue will be a lifelong advantage.

the age of two, and language development often occurs in spurts. But if you suspect that your child's language abilities aren't progressing as they should, then do talk to a health professional. Your child can be referred to a speech therapist if necessary.

ENCOURAGING LANGUAGE

You don't need to "teach" your child to speak, but you can certainly encourage language development.

Talk lots. Studies show that children who are spoken to a lot when they are young have better vocabularies and higher IQs. Talk about what you or your child are doing. When you are out and about, point out things of interest: the red bus, the noisy pigeons and so on. If you have twins, be sure to address them individually.

Listen carefully. Toddlers' pronunciation is indistinct, so you have to concentrate to understand what they are saying. Repeating back what your child says or expanding on it shows that you are listening.

Don't answer for your child. If you ask your child a question, give him or her enough time to respond rather than jumping in. Don't finish your toddler's sentences.

Have fun with word play. Children love songs, nursery rhymes and finger games such as "Round and round the garden" and "This little piggy".

Talk about feelings. Being able to name his or her feelings will help your child to cope with them. Say things like, "Did you feel cross when I took your pencil away?" and "You have a big smile, are you feeling happy?"

If you talk to your child a lot about what he or she is doing or can see, you will naturally introduce useful new words. Older toddlers love counting games: count their toy animals, cars, socks and so on.

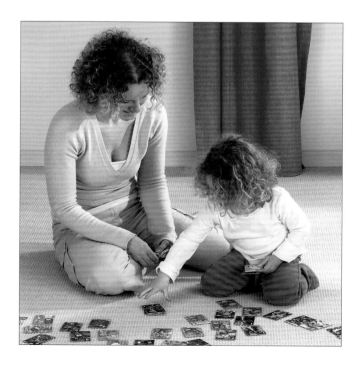

The preschool years

> **❝** It is important to nurture your child's self-esteem, celebrate what is special and help him or her cope with things that they find difficult. **❞**

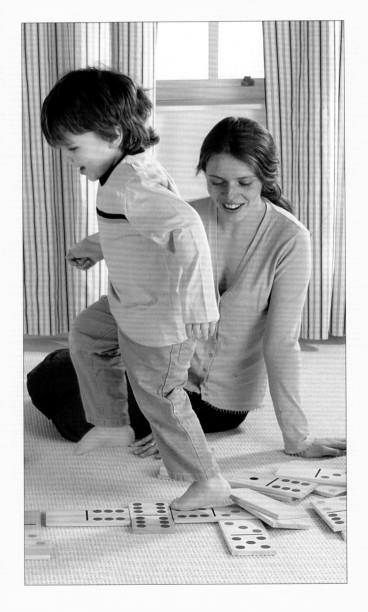

A toddler has very few social graces: when it comes to understanding the needs of other people, he or she is more like a baby than a mini-adult. But, very slowly, he or she starts to blossom into a more reasonable and social little being – someone who can think about other people. From the age of three, toddlers shows the first signs of empathy. He or she is open to persuasion, and any temper tantrums become less frequent.

A four year old realizes that people have feelings that must be respected, and is able to initiate friendships. He or she will share toys, invent games of their own, play for extended periods, and develop favourite pastimes. Preschool children become more aware of the differences between themselves and other people and will start to compare themselves to others. Succeeding or failing, and winning or losing all become more important issues at this stage, and it is important to nurture your child's self-esteem, celebrate what is special and help him or her to cope with things that they find difficult.

Preschool children will still have sudden mood swings, but generally will begin to become more rational and easier to negotiate with.

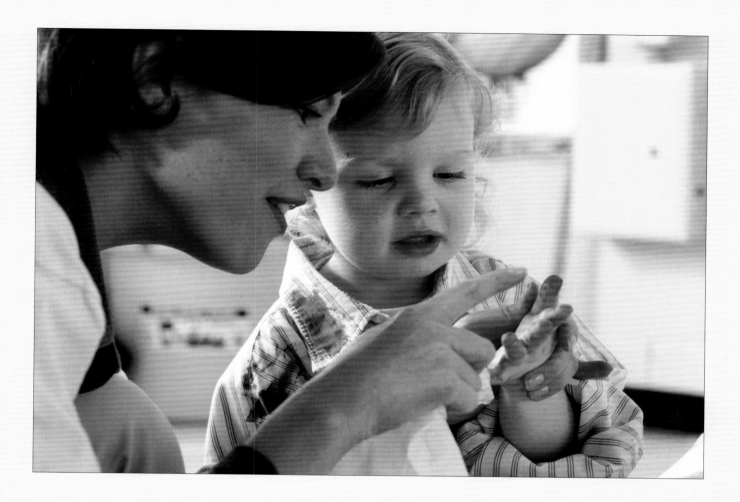

Young children love to learn, and now they have the language skills to help them. These years are a good preparation for the time when your child goes to school. Even the first term at school is a far more structured environment than your child has been accustomed to, so it is not surprising that many children get extremely tired in their first weeks and months in a school-day routine.

Good sleeping habits and a healthy diet, established over these early years, will help your child to cope. Your child will also get a new sense of himself or herself as a member of a group. Mixing with other children in the preschool years helps with this process, and all that play will have given him or her a love of learning that will help in the first steps of formal education.

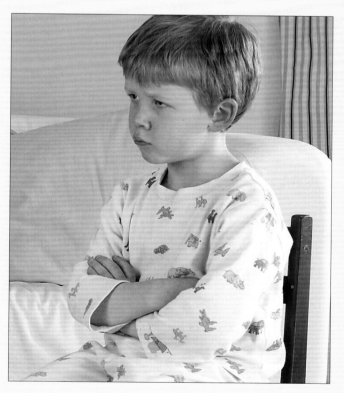

Top: As children's lives develop, people other than you will bring stimulus and interest. Your pre-school child will benefit from these expanding horizons.

A young child is still likely to be unreasonable and grumpy, but uncontrollable tantrums should lessen as he or she becomes more able to communicate.

Food and the preschooler

Young children can be surprisingly sensible eaters. If you offer them lots of healthy foods, they will generally take enough for their needs and select a reasonably balanced diet. So even if your child is one of the many who turns his or her nose up at vegetables, you will probably find that a reliable liking for several types of fruit compensates for this.

Helping your child to develop a positive relationship with food is part of good parenting, but it isn't always easy, especially as your child starts to socialize more. Relatives and friends are bound to offer sweets, crisps and so on from time to time. Three to five year olds will probably be exposed to advertising for junk foods that is deliberately targeted at them. And they are likely to see other children eating these foods, which will naturally make them want to have some too.

The best way to cultivate your child's interest in good food is to involve him or her in choosing or preparing it. Even a trip to a supermarket can be fun.

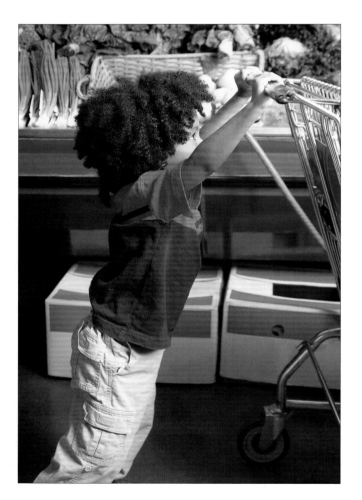

Children learn best by example, so to absorb the rudiments of table etiquette your child should share family mealtimes. Around the age of four, a child learns to handle a knife and fork well, but this is easier if they are special child-sized ones.

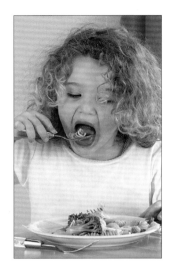

ESTABLISHING GOOD EATING HABITS

To help your child take a sensible and positive attitude to food, you need to set a good example yourself. If choosing and eating good nutritious food is the norm in your household, your children will naturally be inclined to adopt good eating habits. Explain that certain foods are good for you and others aren't, but don't give your child long lectures about healthy eating: he or she will switch off. Instead, get your child involved in choosing and preparing food to help develop an interest in it: let him or her pick out which fruit to buy when you are shopping and do some simple cooking together.

Avoid loading particular foods with emotional significance. People often give children sweets as rewards or bribes for good behaviour or to cheer them up when they are upset. It's better if your child views them just as another pleasant food. Equally, don't ban foods completely or you will make them seem even more desirable. An occasional trip to a fast-food restaurant won't ruin your child's palate.

Choose healthier snack foods: baked low-salt pretzels are better than flavoured crisps; chocolate, which quickly dissolves in the mouth, is better than boiled sweets, which linger. Have plenty of healthy snacks available:

IRON
Some preschool children don't get enough iron. The richest sources are red meat, but eggs, red kidney beans, canned fish, dried fruit and green leafy vegetables are also good. Serve foods rich in vitamin C at the same time to help the body absorb the iron.

BRAIN FOOD

Give your child two portions of fish a week, including one portion of oily fish such as salmon, mackerel, trout or tuna. Fish oils have been shown to help with concentration, social skills and behaviour.

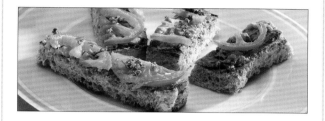

Milk and other dairy foods are still an important part of your child's diet: give three servings a day. A 200ml/¹⁄₃ pint glass of milk, a pot of yoghurt and a chunk of cheese provides your child with enough calcium.

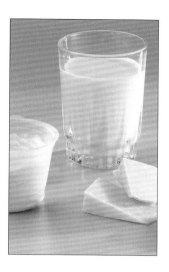

sticks of cheese, fresh fruit, mini-sandwiches, oatcakes, rice cakes and so on, and allow your child free access to these foods.

Give your child lots of water to drink as well as milk. If you want to give juice, dilute it well (one part juice to five parts water) and restrict it to mealtimes. Don't keep fizzy drinks (soda) or sweetened fruit drinks at home. If your child occasionally has these when out, try to make sure they are the ordinary versions rather than diet ones: the latter contain artificial sweeteners (such as aspartame), which are not recommended for young children.

Don't give your child ready-made convenience foods, which tend to be high in salt and made with inferior ingredients. You can make your own, much healthier versions of popular children's dishes: for example make chicken nuggets by dipping organic chicken pieces in whisked egg white then rolling them in breadcrumbs and baking in the oven; grill your own burgers, which are easily made from lean mince, wholemeal breadcrumbs, minced onions and herbs, bound together with egg. Roast thick-cut chips in the oven rather than fry them, and blot off the oil with kitchen paper, if you want to.

CHILDREN AND WEIGHT

Toddlers gradually slim down as they grow up, but you'll notice that your preschool child gets tubbier from time to time. This is because a child's body is designed to put on weight (puppy fat) just before a growth spurt. The energy stored in the fat will be burned off as it fuels the growing process. A small proportion of children put on weight without gaining height. This is the first step towards childhood obesity, an ever more acute problem in modern society. So if your child is overweight, you should address this, but follow these important guidelines.

Don't put a young child on a diet. It is better for a child to grow into the weight than to try to lose it.

Don't talk about losing weight. Don't comment on your child's body in a negative way.

Do increase physical activity. Do something active every day: get out to the park more often, play chasing games, go swimming, get your child a bike.

Do maintain healthy food habits, but still allow your child other treats from time to time.

Do give semi-skimmed milk rather than full-fat milk.

Do give small portions at mealtimes. Give your child another helping if he or she wants it, but never push extra food on your child or insist that everything is eaten.

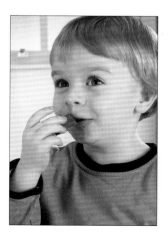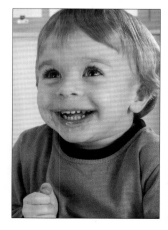

Banning sweet treats altogether is likely to be counterproductive – the occasional piece of chocolate will give huge enjoyment.

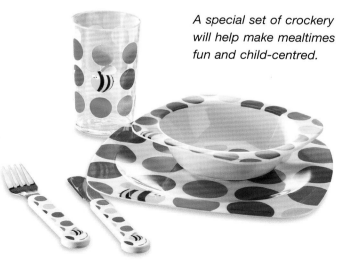

A special set of crockery will help make mealtimes fun and child-centred.

Sleep for preschool children

Many preschool children positively enjoy going to bed. Unlike toddlers, who don't like to be separated from their parents, older children can really appreciate the calm and routine of bedtime.

The need for sleep varies from child to child, but most preschool children need 11–13 hours' sleep a night. If your child doesn't get enough sleep, he or she is likely to be tired and irritable during the day. And your sleep will inevitably be affected, too. To encourage good sleeping habits, stick to a set bedtime and have a consistent bedtime routine. Help your child to wind down by avoiding rough play and noisy games and ruling out television, which can be physically and emotionally stimulating, for the hour before bedtime. Help your child to make a calm transition by giving a warning that bedtime is coming up. While young children probably need a five-minute warning followed by a one-minute

Reading a story together before bed is a wonderful way for your child to wind down and to enjoy being close to you at the end of the day.

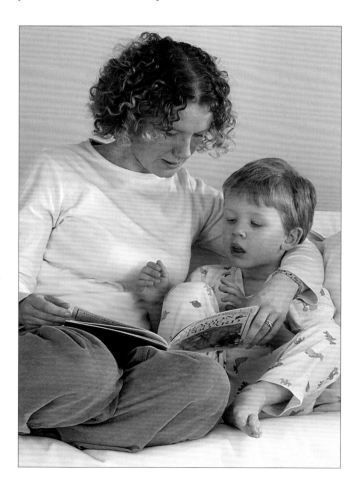

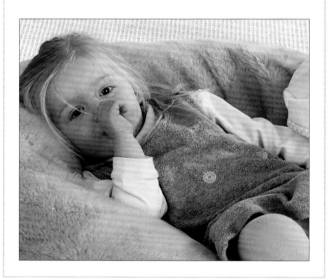

DAYTIME NAPS
Some children continue to have a daytime nap until they go to school, but most have stopped napping by the age of four. When your child first gives up a daytime nap, he or she is bound to get tired and irritable by the end of the day. You can help to manage this fatigue by ensuring that your child has regular meals and snacks and drinks lots of fluid. Balancing physical activities with quieter ones will also help. Some parents find that their preschool children are happy to go to bed for half an hour or so after lunch for some "quiet time" instead of a nap: this is a great habit to instil.

warning, older children benefit from longer warnings (15–30 minutes), and may want to choose a final activity before the bedtime routine starts. Give your child your undivided attention as he or she prepares for bed. Most children love their bedtime story and goodnight kiss. Bedtime is also a valuable opportunity for your child to tell you about the day or confide something that is worrying him or her.

Be clear that lights-out means sleep time, and don't let your child string out bedtime by asking for "one more story". Leave your child to drop off alone, but for reassurance say that you'll be back in five minutes to check if he or she is asleep. If the child is still awake when you go back, say you'll be back in another five minutes. Have a firm rule that once in bed, your child stays there and should call you if he or she needs anything. The exception is needing to go to the bathroom.

SLEEP PROBLEMS

Some sleep disturbances are a fact of childhood: a nationwide survey of American children found that about 70 per cent experienced one or more of the following sleep problems most weeks.

Nightmares. Children between three and five have vivid imaginations but don't yet understand where the boundary lies between the physical world and their own inner universe, so nightmares are common. They need swift comfort and reassurance after a bad dream. It's important to tell your child that dreams aren't real and can't hurt, but you may need to switch on the light so that you can prove that there are, say, no monsters in the room. A small number of children have regular nightmares, which may be triggered by stress, changes in their routine or upsetting events. Helping children to talk about how they are feeling is helpful, and comforters and nightlights provide extra reassurance.

Night terrors. Unlike nightmares, which happen late at night, night terrors tend to occur an hour or two after the child has gone to sleep. They can be scary to witness because the child's eyes are open but he or she appears to be terrified. Don't try to wake your child, but stay with him or her. The child will settle when the dream ends, and won't remember it the next day. Night terrors can be connected with lack of sleep, so making bedtime earlier may help. Factors such as stress and sleeping in a strange environment can also trigger them.

Sleepwalking. Sleepwalking is very common in children. They usually do it an hour or two after going to bed. Don't wake a child who is sleepwalking, but make sure he or

Make sure your child has calmed down before you begin the bedtime routine. If he or she is involved in a game, give a warning that bath time is in five minutes.

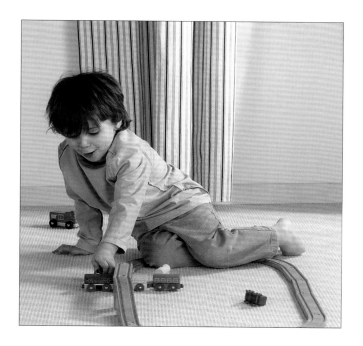

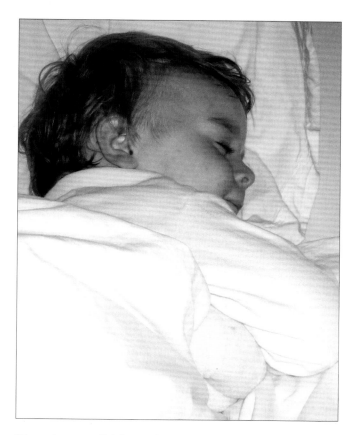

Sleep is essential for maintaining physical and mental health, so it is important to teach your child good sleeping habits from an early age.

she cannot come to any harm. Sleepwalking is associated with lack of sleep.

Snoring. Most children snore from time to time, and around 10 per cent snore often. If your child snores regularly and loudly, and also seems to have difficulty breathing, he or she could have sleep apnoea. In this condition, the child momentarily stops breathing and starts suddenly with a gasp or snort. This stop-start breathing affects sleep, so your child may be cranky or tired during the day. If you think your child may have sleep apnoea, see your doctor for a referral to a sleep specialist.

YOUR CHILD'S BEDROOM

It will help your child to sleep well if he or she sees their bedroom as a pleasant place to be, so don't use it as a place to send them as punishment. A nicely decorated room that is kept reasonably tidy and clean is naturally appealing, and you can choose an attractive bedcover that your child will like – or you can let him or her choose it. Keep a selection of toys and books within reach of the bed, so that he or she can amuse himself when he wakes up. A light that he or she can switch on from the security of the bed can help a feeling of security. If he or she is scared of the dark or has nightmares, then try leaving a dim nightlight on. He or she may have a special soft toy or comfort object that you can suggest they sleep with.

Physical and mental development

Three year olds have mastered the basic physical skills: they can walk, run, jump and climb easily. But can still be clumsy and uncoordinated. Over the next year or two, their balance will improve to the extent that they can walk along a low wall without falling off it. They'll also learn to hop (some time around their fourth birthday), but skipping – a complicated movement – will take longer to master. They may learn to ride a bike if given lots of help.

The upper body gets much stronger and children learn to pull themselves up by their hands. If they are confident in the water, they may learn to swim. It's a good idea to get your child into the habit of having lots of physical activity at an early age, so get out to the park and play plenty of games, chase and so on.

Hand and finger control become more precise: by the age of four, children tend to grasp a pen between thumb and finger as adults do. This allows them to draw with much greater accuracy: a four year old can usually copy simple geometric shapes and colour inside the lines. Everyday tasks such as getting dressed, putting on shoes and washing the face and hands will be achieved more easily, though adult help is often needed. Some children are able to clean their own teeth at four or five, but still need supervision.

Developmental reviews (well-child visits) will check hearing, eyesight and progress, and give you an opportunity to discuss your child's daily life.

Many children learn to recognize numbers from quite a young age and may like to play simple number-recognition games such as dominoes.

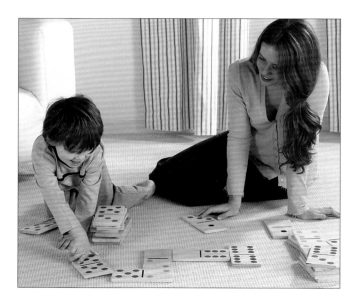

WATCHING TELEVISION
Children over the age of three can benefit from watching some television: research by the American Academy of Pediatrics found that children who watched educational television actually did better in some maths and language tests. But too much television will stop them learning through more active play, so limit your child to an hour's viewing a day, of children's videos or educational programmes.

MENTAL PROGRESS
Preschool children gradually gain much better recall of recent events. Their sense of time is also developing, and their new ability to think about future events means that they can start to plan ahead.

Language develops rapidly now and most young children enjoy learning new words. Your conversations will get more interesting and you'll notice that your child starts to use adjectives and adverbs as well as nouns and verbs. He or she will enjoy all sorts of language play: made-up words, silly songs, jokes, rhymes and stories.

Your child can now express curiosity about the world in language, so prepare to be bombarded with questions. "Why?" is the familiar cry of the preschool child. Answer these questions as simply as you can. Sometimes children ask why? to continue the conversation rather than because they want a specific answer. Encourage your child to frame a genuine query in a whole sentence.

TEACHING NUMBERS AND LETTERS
You don't need to teach your preschool child to read or do sums, but it is helpful to get him or her familiar with letters and numbers. Show your child the letters that make up his or her name: stick magnetic letters or numbers on the fridge. Help your child learn about numbers by pointing out that he or she is playing with two teddies, but only one doll, for example; look at house and bus numbers when you are out and about.

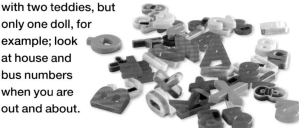

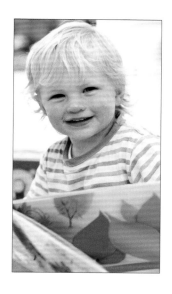

Left: If books are a part of a baby's life right from the early months, it is likely that your developing toddler will entertain himself or herself by looking at the pictures in books, as well as asking you to read the story.

Right: At first, children paint for the fun of it, then they give their art a label. Finally they draw something specific.

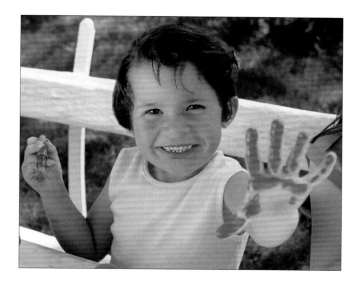

TOYS AND GAMES

Choose toys with long-lasting appeal, which can be used in different ways as your child gets older. Good toys for this age group include dolls, extendable railway sets, small construction blocks, balls, musical instruments and non-toxic felt-tip pens. Avoid buying toy guns: a young boy will almost certainly make his own make-believe weapons using his fingers or sticks, but research shows that having toy guns encourages aggressive play. Preschool children enjoy make-believe. They want to play at being other people, rather than just imitating their parents' actions, as toddlers do. Expect to see your mannerisms exaggerated in games of mummies and daddies and to see some rather sexist divisions of labour.

Three and four year olds can get a lot out of playing board games or simple card games, such as "pairs", in which they have to turn over matching picture cards. These games naturally involve turn-taking, and they also are a good way to introduce the concept of winning and losing. But losing is hard for most children, so it is good to let them win most of the time.

ENJOYING BOOKS AND MUSIC

Your child will get a lot out of story books: look out for books with detailed illustrations that offer more scope for discussion. It's also worth getting a couple of illustrated children's reference books: you are unlikely to be able to answer all the questions that your child has about the world, and it is good for children to see that books offer exciting information they want to know about.

Have fun with music: there's evidence to suggest that active music-making can help with language and mathematical ability, concentration and memory. Sing together (songs that involve movement are particularly good), get your child a musical instrument such as a keyboard, toy piano or xylophone, dance together (a child will love to stand on your feet and hold your hands while you dance), and look for a dance or creative movement class for under-fives in your area. Play recordings at home and seek out live music you can enjoy for short periods.

Your child is now old enough to do some simple cooking, which offers real-life practice in weighing, measuring and pouring.

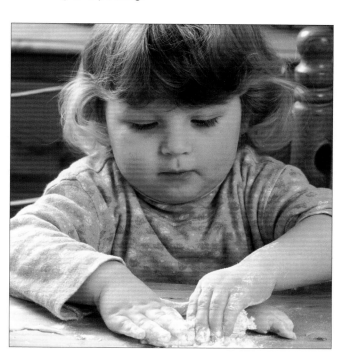

HOW CHILDREN DRAW PEOPLE

Children's representations of the human figure all follow the same progressive pattern. At first, children will draw a circle for the head with two vertical lines representing legs. They may add dots for eyes and marks for the mouth and nose. By four, a torso is usually present and the figure may have arms. By five, the figure has a trunk, arms have hands, legs have feet, and there may be clothing on the body.

Yoga for children

Yoga is a beautiful discipline that involves using the body in a completely different way to other forms of exercise. Children don't have the focus to practise it as adults do: you can't expect a preschooler to sit quietly for long. But they will get a lot out of a short yoga session that focuses on having fun.

BENEFITS OF YOGA

Children are naturally supple, but they start to stiffen up once they go to school and spend most of the day sitting, then spend lots of time watching television or playing computer games. Yoga helps them to stretch their bodies and maintain flexibility, good posture and muscle strength. It teaches good balance, coordination and natural awareness of the body, which can reduce clumsiness. It is non-competitive but can be challenging, so it can increase children's physical confidence.

Lots of the poses are based on animal movements or other elements of nature. Imagining themselves as different creatures, trees or mountains can help children to become more aware of their environment and more sensitive to it.

Yoga works on the mind as well as the body. It induces a feeling of natural calm and relaxation, and may help your child to sleep better. It also builds the mental focus of children, including those who are hyperactive. It teaches that being quiet can be enjoyable. There are lots

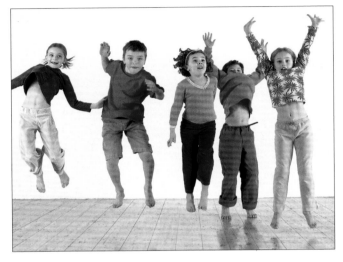

A good yoga class will offer an outlet for youthful exuberance and help children to channel their natural energy in a positive way.

of health benefits, too: yoga encourages good breathing (it may be helpful for those children who have asthma or get chesty), it also helps the digestion and boosts the immune system.

YOGA AT HOME

You don't have to be an expert to teach your child simple yoga poses. Find a quiet area of the home (or go outside), clear away clutter, which can be distracting, and make sure you are both able to stretch out safely. Wear comfortable clothing that doesn't restrict your movements, and have bare feet.

Do a quick warm-up by running on the spot or doing some star jumps to help your child release excess energy. Then try some of these poses: keep the atmosphere playful and move quite quickly from one posture to the next to keep your child interested. Getting your child to make noises (such as barking like a dog) or to imagine what each pose is based on will help him or her to maintain the poses for longer. Try to end the session with a few moments' rest.

CHILDREN'S YOGA CLASSES

A good yoga teacher for children will use the classic postures as the basis for games or to create a magical story: children may swim like fishes or roar like lions. Look for an atmosphere that is creative and dynamic. Some classes take children from the age of two, but most are for the over-threes.

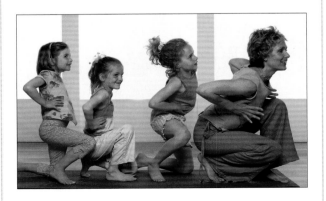

CAUTION

Don't get children doing headstands or shoulderstands – their neck muscles are not strong enough. Never push a child into a posture, or you could cause damage.

Cat stretch

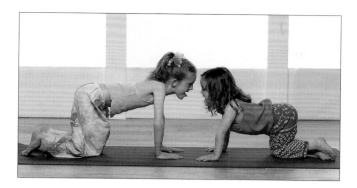

Go on to all fours, on your hands and knees; you are going to be cat who has just woken up. Stretch like a cat – let your head drop down and arch your back and stre-e-e-tch. Now bring your head up, let your back drop down and miaow, miaow, miaow. Do both again. Walk around the room being cats.

Dog pose

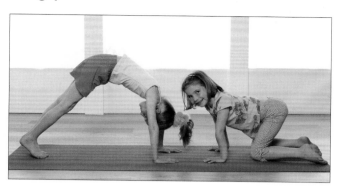

Get on to your hands and knees. Then go on to your toes and straighten your legs: you are a dog stretching after a sleep. Push your hands and your toes into the floor and stre-e-e-tch. Now imagine you see a tiny mouse under your nose: bark to shoo it away. Thank goodness, you can stretch again. Oh-oh, here comes the mouse again...

Roar like a lion

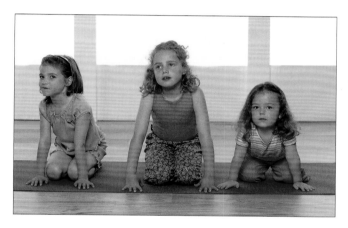

1 Kneel on the floor with your legs together, then sit back, with your hands on the floor in front of you.

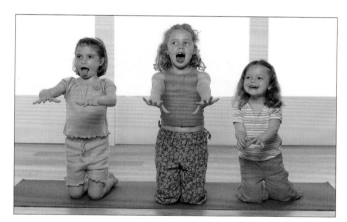

2 Get ready to be a scary lion. Kneel up, stick your tongue out and roar... "Raaaah!" Hold out those sharp claws.

Bridge

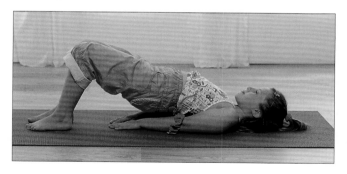

Lie on your back with your arms by your sides. Now bend your knees and bring your heels up to your bottom. Keep your feet and knees apart. Lift up your bottom and turn your body into a bridge: you've got to be really strong so that all the people can walk over you. Keep your bottom up: let the ships sail underneath you. Lower your bridge and repeat a couple more times.

Give yourself a cuddle

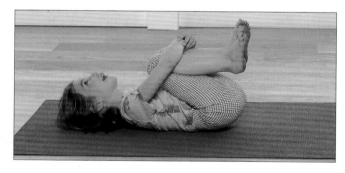

Lie on your back, bend your knees so that you can put your feet flat on the floor. Now bring up your knees so you can hug them. Give them a squeeze – bring them right to your chest: give yourself a lovely cuddle, mmmmmmm. Now try rocking from side to side, like you are a little turtle on its back: ooh this is comfy. Now stretch out your legs again and sl-ee-eeee-p.

Encouraging good behaviour

Small children don't have any real sense of what is right and what is wrong. But they do have a desire to please their parents or carers and they understand that older people have authority over them. You can channel your child's instinct to please you into good behaviour in the following ways.

Set a good example. Children love to imitate, and they naturally think that what you do is right. So you must set an example of good behaviour yourself: if you want your child to speak politely to others, you must do so too; if you don't want your child to shout or hit out at others, don't shout at or hit your child.

Encourage a level of responsibility. Give your child opportunities to help you: wiping up the drink he or she has spilled, fetching your bag when you are going out.

Acknowledge good behaviour. Show that you are pleased when your child is doing things that you approve of, such as giving another child some of his or her apple slices, or playing nicely with toys.

Disapprove of bad behaviour. When your child does something you dislike, say so. Keep it simple: "You kicked Ellie. Kicking is wrong because it hurts people." Talk about the behaviour as being wrong, rather than the child being "naughty" or "bad". Don't unintentionally "reward" bad behaviour by giving your child extra attention because of it.

BEHAVIOUR AND DIET

Lots of parents see a link between certain foods and their child's behaviour. Fizzy drinks (soda), processed foods and lots of sugar can all have a negative impact, while regular meals and healthy snacks help to regulate a child's blood sugar levels and moods. Fish oils have also been shown to have a beneficial effect on behaviour: a children's fish-oil supplement may be worth considering.

Be fair. Give your child the opportunity to learn what is unacceptable. A small child may be confused if you tell him or her off for, say, drawing on the walls when in the child's eyes it is no different from the perfectly permissible business of scribbling on an old newspaper. What is more, small children naturally believe that the naughtiness of a given action is related to the enormity of the consequences, rather than to the intention to do harm. So you need to make a distinction between deliberate acts (such as hitting others) and accidental ones (such as knocking over a vase). It will take time for this to sink in, so be patient, forgiving, consistent and persistent.

Stay in control. If you get angry, or shout at or smack your child, you have lost control. Your child may do what

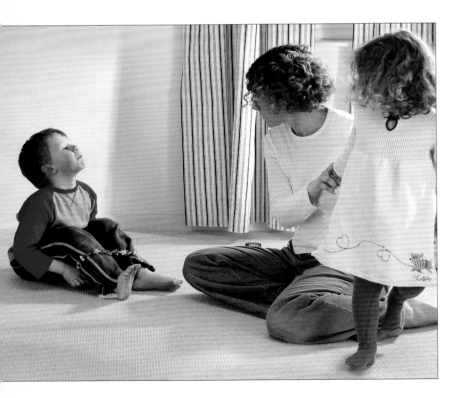

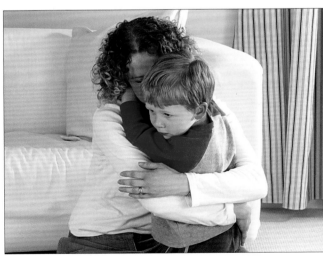

If there has been a dispute between two children, make sure that after you have mediated and reprimanded there is forgiveness. Make space and time for apologies and making up. Don't stay angry for too long on principle. Once you have made your point let everyone recover from it and move on.

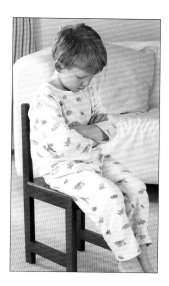

Time out is a great technique to help your child learn that their negative behaviour will have negative consequences. It isn't a punishment so much as a chance for your child to calm down and reflect on his or her actions.

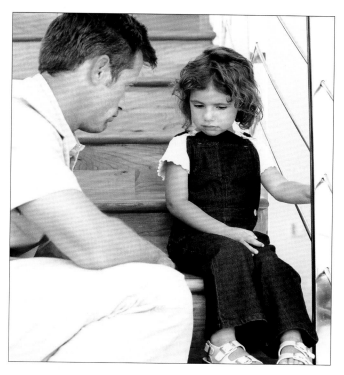

If you need to reprimand your child, squat down so that you are at the child's level. Say the behaviour is wrong in a calm but firm voice. Don't shout from on high.

you say from fear but this won't help him or her to learn how to behave well. If you think you are going to lose your temper, tell your child that you are getting angry and are leaving the room to calm down. And if you do lose it (as almost all parents do at some time), it's best to acknowledge the fact and apologize.

FEELING THE CONSEQUENCES

A good way to help preschool children develop better behaviour is to let them feel the consequences of their actions. If your child refuses to eat dinner, for example, you could try going out and not taking snacks with you. Once a child experiences the consequence of refusing food – being hungry – he or she may be more inclined to eat dinner next time.

The consequence has to be linked to the behaviour, and must be proportionate to it. So, you might let your child go out without food, but you won't keep him or her

out for hours. Keep your attitude calm and sympathetic – "What a shame you are hungry, that's probably because you didn't eat your dinner" will drive the message home.

THE TIME-OUT METHOD

If your child is doing something that he or she knows is wrong, then the time-out method can be very helpful. It involves putting the child in a safe place until he or she is ready to behave reasonably. To make it work, you have to observe all the steps, in the order given here. In particular, don't miss out the warning stage.

1 Tell your child not to do something: "Peter, stop kicking the table." If the behaviour continues, say, "Peter, I told you to stop kicking the table. You either stop now or go for some time out."

2 If the child does it again, remove him or her to your safe place: this could be a room with a door you can shut, the bottom stair or a quiet corner of the house. Tell the child he or she is to sit there until ready to behave nicely. Alternatively, tell your child to sit there for a set period – one minute for each year of age is a good formula: a four-year-old should stay for four minutes, and so on.

3 When your child comes out or time is up, ask him or her to say sorry. If the child does this, have a hug and make up. If the child refuses, put him or her back into the time-out spot and repeat until you get an apology.

5 Some children run out of the safe place immediately. Simply lead your child back again quietly and calmly, as often as it takes. Don't lose your cool.

LYING AND STEALING

Telling lies is very common in the over-threes: it is a sign of their growing imaginations and a normal developmental stage. Young children make up lots of fantastic stories because they have difficulty distinguishing between fact and fiction. They may also lie to get themselves out of trouble. It will help your child to be honest if you are understanding about naughtiness and don't overreact to misdemeanours or accidents.

Similarly, you may find that your child squirrels away things that don't belong to him or her. Young children have only a vague idea about possessions, so your child doesn't understand why this is wrong. Calmly explaining that we don't take things from other people because it makes them sad will help. In older children, stealing can sometimes be a sign that the child feels he or she is lacking attention or love.

Sociability in the wider world

Children gradually develop empathy from the age of about three: they realize that other people not only have feelings but may react or feel differently than they would do themselves in the same situations. Once they have made this intellectual leap, they are able to make proper friendships and their social skills improve. With your help, your child will start to show behaviour that is more cooperative and thoughtful.

ENCOURAGING FRIENDSHIPS

Friends will become increasingly important to your child from now on. Going to nursery or playgroup, or having regular playtimes with other children, will give your child lots of opportunities to interact with other children.

Teach your child to take turns and not to snatch things from another child. If small children are playing a game that involves turn-taking, an adult should supervise.

Your child needs to be able to voice his or her needs honestly. Children with good language skills naturally find it easier to manage in group situations, so set aside time each day to talk to your child without interruptions. Encourage a shy child to speak loudly and clearly. When with other children, try to get him or her to come up with solutions for conflict. Say something like, "You and Mike both want the toy and you are getting cross. How can we make both you and Mike happy?" Suggest taking turns, playing together, and other possible solutions if your child isn't able to come up with any.

Teach your child to stand up for himself or herself when necessary. Young children need to know that they can say "No" to another child or refuse to give up a toy if someone else tries to grab it. Practise ways of doing this in a reasonable way. But don't let your child think he or she has to do this all alone: children need to know that they can ask an adult for help. Help your child feel secure in a new situation, such as preschool nursery, by introducing him or her to it gradually and make sure he or she knows which adult is in charge in group situations.

Encourage empathy – helping children to recognize other people's feelings spurs them to be kind and cooperative. So say, "If you take Joey's tractor, he'll be sad." But alongside this encouragement to behave well, let your child know that you understand that doing things for other people can be difficult.

BOOSTING SELF-ESTEEM

Children who feel good about themselves naturally do well in group situations and will also cope better with the challenges of school. Here are some ways to boost self-esteem in your child.

- Talk to your child about what is special about him or her.
- Point out things that your child is good at.
- Don't tease your child about things he or she finds difficult; be sympathetic.
- Encourage your child to talk about his or her emotions.
- Make sure your child knows that he or she is loved even when behaving badly: it is the behaviour that you don't like, not the child.
- Show your child that his or her opinions are important by listening and acknowledging what he or she says (even if you don't do what the child wants).
- Give your child some sense of mastery over a situation by letting him or her make simple choices between two or three equally satisfactory options.

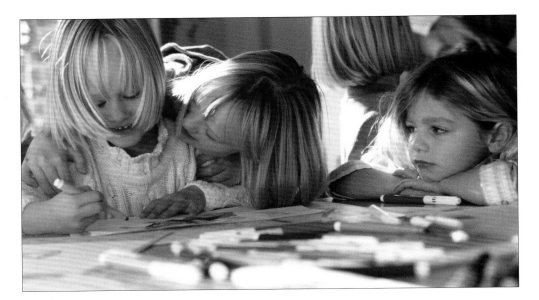

If you feel your child is struggling to integrate at nursery, talk to him or her about ways to start an interaction with someone else: try telling a story about another child who wants to join in a game, and get your child to suggest some strategies.

CHOOSING A NURSERY

Some group care can be beneficial for children over the age of three because it gives them the opportunity to develop good social skills before they go to school. It also sets up a positive pattern for learning. An American study that followed children through their early school years found that those who received high-quality nursery care did better in language and maths. They also tended to have better concentration, were more sociable and demonstrated less problem behaviour. If you are choosing a nursery for your child, look for one where:

• the atmosphere is friendly and happy
• the nursery is clean and well-organized
• the children seem to be enjoying their activities
• the children seem happy to make requests from staff
• the staff speak warmly about and to their charges
• the majority of staff are trained
• the facilities and activities on offer suit your child's personality – for example, for a very active child, look for a nursery with a soft room and outdoor play area.

STARTING NURSERY

If your child has never been to nursery before, it is bound to feel strange at first. It will help your child to cope if he or she is already used to being in groups of children (such as parent-and-toddler groups).

Attend a trial session so that your child can meet the staff and learn where everything is while you are there. Stay in the background as much as possible. If your child seems to be settling happily, then tell him or her you are going out (to visit the shops) and will be back soon. Say goodbye calmly and confidently – it won't help your child cope if he or she can see that you are worried about leaving, and sneaking off without saying you are going will

Learning to manage in a group situation is an essential life skill. Going to preschool can give your child valuable experience of this before he or she goes to school.

MALE ROLE MODELS

Most children are cared for by their mothers, and nursery workers and preschool teachers are also predominantly female. It's important that children spend time playing with their fathers, and that those whose fathers are absent most or all of the time develop strong relationships with other trustworthy male relatives or family friends. This is particularly important for boys. It's also very good for young boys if their fathers read to them and, later on, take an interest in their schoolwork.

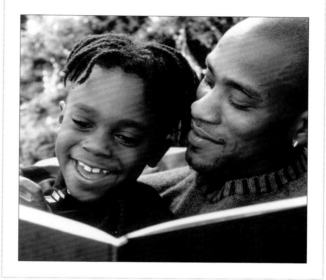

shake your child's confidence. Make a judgment on how long to stay away: err on the side of caution the first time.

Some children need a few trial sessions: gradually increase the length of time you leave the nursery. If your child cries when you leave, call to check whether he or she has settled soon afterwards (most children do). It can be helpful to follow the same "goodbye" and "hello" ritual each day to ease the stress of the transition, and many children like to keep a favourite toy with them.

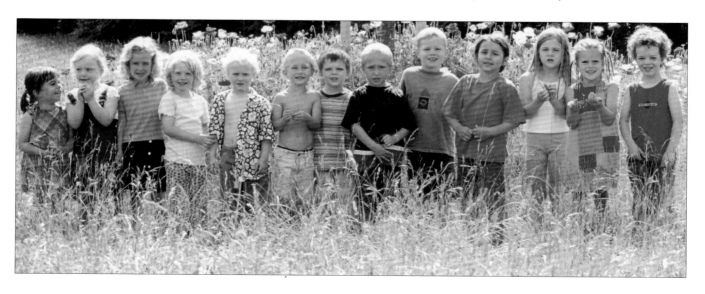

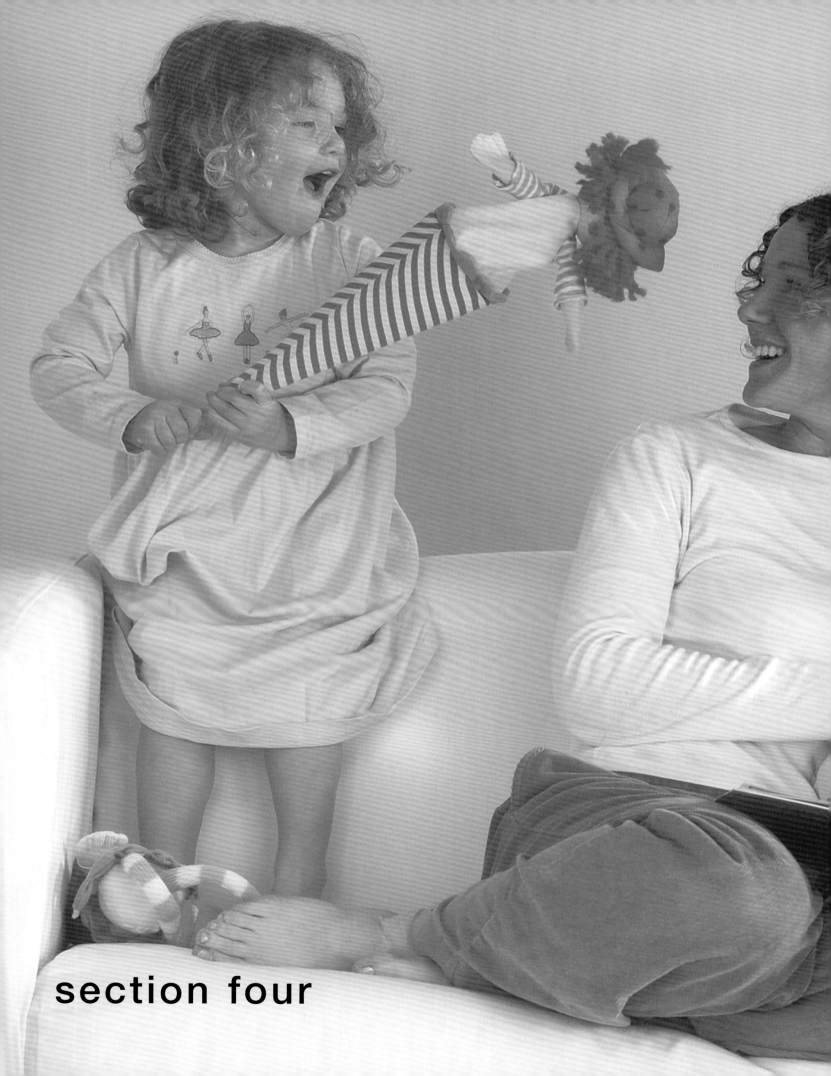

section four

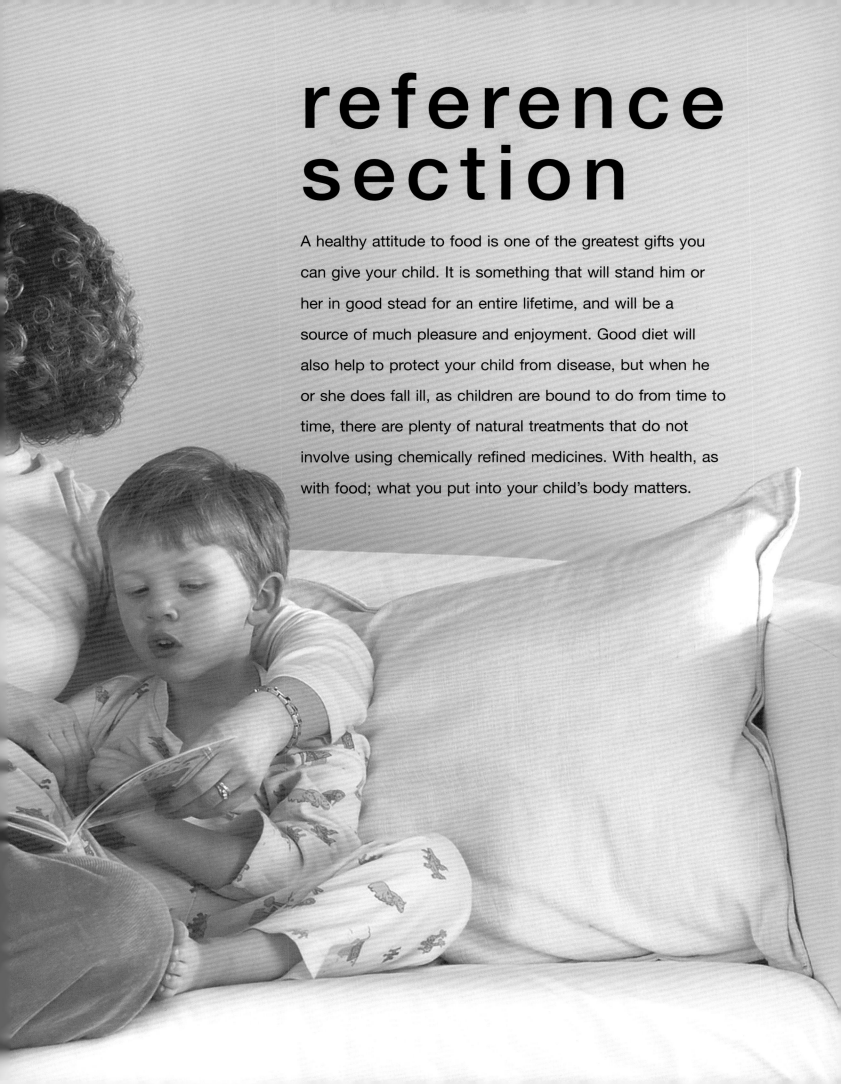

reference section

A healthy attitude to food is one of the greatest gifts you can give your child. It is something that will stand him or her in good stead for an entire lifetime, and will be a source of much pleasure and enjoyment. Good diet will also help to protect your child from disease, but when he or she does fall ill, as children are bound to do from time to time, there are plenty of natural treatments that do not involve using chemically refined medicines. With health, as with food; what you put into your child's body matters.

Health and safety

“ Children need to feel loved and secure in order to develop good mental health, which also contributes to physical well-being. ”

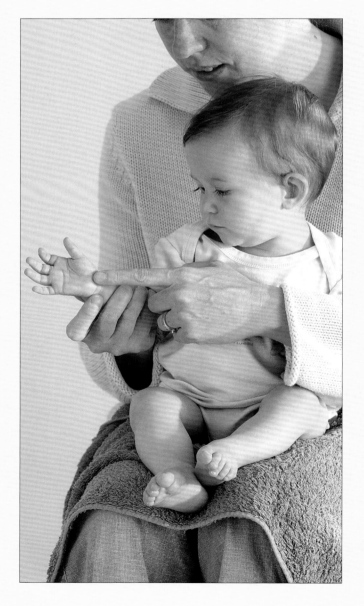

A healthy lifestyle will go a long way towards making your child's immune system strong, so that he or she can fight off bugs and recover from minor ailments quickly.

Give your child a healthy balanced diet of home-cooked food. Using fresh, locally produced, organic produce will minimize the amount of pesticides your child is exposed to and will help to ensure he or she gets as many nutrients as possible. Fresh garlic in the diet is helpful: it has natural antibiotic properties. Encourage your child to drink lots of water. Proper hydration is essential for general well-being, and may help reduce the risk of disease. Filter tap water before giving it to your child if you can.

It's important to facilitate good sleeping habits. Children need a lot more sleep than adults: up to 16 hours for newborns, and around 12 hours for three year olds. And make exercise part of your child's daily life. Most children spend about 90 per cent of their time indoors, so some physical activity outdoors will build muscle strength and get them

Natural remedies such as aromatherapy oils can relieve common symptoms, but check that your child won't react to them by doing a patch test before use.

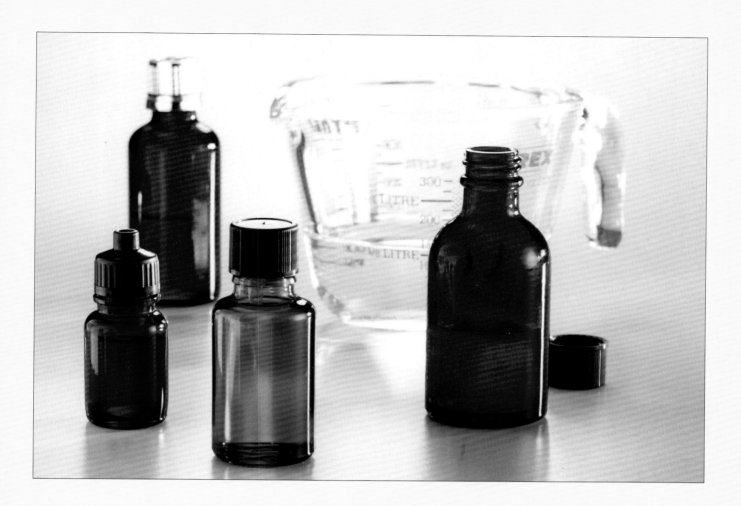

breathing fresh air. Babies benefit from being taken out every day and from spending time on the floor, where they can move their arms and legs freely.

Make your home as healthy an environment as possible, by reducing your use of chemical-laden household products and taking basic safety precautions. Avoid unnecessary risks. Observe basic hygiene when preparing your child's food to prevent stomach upsets, and keep your child away from people with infectious diseases.

Finally, give your child lots of unreserved love and affection. It's known that babies need plenty of physical contact in order to thrive; children, too, need to feel loved, valued and secure in order to develop good mental health, which also contributes to physical well-being.

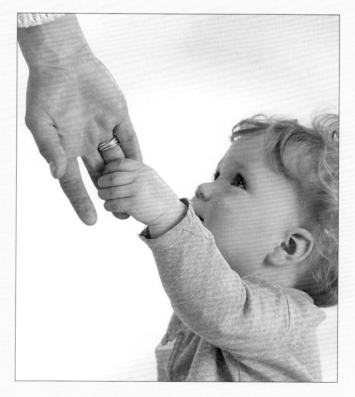

Top: Reducing the amount of noxious chemicals you use in the home is an important aspect of healthy living. For a natural air freshener, try aromatherapy oils.

All parents want to do the best for their children, and an abundance of love and affection lays the foundation for good mental health.

Immunization and supplements

The subject of immunization causes parents a lot of anxiety, but in a sense there is nothing unnatural about it: what you are doing is introducing a small dose of a disease into the body so that the immune system can develop antibodies to it. This is exactly what the body does when it encounters a disease "accidentally", except that with vaccination the body does not go through the dangers and unpleasantness of illness.

There is no doubt that we all have benefited from a widespread vaccination programme: smallpox has been eradicated worldwide, and diseases such as polio and diphtheria are now largely unknown in developed countries. However, there is much debate about the wisdom of vaccinating very young children. Some natural practitioners say that the standard practice of immunizing babies against several diseases at once overloads their immature immune systems and can lead to an increased risk of problems such as asthma, eczema and allergy later on. And parents worry about the possibility of side effects. Controversy over the MMR jab, which was linked to autism in one British study, caused many parents to decide not to give it to their children. This study has been widely discredited and intensive research has not found a link. Generally speaking, the risk of serious side effects from a vaccine is much smaller than the risk from diseases such as measles.

Every parent has to make an individual decision about what is right for a child. There are four options:

Following the standard vaccination programme. This is what the vast majority of doctors recommend.

Delaying vaccinations. Some people prefer to give vaccinations when the child is older, to give the immune system a chance to strengthen. This may make you feel more comfortable, especially if there is a family history

WHEN NOT TO VACCINATE
If your child is ill, you should delay vaccination. Always tell the person giving the vaccination if your child is unwell or is taking medication. Vaccination is not appropriate in the following cases.
• Children who have a high temperature.
• Children who have a weakened immune system.
• Children who have had an allergic reaction to a previous immunization or who are allergic to ingredients used in the vaccine.
• Children who have had fits.

of allergy or allergy-related illnesses. However, your child will obviously not be protected in the meantime.

Having selected vaccinations. Some parents prefer to avoid giving children all-in-one shots, and choose not to vaccinate against certain diseases. It is worth bearing in mind that single-vaccine injections may not have been tested as rigorously as the standard injections.

Not vaccinating. If you feel strongly that vaccination is not right for your child, then you may decide not to do it

VACCINATION AFTER-EFFECTS
Your child may experience some minor side effects after a vaccination: fever, feeling irritable, and redness and soreness in the injection site are common. Call your doctor if his or her temperature goes above 39°C/102°F. Some children have an allergic reaction after the immunization; for this reason, you will asked to wait in the doctor's surgery for a short period after the injection has been given.

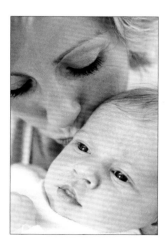

Vaccination jabs are usually given in the thigh. Some children barely notice them; others get upset but can usually be quickly soothed.

Giving children a specially developed multi-vitamin supplement will ensure that they receive the right amount of vitamins and minerals in their diet.

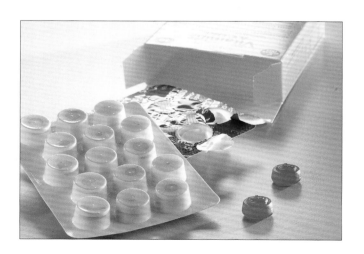

THE IMMUNIZATION PROGRAMME (UK)

2 months	One shot for diphtheria, tetanus, pertussis (whooping cough), haemophilus influenza B (HIB), polio
	One shot for meningitis C
3 months	One shot for diphtheria, tetanus, pertussis, HIB
	One shot for meningitis C
4 months	One shot for diphtheria, tetanus, pertussis, HIB, polio
	One shot for meningitis C
13 months	Measles, mumps and rubella (MMR)
3–5 years	One shot for diphtheria, tetanus, pertussis, HIB
	One shot for MMR

THE IMMUNIZATION PROGRAMME (US)

Birth–2 months	Hepatitis B (1/3)
2 months	Diphtheria, tetanus, pertussis (1/5)
	HIB (1/4)
	Polio (1/4)
	Hepatitis B (2/3)
	Pneumococcal conjugate (PCV7) (1/4)
4 months	Diphtheria, tetanus, pertussis (2/5)
	HIB (2/4)
	Polio (2/4)
	PCV7 (2/4)
6 months	Diphtheria, tetanus, pertussis (3/5)
	HIB (3/4)
	PCV7 (3/4)
12 months	Hepatitis B (3/3)
	Varicella (chickenpox)
	MMR (1/2)
6–23 months	Influenza (annual shot)
15–18 months	HIB (4/4)
	Polio (3/4)
	PCV7 (4/4)
	Diphtheria, tetanus, pertussis (4/5)
2 years +	Hepatitis A, for specific groups only (1/2)
2 1/2 years +	Hepatitis A, for specific groups only (2/2)
2–5 years	Pneumococcal polysaccaride (PPV23), high risk only (1/2)
4–6 years	Diphtheria, tetanus, pertussis (5/5)
	Polio (4/4)
	MMR (2/2)

at all. Ensuring your child is as healthy as possible is vital: a child with a robust immune system is likely to react to infection less severely. Seek advice from a naturopath, nutritional therapist or homeopath on ways to help support your child's immune system.

NUTRITIONAL SUPPLEMENTS FOR CHILDREN

Many nutritionists maintain that you can get all the nutrients you need from a good mixed diet. However, the mineral and vitamin content of fresh produce has dropped in recent years as the soil in which food is grown has become depleted. Giving children a daily multimineral, multivitamin supplement helps to ensure that they get enough health-giving trace elements, such as zinc.

Minerals work in combination inside the body, so it is not a good idea to give single-mineral supplements without professional advice: giving a dose of one mineral could lead to a deficiency in another. Giving high doses of certain vitamins can also be dangerous. If you think that your child needs a particular nutrient, it is best to seek advice from a qualified nutritional therapist or your doctor.

Probiotics work to replenish levels of good bacteria in the gut, which help with digestion. They can be very useful if your child has had a stomach upset or been on antibiotics. Fish oils (omega-3), or a vegetarian equivalent such as flaxseed, can be beneficial if your child will not eat oily fish. A deficiency in omega-3 oils may contribute to behavioural problems (including hyperactivity) and conditions such as eczema and asthma.

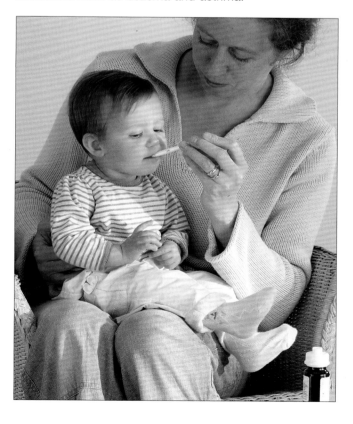

A liquid vitamin formulation, which is gentle on the stomach and suitable for children, can be bought from health food stores; babies can be given vitamin drops.

Natural medication

There's no doubt that modern medicine can be useful when your child is very ill. But it is wise to refrain from giving medication when it is not strictly necessary. Some medicines – such as cough mixtures – interrupt the workings of the immune system. Others, such as antibiotics, tend to be overused to the extent that they can be rendered impotent.

Natural remedies and common-sense measures can be just as good as conventional medicines in soothing certain symptoms and encouraging healing. And complementary therapies can encourage the body's natural ability to mend itself. Parents often feel more comfortable using natural methods to treat their children because they tend to have a gentler action than conventional medicines. But it is essential to take a balanced view. For example, not all natural remedies are gentle: some are toxic if taken in large quantities or are not advisable for babies or young children. And if your child is seriously ill, natural remedies are unlikely to help and urgent medical attention should always be sought.

GIVING MEDICATION

Doctors have different attitudes towards natural remedies and complementary therapies. If possible, find a doctor who is open-minded and try to build a good and respectful relationship so that you can discuss alternative methods. If you know that your doctor generally agrees with a cautious approach to medication, you will also feel more confident about taking advice if he or she urges conventional treatment.

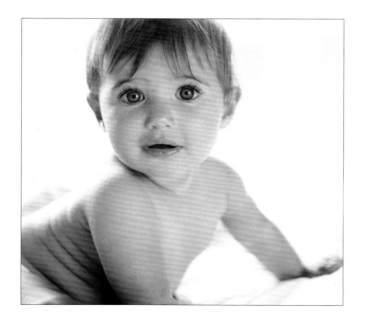

Always ask how a medicine works if you are going to give it to your baby. You should know why you are giving it. Ask whether there are any side effects, so you can be on the lookout for them. If your baby is already on medication – or is taking natural remedies – always mention it to the doctor. Check that the medicine is really necessary in your baby's case. Sometimes a doctor may prescribe medication because that is what most parents expect, not because he or she feels it is essential treatment. Ask whether alternative medicines or approaches could work. Your doctor may be happy for you to delay giving antibiotics, say, for 24 hours to see if your child's condition improves on its own.

When you do give medication, don't forget to give every dose on time. Set an alarm to remind you, and keep a record of every dose you give. Don't stop the medication if your baby starts to feel better. Antibiotics, for example, need to be taken for a set number of days in order to kill the bacteria and prevent infection recurring. On the other hand, sometimes the recommended course is longer than strictly necessary, to allow for a margin of error: check with your doctor whether you could stop a course a day or two earlier.

HIGH TEMPERATURE

The conventional response to a temperature is to give paracetamol (acetaminophen) in order to bring it down again. It is worth considering whether this is necessary, and whether simple natural measures may be sufficient. Fever is part of the body's natural response to infection. It helps to increase the number of disease-fighting white blood cells in the bloodstream, and boosts the level of the antiviral substance interferon. Once the immune system has beaten the infection, the body's thermostat will reset itself and your baby's temperature will return to normal.

A child may have a raised temperature simply because he or she has too many clothes on. Taking off a layer or two and opening a window may be all you need to do to combat a slightly raised temperature. Teething and vaccination may also cause a rise in body temperature.

CAUTION
A very high temperature in a child can cause a fit (febrile convulsion). In the event of a seizure, lay your child on one side and remove anything in his or her mouth. Call an ambulance.

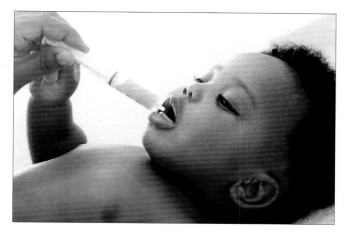

If you need to give a young baby medicine, use a sterilized syringe. Hold it against your baby's bottom lip and depress the plunger slowly so that the medicine doesn't hit the back of the throat hard.

Your child needs a strong immune system in order to cope with all the bugs he or she comes across in daily life. One study found that the more fevers children had in the first year of life, the less likely they were to develop allergies later on. So it may be unwise to give medicines that, in the long term, may interfere with this natural mechanism for dealing with disease.

WHEN TO CALL A DOCTOR
Seek medical advice if a baby under three months has a fever, or if a child has a fever that is over 39°C/102°F, lasts

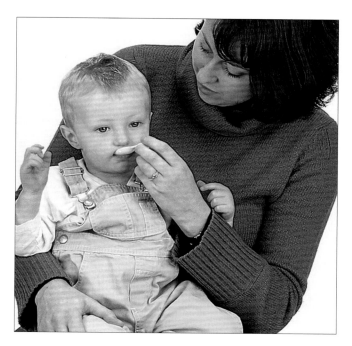

Older babies and children may prefer to take medicine from a spoon rather than syringe; use a proper measuring spoon to be sure of giving the correct dose.

for longer than 24 hours or seems to be steadily increasing. If you do decide to give medication, children's paracetamol (acetaminophen), suitable for babies over two months, is milder than chidren's ibuprofen. Never give a child aspirin, which is linked with the rare and potentially fatal disease Reye's syndrome.

MANAGING FEVER NATURALLY
A fever can be dangerous if it gets very high and a raised temperature can also be uncomfortable. Follow these steps to help to lower a fever naturally.

1 Remove your child's clothing. Turn down any heating and ventilate the room to cool it.

2 Sponge your child down using tepid water; don't use cold water, as this will cause the blood vessels to contract, and so raise the core temperature of the body. Leave the water to evaporate rather than drying with a towel.

3 Dress your child in minimum clothing and, if he or she is in bed, cover with a sheet or light blanket. Give lots of fluid: frequent breastfeeds or extra drinks of cooled, boiled water for a baby; lots of cool drinks for older children. Encourage your child to sip drinks, as gulping could induce vomiting.

4 Check your child's temperature in half an hour, and then every hour or two.

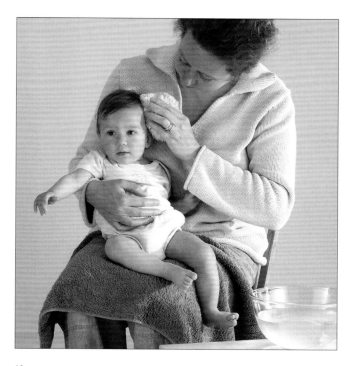

If you are sponging a child down to reduce fever, try adding 2 drops of lavender or chamomile essential oil dissolved in 20ml/4 tsp full-fat milk to the water: these oils reduce fever and encourage sleep.

Complementary therapies for children

Two types of treatment constitute complementary medicine. On the one hand, there are natural remedies that can be used to target particular ailments or symptoms, such as herbal teas and tinctures, essential oils, certain homeopathic pills and herbal creams. On the other hand, there are therapies such as acupuncture, osteopathy and homeopathy.

Natural therapies are holistic – they treat the body as a whole rather than targeting specific parts or symptoms. The body is seen as an organic and complex system in which an ailment may be caused by an imbalance in many parts; conversely many of the body's systems may need to be brought to bear to cure a specific hurt or sickness. For this reason, two children who seem to have the same symptoms may be given different treatments or remedies by the same complementary health practitioner.

There is often an assumption that natural remedies and therapies are always gentle and safe. But any treatment that is effective can be harmful if used incorrectly. Children can be more vulnerable to any side effects than adults, because their bodies are small and still developing. So it is essential to use complementary therapies and natural remedies wisely. Always check unusual symptoms with a doctor first.

USING COMPLEMENTARY THERAPIES SAFELY

When seeking treatment for your child, choose a complementary therapist who is qualified and trained. If possible, find one who specializes in treating children. Ask your doctor or other parents for a recommendation (but don't rely solely on someone else's opinion).

Where possible, pick a practitioner with several years' experience and make sure the therapist you choose is registered with the relevant professional association and that he or she is insured. Follow your instincts. If you do

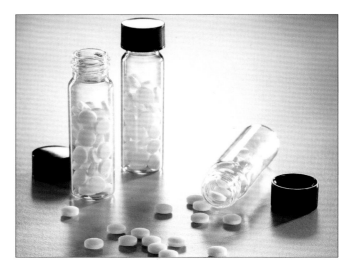

Always check that any natural remedy you buy over the counter is safe for children. If in doubt, or if your child has a chronic condition or severe symptoms, consult the relevant therapist. Check that the dosage is correct for your child.

not feel comfortable with a particular therapist, don't let him or her treat your child. Beware of anyone promising miraculous results.

Tell your doctor about any natural therapies your child is having: some remedies can interfere with conventional medication. Likewise, always tell a complementary therapist about any medication your child is taking. Do not stop your child's medication because he or she is having complementary treatment.

HOMEOPATHY

Homeopathic medicine uses very gentle remedies derived from natural ingredients (plants, minerals and animal substances such as bee venom). The remedies have been

AROMATHERAPY FOR CHILDREN

Age	Suitable oils	Recommended dosage
0–3 months	Do not use essential oils	
3–6 months	Lavender and Roman chamomile	1 drop per 10ml/2 tsp carrier oil or full-fat milk, or use in a vaporizer
6–12 months	Lavender, Roman chamomile, mandarin, neroli, rose	1 drop per 10ml/2 tsp carrier oil or full-fat milk, or use in a vaporizer
12 months–3 years	Lavender, chamomile, tea tree, mandarin, neroli, orange, rose, rosewood	2 drops per 10ml/2 tsp carrier oil or full-fat milk, or use in a vaporizer

diluted many times over, so that only a minuscule part of the active ingredient remains. However, homeopaths say this is enough to stimulate the immune system and encourage the body's natural ability to heal itself. Homeopathy can be used for a wide range of childhood complaints, including teething, sleeplessness, digestive complaints, coughs and colds. Many doctors refer patients to homeopaths, and some are trained in homeopathy in addition to conventional medicine.

Homeopathic remedies are available from health food stores and pharmacists, so home treatment is possible, but homeopathic remedies are prescribed not just on the basis of the symptoms but also according to personality, habits, build and so on. For this reason, it is usually better to consult a qualified homeopath, who can prescribe the correct constitutional remedy for your child.

A homeopath can also advise you on dosage. The paradox at the heart of homeopathy is that the more diluted the remedy the more powerful its effects: a remedy marked 200c is more dilute than one marked 6c. As a general rule, you should stick to remedies of 6c and 30c when treating at home. These are usually given three to six times a day, depending on the severity of the symptoms. Give 30c for no more than three days, 6c for up to a week, but stop when symptoms improve. Give one remedy at a time.

AROMATHERAPY

Essential oils, distilled or pressed from the flowers, leaves, bark or other parts of plants, have therapeutic properties, and can be helpful for skin problems, anxiety and sleeplessness. But they are highly concentrated so only a few are suitable for children. The best ways to use

Natural and conventional approaches to health are not mutually exclusive and are often used side by side.

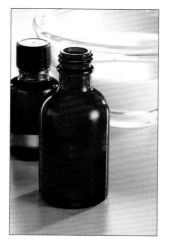

Essential oils should never be applied neat to a child's delicate skin. Always dilute them in either full-fat milk or in a suitable carrier oil before using.

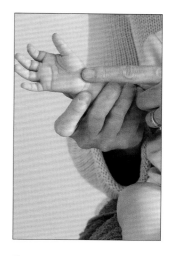

Do a patch test before using an aromatherapy oil in a massage oil: add a drop of the diluted oil to your child's wrist and wait 24 hours to see if any reaction occurs.

them is to dilute them well in a carrier (such as olive oil, sunflower oil or full-fat milk) and then apply the aromatic oil to the skin or mix into the bathwater. Another very gentle way of using them is in a vaporizer.

Always use pure essential oils, preferably those that are made from organically grown plants. Do a patch test on your child before using aromatherapy oils in massage oil: if there is a reaction, it is best to avoid using that essential oil on your child for now. If the skin is fine, that particular oil is safe to use but you will have to test any others in the same way

Lavender and chamomile are very gentle essential oils and can be used on children over three months.

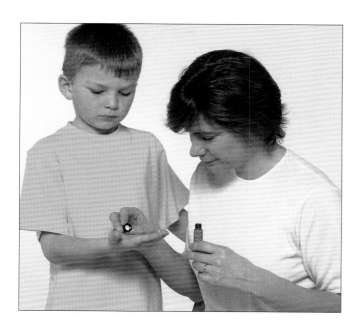

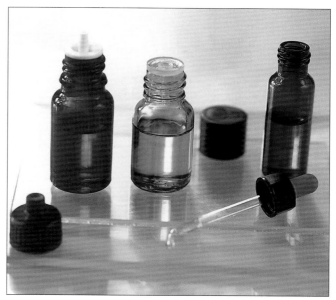

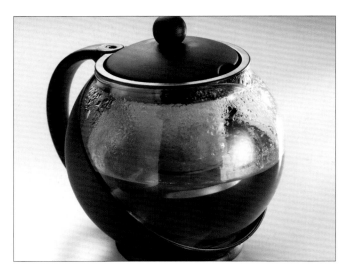

Herbal infusions are a gentle way of giving herbs to a child. The tea should be weak enough to be palatable, you can sweeten it with honey for an older child.

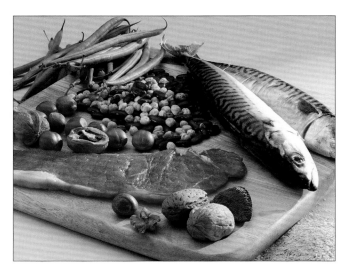

A nutritional therapist can help you to ensure that seemingly healthy food in your child's diet is not the root cause of a lingering health problem.

MEDICAL HERBALISM

Herbal medicine is the oldest form of medicine. Many conventional medicines are based on isolated plant ingredients, but herbalists believe that it is better to use whole parts of the plant – roots, leaves, berries, seeds and so on. The idea is that the many active ingredients in plants work together to promote healing in a gentle and holistic way.

Childhood complaints such as skin problems, asthma, coughs and colds can all be helped with herbal medicine. As with homeopathy, a herbalist will take into account your child's personality and behaviour traits as well as the symptoms when prescribing a remedy.

Herbal remedies come in the form of creams, tinctures, syrups and capsules. Some have well-known effects and can be used in home treatment. But many herbal

remedies can be toxic so it is essential that you do not give one to your child unless you know it to be safe. If your child suffers any ill effects when taking a herbal remedy, stop giving it immediately and contact your herbalist and your doctor.

ACUPUNCTURE OR ACUPRESSURE

These Chinese therapies are based on the idea that well-being depends on the free flow of life energy (chi) through the body. In acupuncture, fine needles are inserted – usually painlessly – into specific points on the body in order to release blockages or quicken a sluggish flow. However, the points can also be stimulated by finger pressure (acupressure), and most acupuncturists would treat children in this way rather than with needles.

The principles that underlie acupuncture are very different to those that inform western medicine, but scientific research has shown it to be highly effective in easing pain and reducing the symptoms of common problems such as constipation, sleeplessness or anxiety. Many doctors are now happy to refer patients to acupuncturists for treatment.

NUTRITIONAL THERAPY

Good diet is fundamental to a healthy life, but particular foods can sometimes be the underlying cause of many childhood complaints: for example, a series of ear infections may be linked to an intolerance of dairy foods. A nutritional therapist will help you to ascertain whether your child is intolerant of particular foods, or deficient in certain nutrients.

You will usually be asked to complete a diet and lifestyle questionnaire before the first appointment. A nutritional therapist may carry out tests, and will come up with an eating plan tailored to your child's particular

---

MAKING A HERBAL INFUSION

To make a herbal tea for a child over one year, put ¼ tsp dried leaves or ⅓ tsp fresh leaves in a cup or small teapot. Pour over 200ml/⅓ pint boiling water and cover. Leave to steep for 10 minutes, then strain. Give a small cupful (about 50ml/2fl oz) to your child.

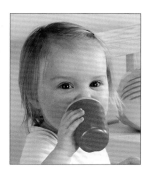

Store the rest in a sterilized screwtop jar in the refrigerator and use within 24 hours. Give no more than three cups a day.

If you want to add the infusion to your child's bath, make ten times the quantity.

NATUROPATHY

Naturopaths use a wide range of natural treatments, including nutritional therapy, herbal remedies and water treatments (hydrotherapy). Some naturopaths may also be trained in homeopathy or osteopathy.

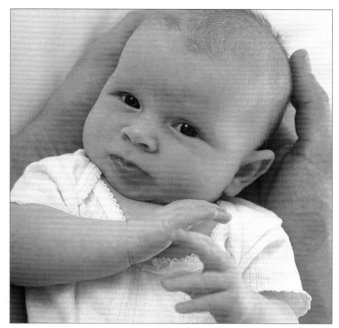

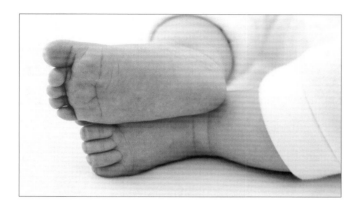

Children can respond well to reflexology, and it is helpful to start when they are young and to have the therapist come to your home so that your child is in a familiar environment.

A cranial osteopath lays his or her hands on a baby's skull and uses featherlight touch to manipulate it. If you have this treatment yourself, you will find that you are barely aware of what the practitioner is doing.

needs. He or she may recommend eliminating certain foods for a while and then re-introducing them to check for intolerances. You will usually have to return for several appointments during this process. You may also be given natural supplements such as grapefruit-seed extract for your child to take.

CRANIAL OSTEOPATHY

Cranial osteopaths believe that many physical health problems can result from tiny misalignments in the bones of the skull. They use very gentle touch to manipulate the bones and surrounding tissues into their correct place. Some also practise cranial-sacral therapy, which involves working on the spine and sacrum as well as the head.

SEEING A PRACTITIONER

A complementary health practitioner should take a full medical history of your baby or child from you before starting any treatment. He or she will also ask about various aspects of your child's daily lifestyle and habits: such as bowel movements, sleep patterns, diet, likes and dislikes, and general behaviour. The treatment should always be gentle, and you should be able to stay with your child throughout. After the treatment, symptoms may occasionally get worse for a day or two before they start to improve. Call the therapist or your doctor if anything unusual occurs that worries you. Most therapists recommend several follow-up treatments.

Cranial osteopathy and cranial-sacral therapy are particularly good for babies, especially those who have had difficult births. A baby's head is naturally compressed as it travels down the birth canal, and then gradually regains its normal shape over the next few days. Cranial osteopaths say that sometimes this process leaves slight distortions in the skull that cause tension in the body and may be a root cause of sleeplessness, colic, wind and other digestive problems in babies. They believe that it can also be the cause of problems such as recurrent ear infections, frequent blocked-up noses and headaches in young children.

Cranial osteopathy and cranial-sacral therapy are widely used on babies and young children. These treatments are very safe in the hands of a qualified practitioner. However, always go to a qualified osteopath for treatment; not all cranial-sacral therapists have had the rigorous training that osteopaths have.

REFLEXOLOGY

Like acupuncture, reflexology works on energy points. It is based on the idea that the body is divided into ten energy zones, which run from head to feet, and that all the parts of the body can be influenced by working on the feet. Practitioners use a variety of gentle massage techniques to stimulate energy points here, and the effect is generally very soothing.

Reflexology can be good for colic, bowel problems and digestive complaints, skin problems, breathing disorders, sleeplessness and hyperactivity.

Natural first aid

All children have tumbles and minor accidents, and you are bound to have to deal with grazed knees, burns and cuts. Natural remedies help speed healing and can also soothe an unhappy child. But don't hesitate to get medical attention if your child has had a bad fall or if you cannot easily treat the injury yourself.

A NATURAL FIRST-AID BOX

These are some of the most useful natural remedies to have to hand.

Aloe vera gel. A herbal remedy for burns and rashes. Aloe vera has natural antiseptic, antibiotic and anti-inflammatory properties. You can also use the fresh sap of an aloe vera leaf.

Arnica. This homeopathic remedy

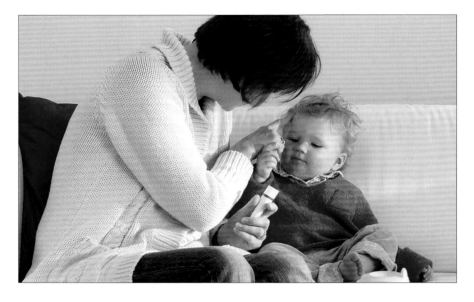

comes in cream and tablet form, and it is worth getting both. The cream is good for bruises; the tablets are also helpful for bruises as well as sprains, shock after an injury, and nosebleeds.

Calendula cream. A natural antifungal and antiseptic cream that fights infection. Calendula is good for minor skin complaints such as burns, blisters and insect bites and stings.

Chamomilla. A homeopathic remedy for teething pain and sleeplessness. Diluted chamomile tea can also be useful, both to sip and for compresses.

Distilled witch hazel. A widely available liquid herbal remedy that is good for bites, stings, bruises and sprains.

Lavender oil. A multipurpose essential oil that has antibacterial and anti-inflammatory qualities; it is good for sleeplessness, minor skin problems and headaches.

Rescue Remedy. This gentle blend of flower essences is great for calming upset children after an accident. Put four drops in water and give to your child to sip.

Most children enjoy having a "magic" cream smoothed over their hurts. Arnica will help to speed healing from bruising.

Roman chamomile oil. A soothing essential oil that helps with sleeplessness, muscle strain and skin problems.

Tea tree oil. An antibacterial and antifungal essential oil that helps to prevent infection.

Honey has been used for centuries as a natural antiseptic, it also has anti-inflammatory qualities, and is a natural antihistamine.

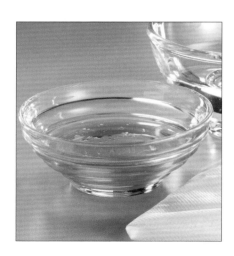

STANDARD FIRST-AID ITEMS

You can buy a first-aid kit from pharmacists, but it is easy to make your own. Get a rigid, closable box and fill it with the following basic items: scissors, safety pins, tweezers, cotton wool, bandages, absorbent dressings, gauze dressings and assorted plasters.

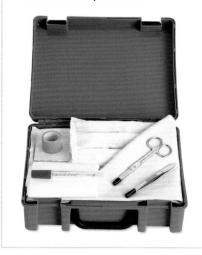

MAKING A LAVENDER COMPRESS

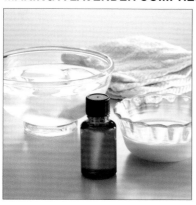

1 Fill a bowl with very cold water and add a handful of ice cubes.
2 Add a few drops of lavender oil diluted in 15ml/1 tbsp full-fat milk.
3 Dip a clean facecloth into the scented water.
4 Squeeze out excess water and apply to the bruised area. Dip the cloth frequently to keep it cold. Apply for a maximum of 10 minutes in total. Reapply every few hours as necessary.

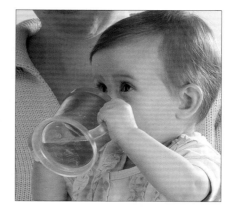

A few drops of Rescue Remedy added to a cup of water can help soothe minor shocks and upsets.

CUTS AND GRAZES

Most cuts are minor wounds that heal quickly but you should always clean the damaged skin to prevent infection. Grazes often occur when the child has slid along the ground after a fall, so they may contain bits of dirt or grit, which will all need to be removed.

What to do. Fill a small bowl with warm water, add a couple of drops of tea tree oil and use to bathe the wound, or simply wash under running water. Press a folded pad of gauze or similar over the area to stop bleeding (don't use cotton wool (cotton balls) as the fibres may stick). Smooth a little Calendula cream over the cleaned area before covering with a plaster. You can also apply honey: ideally use manuka honey, which has a marked antibacterial and anti-inflammatory action.

When to seek help. Seek medical attention if the cut is very deep, there are objects embedded in it that you cannot easily remove, it doesn't stop bleeding when a dressing is applied or if it covers a large area.

BRUISES

When the blood vessels under the skin are damaged, blood seeps out into the surrounding tissues, causing bruising. Some children bruise more easily than others. Including more fruits and vegetables in the diet can help, since these foods are known to contain vitamin C and bioflavonoids, which help to strengthen the walls of blood vessels.

What to do. Apply a cold lavender compress to the skin for a few minutes to reduce swelling. A packet of frozen peas wrapped in a towel will also work well. Don't hold a compress against your child's skin for longer than 10 minutes. To encourage healing, smooth Arnica cream on the bruise three times a day. You can also give an Arnica tablet immediately after the injury to help with the shock, and every two hours during daytime for the next 48 hours.

When to seek help. See a doctor if you suspect a broken bone, or if the pain is worse 24 hours later. Frequent bruising is occasionally due to a problem with blood clotting: see your doctor if your child bruises very easily and unusually.

NOSEBLEEDS

A nosebleed happens when the delicate blood vessels that line the nose are damaged by a blow, frequent nose-blowing or picking, or inflammation caused by a cold. If your child has nosebleeds often, try giving more fruits and vegetables to increase his or her intake of vitamin C and bioflavonoids.

What to do. Get your child to lean forwards (not backwards), and gently pinch the fleshy part just under the bridge of the nose for 10–15 minutes. Release, repeat if bleeding continues. Arnica tablets can be given after a nosebleed, or daily for frequent bleeds. Rescue Remedy helps soothe any shock.

When to seek help. Take your child to hospital if a nosebleed occurs after a blow to the head, or if the bleeding doesn't stop within half an hour. See a doctor if your child has frequent nosebleeds.

A pack of frozen peas wrapped in a muslin makes a makeshift icepack.

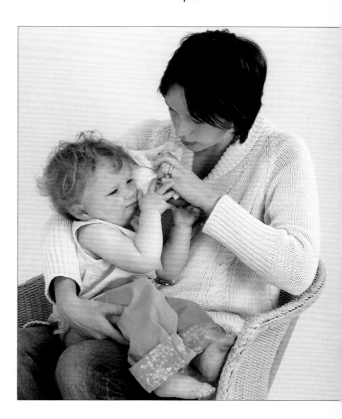

CHOKING

A sudden fit of coughing may mean your child is choking on a piece of food or other small item. The natural instinct to give someone who is choking a slap on the back is a good one, but encourage a child to cough first – this is often enough to remove an obstruction. Check the mouth and remove the obstruction if you can see it: don't feel for it with your fingers – you may damage the throat or push the obstruction in further.

If you do need to slap the child on the back, get him to bend over (or bend him over your knee) and slap between the shoulderblades. If a baby is choking, hold him face-down along your forearm so that the head is facing downwards and use two fingers to tap sharply between the shoulder blades.

All parents worry about choking and it is worth learning how to do chest compressions and life-saving procedures in the very unlikely event that back slaps don't clear the obstruction. You can do a simple first-aid course specifically for babies and children; this usually involves practising the techniques on a life-sized model. Courses are run by voluntary organizations such as St John Ambulance (Red Cross) and are aimed at parents and carers. Often there are child care facilities.

SPRAINS AND STRAINS

A sprain is an injury to the ligaments of a joint, while a strain is an injury to a muscle. It's quite difficult to tell the difference between a strain or sprain and a fracture, especially in young children, whose bones may bend rather than break. If in doubt, seek medical advice.

What to do. Get your child to sit or lie down. Apply a cold lavender or chamomile compress or ice pack for up to 10 minutes. Place a thick wad of cotton wool or other soft pad against the injury and bandage firmly, or put on an elastic bandage to compress. Then elevate the

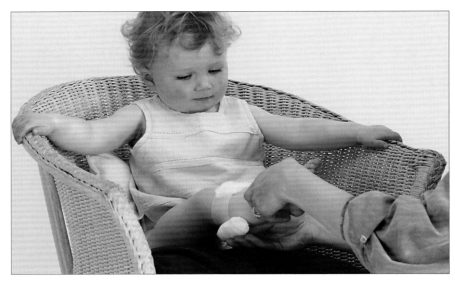

injured part to reduce swelling. Give Arnica for shock and to encourage healing; Rhus tox is another good homeopathic remedy for sprains and strains. Apply Arnica cream or comfrey ointment over the area (only if the skin is unbroken). Rescue Remedy will help soothe any upset.

Caution. Be sure that you do not bandage so tightly that you cut off the circulation. To check, press on an uninjured area of skin below the bandaged area. If it takes more than three seconds for colour to return, your bandage is probably too tight.

When to seek help. Get medical advice if you suspect a fracture or if the pain doesn't subside at all after the treatment.

WASP AND BEE STINGS

These stings can be very painful.
What to do. If you can see a sting in

Arnica cream and tablets help to speed healing for a strain or sprain.

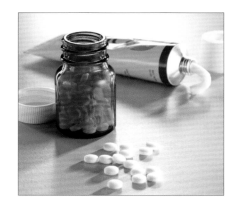

If you need to bandage a sprain, use a thick wad of gauze or cotton wool to cushion the wound first.

your child's skin, remove it carefully. Put a little iced water in a bowl and add a few drops of lavender or tea tree oil diluted in 15ml/1 tbsp full-fat milk. Dip cotton wool in the water and apply to the area every 10 minutes or so until the pain subsides. Other easily available natural remedies for bee stings include witch hazel, bicarbonate of soda or crushed garlic; wasp stings can be helped by applying witch hazel, cider vinegar or lemon juice. The homeopathic remedy Apis can be given to help with the after-effects of a sting.

When to seek help. If your child is allergic to wasp or bee stings, he or she may go into anaphylactic shock, needing urgent medical attention.

INSECT BITES

Gnat, ant or mosquito bites can be very itchy.
What to do. Witch hazel is a good treatment for insect bites. Rescue Remedy can be applied to the bite. Mosquito bites can be soothed with cider vinegar or lemon juice.
Prevention. Before dusk, when mosquitoes are most active, cover up your child in clothes of closely woven, lightly coloured fabric. You can get eucalyptus-based repellents

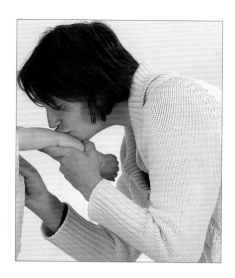

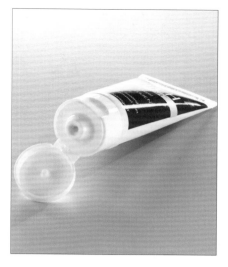

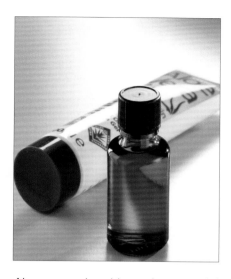

Remove a bee sting by scraping it off with a credit card or by pressing your thumb into the neighbouring skin and pushing it sideways. Don't try to pull it out with tweezers: this can squeeze any poison left in the sting into your child's skin. Suck out any poison before treating.

suitable for children from health food stores. Burning citronella oil in a vaporizer or using citronella candles is also helpful.

BURNS
Minor (first-degree) burns affect only the top layer of skin, which reddens but does not blister or swell. They can be treated at home.

What to do. Place the burned area under cold, running water for 10 minutes. Apply aloe vera gel, Calendula cream, or lavender oil

Acidic lemon juice or cider vinegar can take the sting out of a mosquito bite.

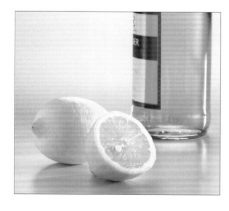

You can get witchhazel in the traditional tincture form or in handy tubes of gel.

diluted in full-fat milk to ease pain and speed healing. Give Rescue Remedy or Arnica for the shock.

When to seek help. If the burn is larger than the child's palm or if the pain gets worse after treatment, seek immediate medical advice. If the skin is moist, swollen or blistered, the burn may have reached underlying areas of skin (second-degree burn); if the child feels no pain after a burn but the area is red, white, yellow or darkened, the nerves may be damaged (third-degree burn). Seek urgent medical advice.

SUNBURN
It's important to protect your child's delicate skin from the sun. If it gets too much sunlight, the skin will be red, hot and sore.

What to do. Bathe the skin in cool water to which you have added a couple of drops of lavender oil diluted in full-fat milk. Add a few drops of lavender oil to aloe vera gel and smooth over the affected area. The homeopathic remedy Sol is good for mild sunburn.

When to seek help. Seek immediate medical advice if the skin has blistered, or if your child develops a high temperature (39°C/102°F or above).

Aloe vera gel and lavender essential oil are two natural remedies for minor burns.

SUNSTROKE
A sunburned child may also develop heatstroke, with a raised temperature, headache, nausea, dizziness and general aches.

What to do. Cool your child down by sponging with tepid water. Give plenty of cool drinks to sip: water, diluted fruit juice or a rehydration drink (available from pharmacists). The homeopathic remedies Sol or Belladonna may be given.

When to seek help. Get immediate medical help if your child's temperature is very high (39°C/102°F).

FOREIGN OBJECTS IN THE EYE
Children can easily rub grit or other irritants into their eyes.

What to do. If you can see a piece of grit in your child's eye, get the child to put his or her head on one side with the affected side uppermost. Holding the eyelids open with your fingers, very slowly pour tepid water into the upper corner of the eye so that water covers the whole eye. If the grit doesn't move, try lifting it off with the corner of a damp handkerchief.

When to seek help. Seek immediate medical attention if something is stuck to the surface of the eye or embedded in it.

When your baby is sick

Babies can't tell you when they are sick, but as a parent you quickly become adept at reading the early signs. The first hint of illness is usually clinginess: your baby may want to be held all the time. This is a very natural response: the baby knows that something is wrong and wants you to take care of him or her. Babies are usually listless when they are ill: yours may be content to lie quietly in your arms and may be needing to sleep more than usual.

Other signs of illness include:

Looking unwell. A sick baby usually looks poorly, with a pathetic expression and dull eyes.

Reduced appetite. Sick babies tend to feed a lot less than normal: this won't harm your baby so long as he or she is taking enough fluid to prevent dehydration.

Irritability. Your baby may cry more than usual or in an unusual way. This can be a sign of pain.

Fever. Illness usually (but not always) goes hand-in-hand with a raised temperature, which causes babies to breathe more quickly than usual.

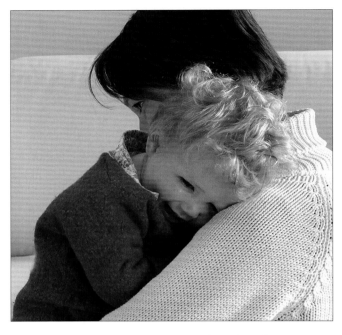

An unusual clinginess may be the first sign that your baby is ill. He or she instinctively knows that he needs to stay close to you.

WHEN TO SEEK HELP

It can be difficult to assess a baby's condition. Similar symptoms occur in serious and non-serious illnesses, and although symptoms are often more severe in a very sick baby, this is not always the case. It is best always to seek medical advice if you think your baby is ill, is refusing feeds or has unusual symptoms. Always see a doctor if a baby under three months has a fever.

Seek immediate medical help if your baby:

• has a seizure (fit)

• is limp and seems unaware of your presence

• is unusually drowsy and hard to wake up

• seems to be getting weaker or sicker by the hour

• is breathing very fast or noisily, or with difficulty, or if the skin between the ribs is sucked in as he or she breathes

• has a temperature over 39°C/102°F, especially if there is also a rash

• turns blue or becomes very pale, blotchy or ashen (if your baby is dark-skinned, check the palms)

• has a bulging or sunken fontanelle (the soft spot on the top of the head)

• has a purplish-red rash that doesn't disappear when you press a glass to it.

Rash. Skin rashes are a symptom of many illnesses and other conditions such as food sensitivity. Occasionally, they may have a serious cause, so it is essential to have an unexplained rash checked by a medical practitioner.

Diarrhoea and vomiting. Babies can be sick when they have an ear, chest or throat infection, and they may pass loose, smelly stools when they have a viral infection. Vomiting and diarrhoea occurring together usually indicate food poisoning or gastroenteritis.

TAKING YOUR BABY'S TEMPERATURE

A normal body temperature is 37°C/98.6°F, when taken by mouth. But it varies slightly depending on the time of day: a temperature taken in the morning will usually be slightly lower than one taken in the afternoon.

Poorly children need lots of fluids to prevent dehydration. A refreshing squeeze of lemon adds a little natural antiseptic to the drink.

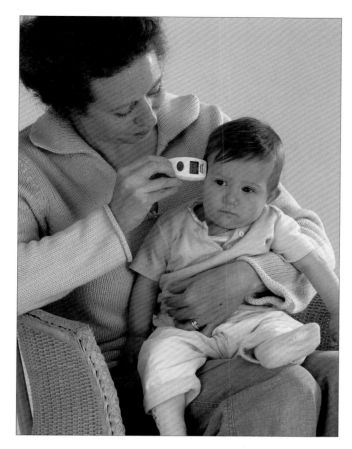

A digital thermometer gives you an accurate reading of your child's temperature in an instant without your having to disturb him or her.

You can often tell that your child has a temperature simply by feeling the forehead. But it is best to get an accurate reading using a thermometer. Get a digital one that bleeps when an accurate reading has been taken: glass thermometers contain mercury, which is highly toxic if released into the atmosphere.

Under the arm. This is an easy way to take a baby's temperature. A normal temperature here is 36.4°C/ 97.4°F; anything over 37°C/98.6°F is a fever. Put your baby on your lap, place the thermometer under his or her arm and hold the arm against the baby's body to keep it in place.

Ear sensor. A digital ear thermometer takes a reading by measuring heat in the ear canal. It only takes a second and is not intrusive, but it is expensive.

Indicator strips. An indicator strip gives you the temperature of your baby's skin – not the body – so it is not an accurate measure.

CARING FOR A POORLY BABY

Sleep is a wonderful cure-all, and babies are naturally inclined to sleep more when poorly. But your baby

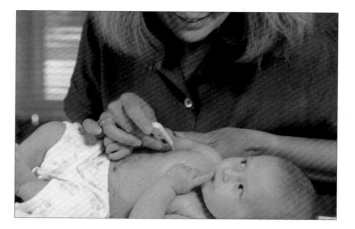

Using a digital thermometer under the arm is a safe and accurate method of reading your child's temperature.

probably won't want to be far from you. Be patient and keep the baby in your arms as much as possible: let the baby doze on you if that is what he or she needs. If your baby normally sleeps in a different room to you, then it is often a good idea to move the cot back in to your room so that you can monitor his or her condition more easily. Alternatively, sleep in the baby's room for a night or two.

Take steps to manage any fever and give frequent fluids to prevent dehydration: fever, diarrhoea, vomiting, coughing, crying or loss of appetite can all make your baby dehydrated. It's best to give fluids in small amounts to prevent your baby from vomiting it back up again. If you are breastfeeding, nurse often. Otherwise, give cooled, boiled water in addition to feeds (unless otherwise advised). If your baby is over six months, you can add a squeeze of lemon juice to the water – it has naturally antiseptic properties.

Don't feel that you have to keep your baby indoors: fresh air can be beneficial even if with a fever. Wrap the baby up well and go out for short periods.

Let a poorly child sleep as much as he or she needs: rest is one of the best natural medicines we have.

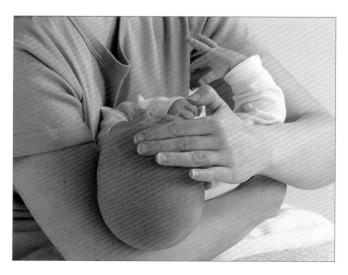

When your child is sick

As your child gets older, it becomes easier to assess what is wrong: now he or she can point to a sore throat, or tell you exactly where it hurts or how they feel. You will still have to rely on the outward signs of illness, too, however. If your child is unusually irritable, not interested in eating or suddenly drinking more than usual, something may be wrong.

You will probably have a good sense of how poorly your child is. Don't hesitate to contact your doctor if you think the child may be seriously ill or if you are not sure what is wrong. If you think the illness may be infectious, tell the reception staff who can arrange for you to sit away from other patients.

CARING FOR A POORLY CHILD

Rest is the best way of managing most illness. If your child doesn't want to stay in bed, then let him or her sit with you: read stories, do jigsaws or simply let the child nap on the sofa. Put light, comfortable clothing on your child: pyjamas and a light cardigan or dressing gown. If the child is in bed, change the sheets regularly. Open the window from time to time to air the room. Disinfect the room using a natural spray (see box).

Be prepared for your child to revert to babyish behaviour traits: a young child who is just potty-trained, for example, may revert to nappies. Be patient if he or she is fractious and irritable.

SYMPTOM SORTER

Symptoms with or without fever	Could be
Runny nose, cough or sneezing	Cold
All the above plus aches and pains	Flu
Sore throat and pain on swallowing	Throat infection
Runny or blocked nose, pain in ear or (in young child) crying and pulling on ear	Ear infection
Cough, phlegm	Bronchitis
Cough, phlegm and or rapid or difficult breathing	Bronchiolitis
Itchy red spots that blister	Chickenpox
Frequent urination and pain or burning when passing water	Infection in urinary tract
Diarrhoea and/or vomiting	Food poisoning or gastroenteritis

If your child has a fever, take steps to reduce it. Give lots of fluids, preferably water with a little added fresh lemon juice. Failing this, try diluted fruit juice even if you don't usually give it: juice is a good way to get vitamins into your child and encourage him or her to drink.

Children who are poorly often don't want to eat. This won't harm your child, and it's best not to encourage

WHEN TO SEEK HELP

Contact a doctor if your child:
- has an unexplained rash
- has a high or persistent fever
- is breathing very fast or noisily
- is unusually sleepy and cannot be roused
- is making you feel concerned.

Go to hospital or call an ambulance if your child:
- cannot breathe properly
- has a fit or is unconscious
- has severe leg pain, cold hands or feet with a high body temperature, very pale skin or blue-tinged skin around the lips (early signs of bacterial meningitis)
- has a headache, stiff neck, aversion to bright light or a purplish-red rash that does not disappear when pressed with a glass (later signs of bacterial meningitis)

AIR FRESHENER

For a natural room spray to refresh the air in your child's room, use 5 drops each of lavender, thyme linalol and eucalyptus smithi essential oils to 150ml/$\frac{1}{4}$ pint water. Pour into a plant spray bottle, shake well, and spray into the air.

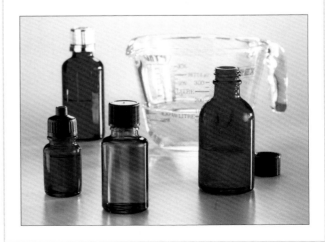

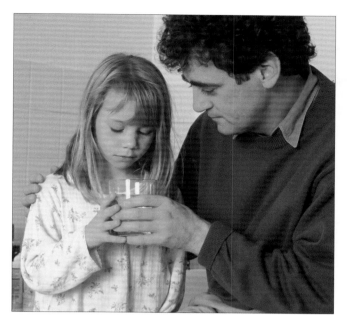

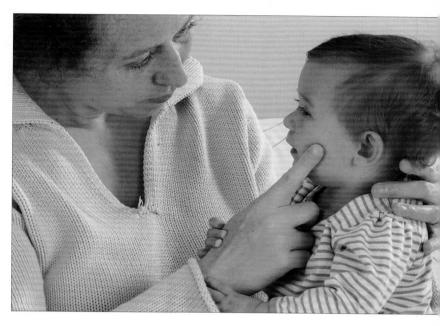

Being sick and having diarrhoea dehydrates the body, so make sure your child drinks enough water after vomitting. Encourage them to take small sips of cooled, boiled water and repeat at intervals.

Trust your own instincts: if something tells you that your child is seriously ill, act on your intuition. You know your child better than anyone else, so you may pick up on clues that may not be obvious to other people.

eating: his or her body may need to put all its energy into fighting off an infection. Once your child starts to feel better, the appetite may return. Give foods that are easy to eat and gentle on the stomach: a thick, smooth home-made vegetable or chicken soup, mashed potato, natural yoghurt with mashed-up banana, or a smoothie made with fruit juice, yoghurt and honey.

A HOSPITAL STAY

A stay in hospital is bound to be disorientating and intimidating for a young child. Prepare your child as much as you can by talking about what will happen. Sharing a book about a child who has to go to hospital could help. If possible, go on a visit to the ward where your child will be staying – see if he or she can meet some of the nurses and other staff who work there and see some of the fun things – such as the television above each bed. Be as

matter-of-fact as you can: it is important that your child doesn't pick up on your anxiety. But do acknowledge any feelings of fear or worry your child may have.

Take familiar items with you: your child's favourite toy or comforter, pyjamas, bowl and spoon, as well as the essentials. Take snacks, water, a book and comfortable clothing for yourself as well. Stay with your child in hospital: even if you have to sleep in an armchair, it will make your child feel much better if you are there. If you cannot be there all the time, ask another trusted relative or friend that the child knows well to fill in for you. Make sure that you are present when your child is examined by a doctor. Even if your child seems to cope well with being in hospital, don't be surprised if he or she displays some signs of disturbance once you get home. It is common for children to be clingy or naughty, even aggressive, after an unsettling experience. Be patient and this will pass.

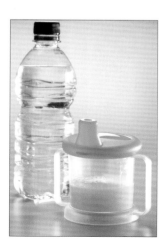

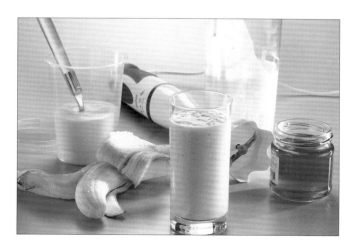

Left: Diluted juice is a good way of boosting a poorly child's energy levels. Use freshly squeezed juice if you can; it has more nutrients.

Right: During illness or convalesence, tempt a poor appetite with food that is easy to eat – a banana and yoghurt smoothie is ideal.

Common problems: colds, coughs and breathing disorders

Children get more coughs and colds than adults. Most children catch between six and eight colds a year until they build up immunity. And as the airways of a child are much smaller than those of adults, they are more vulnerable to infection.

COLDS

It is viruses that cause colds, so antibiotics do not help. A cold usually lasts a week or two, but can go on for longer in young children. Symptoms include a blocked-up or runny nose, sticky eyes, sore throat, a tickly cough (especially at night) and slight fever.

What to do. You can't hasten a cold's progress, but you can make your child more comfortable. Keep him or her warm, but open windows regularly to get fresh air circulating. Take your child out (well wrapped up) on short trips. Increase the humidity in the child's room to help with breathing: put a damp towel on the radiator, place a bowl of water near the radiator or other heat source or use a vaporizer.

Give lots of fluids. Children over a year old can have hot honey and lemon, which is soothing for the throat and a good source of vitamin C. Weak elderflower tea acts as a decongestant. Dilute fruit juices can also be a good way of encouraging a child to drink. Unsweetened blackcurrant diluted with warm water is good if your child has a cold: it is packed with vitamin C.

- If your child is eating, cut out dairy products (which are mucus-forming) while symptoms remain, but give alternative sources of calcium such as tofu, ground nuts and seeds, and leafy green vegetables. Babies will still need their usual milk.
- Get older children to blow their nose regularly, to stop mucus dripping down the back of the throat.
- Consider giving a homeopathic remedy to soothe symptoms. The following are common cold remedies: Aconite, given in the first 24 hours; Allium cepa, when there is lots of watery discharge from the nose and eyes; Pulsatilla, when there is thick, greenish mucus

When to seek help. Seek medical advice if you spot other unusual signs, such as wheezing or earache, if the symptoms are very severe or if your child gets more poorly after a few days.

COUGHS

Coughing is how the body removes irritants or mucus from the breathing apparatus, so it is best to avoid over-the-counter medications that are designed to suppress this natural mechanism. If your child suddenly starts coughing violently, consider whether he or she may have inhaled a foreign object. Take steps to remove it from the airway (see first aid for choking).

What to do. If your child is coughing, the suggestions given for colds above are helpful, together with the following:

- Humidify all rooms by placing a bowl of water under the radiator or heat source.
- Avoid taking your child outdoors if the weather is cold and damp.
- For babies over three months, put a drop of essential oil of

For colds, give drinks of diluted blackcurrant, orange or lemon juice sweetened with a little honey.

There are many homeopathic remedies for different types of cough and cold symptoms.

Eucalyptus oil is a good natural decongestant, but you need only a drop on a tissue.

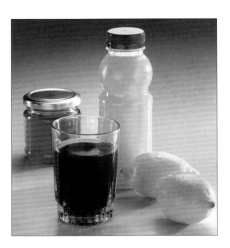

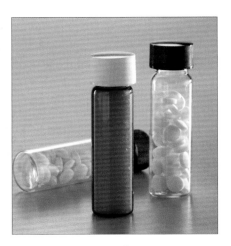

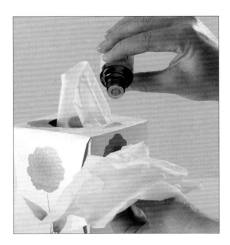

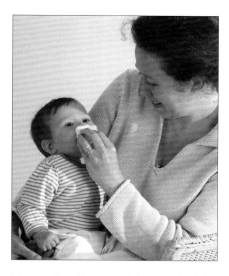

Use soft cotton wool (cotton balls) rather than tissues to wipe a child's nose to stop it getting sore.

eucalyptus smithi (not eucalyptus globulus, which is stronger) on a handkerchief and leave it in your child's room, out of reach.

- For children over one year, give diluted warm blackcurrant juice to soothe a sore throat, or thyme tea remedy (see box). If children are eating, include mild spices such as cinnamon or ginger in their food to help loosen mucus. Pineapple is also good because it contains bromeline, which is a natural anti-inflammatory.

- Consider giving one of the many homeopathic remedies used to relieve symptoms. A homeopath will help you pinpoint the right one for your child. Common remedies include: Aconite, for a dry cough that comes on at night; Bryonia, for a dry, painful cough (worse on inhalation) that follows a cold; Ipepac, for a cough that is accompanied by vomiting up phlegm; Phosphorus, for a dry, tickly cough that is worse at night; Pulsatilla, for a cough that produces yellow or green phlegm

When to seek help. Coughing can be a minor ailment or a symptom of some much more serious illnesses such as bronchiolitis and bronchitis. Always see a doctor if a cough occurs in a young baby, or if it is

severe, prolonged or accompanied by wheezing, noisy breathing or fast breathing.

CROUP

A barking cough and noisy breathing on inhalation are the key signs of croup, which is most common among children aged between six months and three years.

What to do. There are two ways to improve the breathing: take your child into a steamy room (run the hot shower and taps in the bathroom to create steam) or wrap the child up well and go outside into the cold air. Different approaches work for different children, so do which works best for your child.

THYME TEA REMEDY

This traditional remedy can help to ease a dry cough and loosen mucus. If possible, use New Zealand manuka honey, which has particular therapeutic properties.

Add a small handful of finely chopped thyme leaves to a cup of boiling water, steep until cool, then strain. Add honey to sweeten, then pour into a sterilized jar. Give 1 tsp three or four times a day. Keep in the refrigerator for up to 3 days.

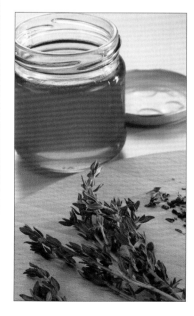

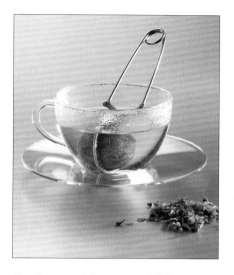

For flu, try giving your child weak lime flower tea, which helps to treat fever and reduce nasal catarrh.

BRONCHIOLITIS

This viral infection is most common in babies under twelve months, and affects the smallest airways in the lungs (the bronchioles). It starts as a cold and fever and develops into coughing, fast breathing (more than 50 breaths a minute) and wheezing.

What to do. See your doctor quickly: sometimes hospital treatment is needed.

BRONCHITIS

This infection of the large airways (bronchi) is common in toddlers and children. The symptoms are similar to those of bronchiolitis. Deficiencies in vitamin C and zinc can be an underlying cause for recurrent lung problems such as bronchitis.

What to do. Medical advice should be sought. Giving a multivitamin multimineral supplement in addition may help.

FLU

The symptoms of flu include a high temperature, aches and pains, cold symptoms, vomiting and/or diarrhoea and general malaise.

What to do. See your doctor for a diagnosis. Lime flower and elderflower tea – or a combination of both – are good for flu. They should be drunk warm, well diluted.

Common problems: asthma and eczema

Asthma and eczema are now very common in young children. Both are the result of oversensitivity of the immune system, which cause it to react to substances that have no effect on other people. They often occur together, and affected children are also more likely to suffer from food allergies.

Nobody quite knows why asthma and eczema have become so prevalent, but it may be because improved living standards have reduced the amount of germs children come into contact with, with the result that their immune systems are less robust. The increase in pollution, both outdoors and indoors, is also a likely factor. One Australian study found that exposure to the volatile organic chemicals (VOCs) found in paint and other

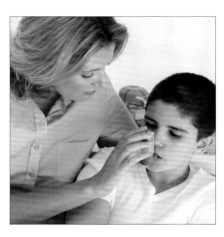

Asthma medicine is given via an inhaler and can quickly reduce symptoms of an attack. Children using inhalers need supervising by a responsible adult.

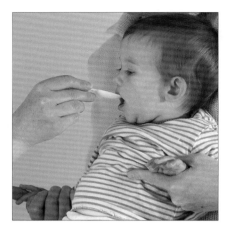

Fish oils have been shown to ease symptoms of both asthma and eczema. In one study, three out of four children given fish oil found that their symptoms improved.

products increased the risk of childhood asthma. Exclusive breastfeeding in the first months of life can reduce the likelihood of both asthma and eczema developing.

ASTHMA

Growing numbers of children suffer from the recurrent attacks of breathlessness and wheezing that characterize asthma. In asthmatic children, the small airways in the lungs are hypersensitive: they narrow when they come into contact with, say, small amounts of smoke or pollutants. Asthma usually gets better as the child gets older. A child who is diagnosed with asthma will be given inhalers to prevent attacks and relieve symptoms. Natural therapies can help to support conventional medical treatment.

What to do. Try to identify possible triggers for your child's asthma and take steps to avoid them. Your doctor can arrange tests to check for allergy to substances such as dust mites. Improve the air quality in your home and keep it free of dust (but

vacuum when your child is out of the way). Choose a synthetic pillow and duvet with allergen-proof covers for your child's bed, and wash the bedding often in hot water. Limit toys in the cot to one or two, and wash them each week at 60°C/140°F or put in a plastic bag in the freezer overnight to kill dust mites.

Make sure that your child has a healthy diet including lots of fresh fruits and vegetables: this has been shown to be good for lung function. Choose organic produce wherever possible to reduce your child's exposure to pesticides. Do not put salt in your child's food, and avoid processed foods that contain added salt and additives such as tartrazine, which may exacerbate asthma. Consider consulting a nutritional therapist to help you uncover any possible food intolerances, and give a multivitamin, multimineral supplement: low levels of vitamin C, vitamin B6, vitamin B12, magnesium and zinc can exacerbate the symptoms. Homeopathy may help. Arsenicum, Ipecac, Nat sulph and

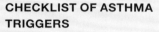

CHECKLIST OF ASTHMA TRIGGERS
- Dust mites
- Pollen
- Pet dander (animal hair and skin scales)
- Certain foods, especially eggs, dairy products, chocolate, wheat, citrus fruits and corn
- Mould spores
- Colds and other respiratory infections
- Cigarette smoke or exhaust fumes
- Fumes from air fresheners, household cleaners, perfumes, dry-cleaning solvents, paints, glues and pesticides
- Cold air
- Exercise
- Stress and anxiety.

Pulsatilla are all prescribed to relieve mild asthma attacks, but you should see a homeopath for a specific remedy for your child. Herbal medicine has several remedies for asthma. A medical herbalist can advise you on the best herbs to use (alongside conventional treatment). Acupuncture may be helpful for some asthma sufferers, and yoga or breathing exercises may help.

ECZEMA

There are different types of eczema: those that usually affect children are seborrhoeic eczema (cradle cap) and the itchy atopic eczema, which one child in five develops. Atopic eczema can affect any part of the body, but is most common on the face, armpits, elbows, hands and knees. During an acute attack, the skin reddens, becomes extremely itchy and can blister and weep. It may be thick, dry and flaky at other times.

What to do. See your doctor, as it's essential to manage your child's eczema to prevent infection. Eczema reduces the skin's ability to act as a barrier, and bacteria are more likely to stick to dry, flaky skin.

Avoid irritating the skin. For example, choose clothing or bedding made from cotton, launder

Keep your child's fingernails short to stop him or her scratching areas of skin affected by eczema and causing infection.

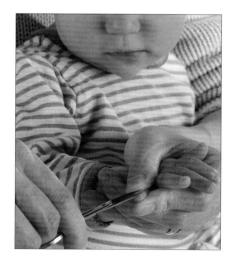

OILS FOR ECZEMA
Aromatherapy oils may help with mild eczema symptoms. Try this simple recipe. You can also make a cool compress using the same oils to soothe itching.

2 drops chamomile essential oil
2 drops lavender essential oil
45ml/3 tbsp hypoallergenic lotion

Mix together all the ingredients and then apply to the affected skin in a thin layer. Be sure to do a patch test 24 hours before you first use the lotion.
You can also make a cool compress using the same oils diluted in a simple carrier oil such as olive oil to soothe itching.

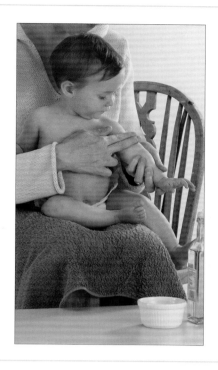

with non-biological washing powders and use an extra rinse cycle on your washing machine. Avoid soap and bath products. Keep your child as cool as possible, as heat and sweating exacerbate eczema. Cut his or her fingernails short to help prevent scratching (put cotton mittens on babies and young children at night).

Keep your child's skin clean and moisturized. Give lukewarm (not hot) daily baths to remove dry skin scales and cleanse the skin. Use an emollient such as a handful of oatmeal tied in a muslin square (you can add a drop of lavender or chamomile essential oil). Different creams work for different children. Hemp seed oil cream is one good natural alternative to try, as is olive oil. Apply a thin layer and let it soak in rather than rubbing it in (which can increase itching).

Increase oils in your child's diet. Add a spoonful of hemp seed oil to your child's food each day and give oily fish or a supplement. Give lots of water to keep your child well hydrated. Consider food sensitivity as an underlying factor, and see a qualified nutritional therapist to help

you pinpoint any problem foods. Milk, wheat, nuts, citrus fruits, fish and eggs are the most likely culprits, and sugar can exacerbate eczema. As with asthma, a multivitamin, multimineral supplement may be helpful, and a child-friendly probiotic will help to improve the balance of good bacteria in the gut, which can also be beneficial.

A probiotic drink that is suitable for children may help with eczema.

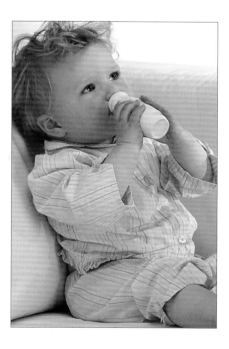

Common problems: digestive disorders

Children have sensitive digestive systems that react quickly to get rid of unwanted substances: they are much more prone to diarrhoea and vomiting than adults. These unpleasant symptoms are basically the body's way of cleansing itself, so medications to stop them are generally unhelpful. Your main aim should be to reduce discomfort and prevent dehydration.

Tummy ache is unusual in very young children, so it is best to report it to a doctor to rule out the possibility of appendicitis. In older

Most children become distressed after vomiting. Give your child a glass of cool water to sip: add a few drops of Rescue Remedy to calm and reassure.

children, it can have a physical or emotional cause: gastroenteritis, overeating or anxiety can all be responsible. Sometimes it can be triggered by other infections, such as tonsillitis. Call a doctor if your child is in severe pain, there is blood in his or her stools or if tummy ache and fever occur together.

DIARRHOEA

Your child may get a short bout of diarrhoea (frequent, loose, unpleasant-smelling stools) after having a lot of fruit or fruit juice, after eating a food he or she is intolerant to, when teething or with a cold. A course of antibiotics can also be a trigger. Diarrhoea can be a sign of food poisoning or gastroenteritis, especially if accompanied by

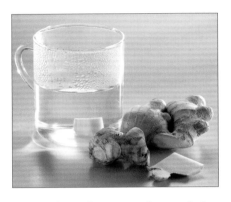

Fresh ginger is a natural remedy for nausea. All you need do is steep a piece of the fresh root in a cup of hot water for a few minutes.

vomiting. In most cases, it lasts 24 hours or less and clears up by itself. **What to do**. Give frequent drinks for sipping. Let a nursing baby breastfeed on demand and give a bottle-fed baby extra drinks of cooled, boiled water. Plain water should be sufficient in mild cases, but you can also give a rehydration drink (available from pharmacists) if necessary. Antispasmodic herbal teas, such as chamomile or fennel, can ease abdominal pains. Diluted unsweetened blackcurrant juice helps to fight infection in the gut.

For a soothing tummy massage, add one drop chamomile essential oil to 15ml/1 tbsp olive or sunflower oil. Gently massage the tummy, with clockwise circular strokes.

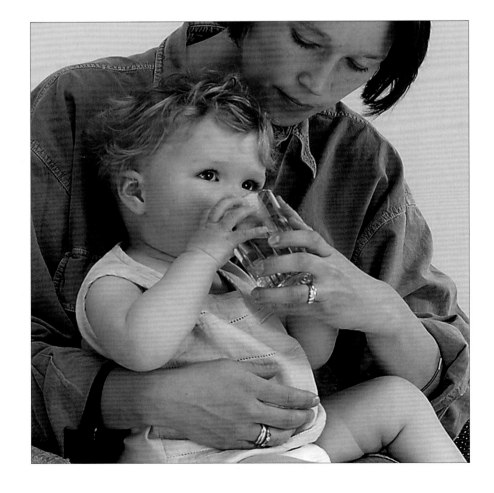

DEHYDRATION
Seek immediate help if your child shows signs of dehydration: dry mouth, sunken eyes, loose skin and dry nappies. The soft spot on the top of a baby's head (the fontanelle) may become depressed.

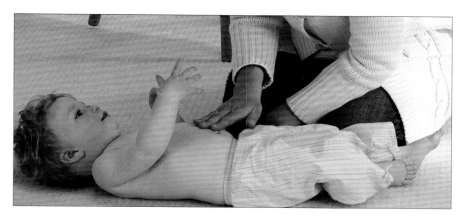

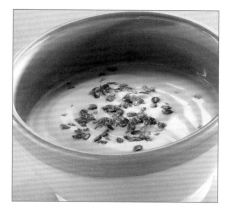

A gentle tummy massage, following the path of the intestines, can help to get the bowels moving.

Consider giving a suitable probiotic to help balance the bacteria in the gut. This can help reduce the duration of a bout of diarrhoea. If the diarrhoea occurred after you introduced a new food into your child's diet, make a note of it. If the symptoms re-occur the next time you give the food, then your child is almost certainly sensitive to it and it is best avoided.

When to seek help. Contact a doctor if a baby has diarrhoea for more than a few hours or if it lasts longer than 24 hours in an older child. Also, seek medical help if the diarrhoea is very severe, if there is blood in the stools, if your child seems dehydrated or has persistent stomach ache or if you think he or she has taken something toxic.

VOMITING
Like diarrhoea, vomiting can have many causes. If your child is doing both, the most likely cause is gastroenteritis or food poisoning. Vomiting on its own can be the result of the child having eaten too much (or a baby having taken too much milk) or can be part of a feverish illness. A baby with a cold may be sick, to expel phlegm from the body. **What to do**. Treat as for diarrhoea (but avoid giving a tummy massage). Encourage your child to sip rather than to gulp liquid to help it stay down. Ginger is particularly good for

nausea and vomiting: you can make a simple ginger tea by steeping a block of peeled, bruised garlic in a cup of hot water.

When to seek help. Contact your doctor if a baby vomits repeatedly or violently, or if vomiting and diarrhoea occur together. Seek medical advice for an older child if vomiting is very frequent, lasts longer than 24 hours, or if there is blood in the vomit.

CONSTIPATION
If your child suddenly goes for longer than normal between bowel movements, and then produces hard, dry, pebble-like stools, he or she is constipated.

What to do. Increase the vegetables and fruits in your child's diet (but cut out bananas): broccoli, leafy green vegetables and dried apricots are particularly helpful. Give older children whole grains: porridge oats and rye bread are better than wholewheat bread, which can irritate the lining of the gut. Most important

If your child is hungry after vomiting or diarrhoea, plain boiled rice is very gentle on the stomach.

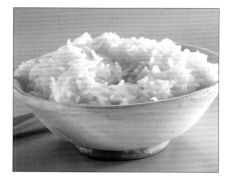

Fibre-rich ground flaxseed can help with constipation. Add a little to natural yoghurt or in a smoothie.

of all, make sure your child is well hydrated: give extra cups of water and remind the child to drink them.

Consider sprinkling a little ground flaxseed (available from health food stores) on your child's cereal, or put 5ml/1 tsp flaxseed oil into your child's food or in a fruit smoothie. Flaxseeds are rich in fibre and are a natural lubricant. Give live yoghurt if the balance of the intestinal flora has been upset by a bout of gastroenteritis or a course of antibiotics. Or consider giving a child-friendly probiotic supplement.

Massage can soothe cramping and encourage the bowels to move: stroke your hand over the abdomen, making an arch shape in a clockwise direction so that you are following the line of the intestines. For children over one year, you can use a massage oil of orange essential oil diluted in a carrier oil. Reflexology treatment can be helpful: one Scottish study found that regular treatment helped to relieve chronic constipation in children.

If constipation is a recurring problem, consider whether food sensitivity could be a root cause. An Italian study found that sensitivity to cow's milk caused chronic constipation in some children.

When to seek help. Seek medical advice if your child does not have a bowel movement for several days, or if the problem is recurrent.

Common problems: skin rashes and ear infections

Rashes are a feature of many childhood infections, both non-serious and serious. It's quite hard to distinguish between different rashes, so it is best to check them out with your doctor.

CHICKENPOX

The first symptoms of chickenpox are usually tiredness, fever and loss of appetite. Within a day or two, small, flat red spots appear, usually on the back, stomach and chest. They can spread to the face and head in a day or two. The red spots join up and blister, becoming intensely itchy. They scab over within 24 hours, as more spots appear.

Chickenpox is infectious from two days before the spots appear until scabs have formed on all the spots. It takes 10–21 days for the symptoms to appear after infection. One attack usually confers lifelong immunity. Chickenpox can be very dangerous for unborn children if the mother is not immune, so if your child has been in contact with a pregnant woman, let her know, so that she can contact her doctor.

Chickenpox spots blister and then scab. They are itchy, but discourage your child from scratching in case of infection and scarring.

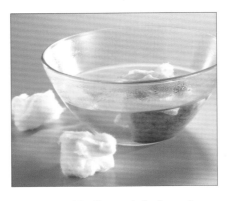

Make an elderflower infusion, dip cotton wool in the bowl and dab on the spots for relief from itching.

What to do. Encourage your child to rest as much as possible and take steps to manage any fever. Use calendula cream or calomine lotion on the spots to relieve itching, or dab them with elderflower tea or a solution of 5ml/1 tsp distilled witch hazel in a cup of warm water. Give lots of fruits and vegetables to boost your child's immune system, and add raw garlic to food if your child will eat it. Consider giving the following homeopathic remedies:

- Aconite, for the initial symptoms of tiredness and fever
- Belladonna, for the early stages if temperature is high and the child is flushed and very thirsty
- Rhus tox, for itching and any restlessness

RELIEVING ITCHING CHICKENPOX SPOTS

A lukewarm oatmeal bath can be soothing. Place a handful of oatmeal in a muslin square or the foot of a nylon stocking, add 2 drops each of chamomile and lavender essential oils, tie up and place in the water. Give several baths a day.

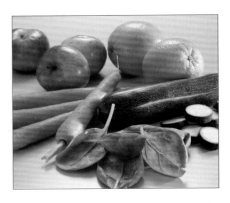

Encourage your child to eat lots of healthy fruits and vegetables to promote healing.

Protect your child's skin from direct sunlight for a couple of weeks after the scabs fall off, to avoid any danger of scarring.

When to seek help. See your doctor if a baby is affected, if the attack is severe, if the spots become inflamed or if you are pregnant and are not sure that you are immune.

HEAT RASH

Young children have immature sweat glands, which are easily blocked. Heat rash usually appears as small red bumps, sometimes with a blister in the centre, that appear on areas exposed to sunlight or areas that sweat a lot.

What to do. Cool your child down: remove clothing, sponge down or give the child a tepid bath. Good topical treatments include aloe vera gel, distilled witch hazel, Calendula cream or a lavender or chamomile compress. The homeopathic remedy Sol can also be helpful.

IMPETIGO

This infectious skin condition usually starts off around the mouth or nose. It takes the form of red blisters, which soon burst and form a golden crust on reddened, weeping skin.

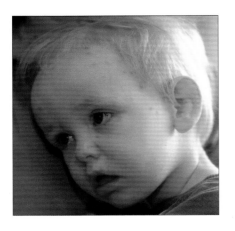

GLUE EAR

This is a condition in which thick, sticky fluid accumulates in the middle ear, leading to hearing problems. It can be linked to repeated ear or throat infections, which block the Eustachian tube. If it is persistent, the conventional treatment is the insertion of a plastic grommet to allow fluid to drain. But the procedure involves a general anaesthetic and has itself been linked to hearing problems. Repeated ear infections are often a cause, so take steps to avoid them (see above). Many complementary health practitioners believe that glue ear is linked to food sensitivity, particularly an intolerance of dairy foods, or to passive smoking.

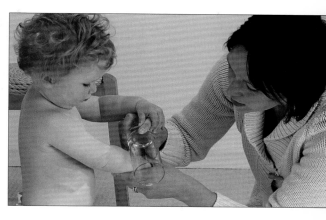

What to do. Bathing the skin with warm salt water can help to reduce itching; tea tree oil added neat to water can also help with itching and can limit the infection. Give garlic perles every two hours for a day or two, then reduce to three times a day, to help resolve the infection. The homeopathic remedies Ant crud or Arsenicum can be useful.

Be scrupulous about hygiene: do not share face towels or pillows and keep your child away from other children while infectious.

EAR INFECTIONS

Children are prone to ear infections, particularly after a cold or throat infection. The Eustachian tube, the drainage canal that links the nose, ear and throat, is very narrow. If it becomes blocked, fluid accumulates and viruses and bacteria multiply. The main symptoms are pain, hearing loss and fever. A small child

Warmth can soothe the pain of an earache; use a covered hot water bottle or a lavender compress.

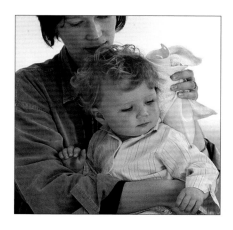

may tug on the ear, but most simply cry and seem unwell.

Seek medical advice straight away if you suspect your child has an ear infection. It needs prompt treatment – usually antibiotics – to prevent the infection spreading. Take steps to prevent recurrence, so your child does not have to take repeated courses of antibiotics.

What you can do. Warm the affected ear by holding a warm lavender compress or a covered hot-water bottle against it. Dilute lavender essential oil in olive or sunflower oil and smooth into the skin around the ear and neck.

For children over one year, give plenty of warm drinks such as honey and lemon and fresh blackcurrant juice; you can give a herbal tea combining chamomile (antiseptic and relaxing), elderflower or lemon balm (to reduce mucus) and lime flowers (to bring down fever) three times a day. Garlic can help relieve infection: add fresh garlic to your child's food if possible, or give garlic perles. If your child has taken antibiotics, give live yoghurt every day for a month to help rebalance the bacteria in the gut.

Raise the head of the cot or bed to help fluid drain from the Eustachian tube. Avoid washing your child's hair or going swimming while symptoms persist. Consider giving a homeopathic remedy, such as:

- Aconite, at the onset of symptoms, especially if the child has a blocked nose, fever and is thirsty
- Belladonna, for earache that is

To test for a meningitis rash, press a clear glass against it, if the spots do not disappear seek immediate medical aid.

worse at night and better when the child sits upright
- Chamomilia, for earache that accompanies teething, is causing extreme pain and irritability
- Pulsatilla, for earache with a cold that is worse at night.

If your child gets repeated ear infections, keep his or her ears, throat and neck warm at all times: wrap the child up well in cold weather. Give the remedies mentioned above at the first signs of a cold, to try to head off infections, but seek advice from a homeopath for a remedy specifically tailored to your child. Consider food sensitivity as a possible cause. Dairy products are the most common culprits, but wheat, eggs and chocolate could also be triggers in some children.

Make sure your child is eating a healthy, balanced diet, with plenty of fresh fruits and vegetables, zinc-rich foods such as meat and poultry, and lots of garlic. Do not give sugar, which depresses the immune system. Warm drinks of honey and lemon or diluted fresh blackcurrant juice support the immune system and encourage mucus to clear. Consider giving a multivitamin, multimineral supplement.

When to seek help. See a doctor if you suspect an ear infection, or if blood or clear liquid is discharged from the ear.

Food allergy and intolerance

Though often confused, food allergy and food intolerance are two different things. In food allergy, the immune system mistakenly identifies the food as a foreign invader. This can cause an extreme and sometimes life-threatening reaction. Food allergy may affect up to 8 per cent of children, but most grow out of it: just 2 per cent of adults are affected. Children with a food allergy are more likely to suffer from other allergy-related problems such as eczema or asthma, which also tend to diminish with age.

Food intolerances are harder to pin down. Symptoms vary widely, even in the same individual. They are usually milder and can occur hours or days after the food is eaten. Some may be delayed reactions by the immune system, others are caused by the body's inability to digest the food properly. For these reasons, many doctors are sceptical even about the existence of many food intolerances, while many nutritional therapists believe them to be a factor in a wide range of common childhood ailments.

WARNING

Children with severe allergies can go into anaphylactic shock, in which their blood pressure drops and they become unconscious. Anaphylaxis can be fatal unless the victim is treated with a shot of adrenaline (epinephrine): call an ambulance immediately. Parents and teachers of children with a severe allergy need to carry an adrenaline shot with them so it can be administered at any time.

COMMON FOOD ALLERGENS

Any food can trigger a reaction, but about 90 per cent of food allergies are caused by one of the following eight foods:

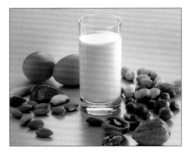

Cow's milk; eggs; peanuts; wheat; soya; tree nuts (such as walnuts, brazil nuts, hazelnuts, almonds and pecans);

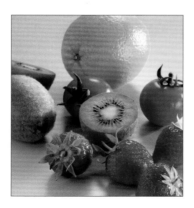

Fish and shellfish.

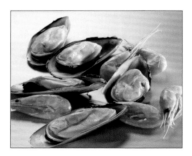

Other common allergenic foods include strawberries, kiwi fruit, tomatoes, oranges, chocolate and soya.

SYMPTOMS

Common symptoms of food allergy include:
- swelling of the lips and throat
- skin rash, eczema or itching
- swelling of the eyelids
- vomiting or diarrhoea
- wheezing or breathing difficulties.

If a child is intolerant – as opposed to allergic – to a food, the symptoms are usually more general, though some are similar to those of an allergic reaction. They include:
- fatigue
- vomiting and diarrhoea
- bloating and wind
- eczema or skin rashes (especially around the mouth)
- wheezing
- muscular aches and pains
- frequent colds or ear infections
- temper tantrums or behaviour problems
- sleeplessness
- cravings (perhaps for the very food the child is intolerant of).

WHAT TO DO

If you suspect that your child may be allergic to a food, the first step is to visit your doctor to arrange for a test. Tests usually take the form of a blood test or a prick test (in which the skin is scratched and a tiny amount of the allergen introduced to see if a reaction occurs). If your child tests positive for an allergy, the only option is to cut the food out of the diet and replace it with healthy alternatives. If there is any doubt, an elimination diet can determine the suspect food. Cutting a food out of the diet is not as easy as it sounds. Someone with an allergy to soya, for example, will also need to avoid foods labelled tempeh, tamori, textured vegetable protein, and so

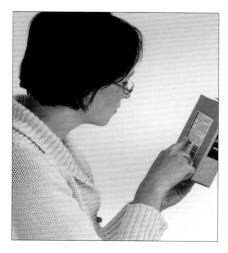

If your child has a food allergy, you will get used to reading the lists of ingredients on food labels: many problem foods crop up in a surprising variety of forms and names. You can find information on food labelling on food allergy websites.

on. A dietician can tell you what you need to look for on food labels.

It is more difficult to test for food intolerances than allergies As a starting point, try keeping a food diary for two weeks, listing everything your child eats and any symptoms. This can sometimes help you to get a better idea of whether

Sweets are full of colourings, preservatives, sugars and artificial sweeteners, all of which can cause behavioural reactions, and certainly have no nutritional value.

your child does indeed have a food intolerance.

If you think this is the case, see your doctor and asked to be referred to an allergy specialist or a dietician. An allergy specialist can help you to check for intolerance by removing the suspect foods from your child's diet for five to ten days, and then re-introducing them. The short period of abstinence should be scrupulously observed in order to be sure that all traces of the food have passed through the digestive system. This has the effect of making any reaction when the food is re-introduced stronger and more immediate, making diagnosis easier.

Although the process sounds simple, it is best to have professional advice when you undertake it: it is very easy to make the mistake of assuming a child has a food intolerance when this is not the case, which could lead you to restrict his or her diet unnecessarily. A specialist will also help ensure that your child is getting essential nutrients while following an exclusion diet.

Where an intolerance is diagnosed, eliminating the problem food is the usual remedy, as with allergies. However, in the case of intolerance, when a food is excluded from the diet, the body tends to build up tolerance to it. This means that the child may be able to eat it again in small quantities not too frequently.

ELIMINATING FOODS
Don't be tempted to exclude important foods such as milk from your child's diet without professional advice. It can be difficult to provide alternative sources of, say calcium. Children can become malnourished while following a severely restricted diet.

If your child does have a food sensitivity, make sure he or she has a good balanced diet, and takes regular meals and snacks to keep blood-sugar levels steady. Consider giving a multivitamin, multimineral supplement and a suitable probiotic drink to encourage good digestion. It's important to get your child to chew food properly (this makes it easier to digest).

You can help to build your child's tolerance to a problem food such as wheat by eliminating it from the diet for a couple of months. After this, the child may have no trouble eating occasional pieces of bread.

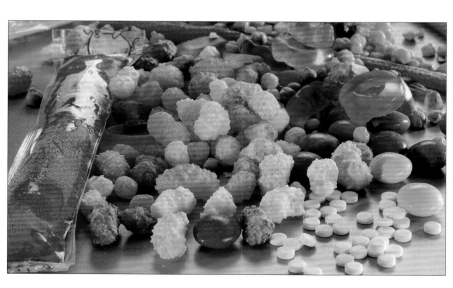

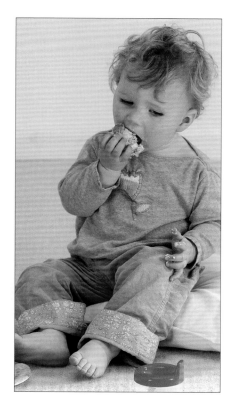

A healthy home

We are all exposed to toxic chemicals every day: they are in the air we breathe, our food and drink and the toiletries and household products we use. Because our homes are enclosed spaces, toxin levels can build up and the air can actually be more polluted than it is outdoors. Ordinary household dust can contain a mixture of solvents, hormone-disrupting chemicals, heavy metals, solvents, pesticides and flame retardants. Children spend a lot of their time indoors and they are more likely to be affected by pollution than adults. So it is important to ensure that your home is a healthy environment for your child to grow up in.

Here are some basic steps for a healthy home.
• Ban smoking at home.
• Open your windows regularly.
• Keep pets out of sleeping areas. If your child is allergic to your pet, you may have to keep it out of all living areas or find it a new home.
• Wipe your feet when you come in, and leave your shoes by the door to avoid bringing dirt, heavy metals and toxic chemicals indoors.
• Choose furniture made from untreated natural materials.
• Wash curtains, other soft furnishings and bedclothes regularly.

Keeping your home dust-free will help to protect your child from inhaling pollutants. But use natural products rather than spray polishes and carpet cleaners.

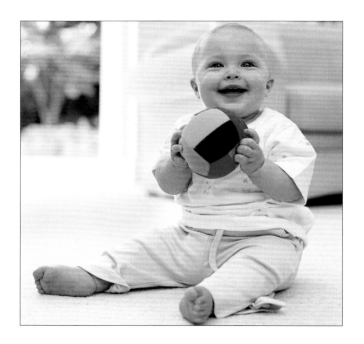

NATURAL CLEANING PRODUCTS

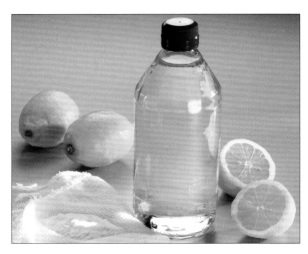

You can use ordinary ingredients to tackle many cleaning jobs around the home.

Bicarbonate of soda (baking soda). Sprinkle this on a damp sponge and use to clean surfaces. For stubborn stains, mix it with a little water and leave for 20 minutes before wiping off. Add 30ml/2 tbsp bicarbonate of soda to a cup of vinegar and add to the toilet bowl. Leave for at least 15 minutes, then clean with a brush. To clean a drain, add half a cup of bicarbonate then half a cup of vinegar. Leave for 15 minutes, then pour down a kettle of boiling water.

White vinegar. This is great for cleaning windows. Add half a cup of vinegar to 1 litre/2 pints warm water and apply with a soft cloth, then buff with crumpled newspaper. Vinegar can also be used for descaling appliances: add equal parts of vinegar and water to a kettle and leave overnight. Throw out the vinegar, boil the kettle and discard the water before using again.

Lemon juice. Lemon is an excellent natural brightening agent and cleanser. Add half a cup of lemon juice to a bucket of water and soak white or coloured clothes overnight before washing as usual.

• Keep your home as dust-free as possible. Consider buying a vacuum cleaner with a high-efficiency particulate air (HEPA) filter. Keep children out of the way while you dust and vacuum.
• Dry clothes outside or in a properly ventilated space. Avoid putting them around the house (on radiators and so on); the moisture will be released into the air and may cause the growth of mould spores in your walls.

DECORATING

If you are planning a nursery for your baby or revamping a child's bedroom, seek out non-toxic decorating products and furnishings. Babies and children spend a lot of time on or near the floor, so choose a natural covering such as wood or cork rather than laminate or vinyl, which may contain harmful chemicals. Hard flooring is the best option because carpet traps dust, which can lead to a build-up of airborne toxins and dust mites. But if you want to use carpet for warmth, choose wool, sisal or coir with a natural backing, and vacuum regularly.

Regular paints contain volatile organic compounds (VOCs), which give off noxious vapours after being applied. Choose water-based low-VOC paints, keep the room well ventilated during and after decorating and don't let your child sleep in the room for a few days after painting it. Better still, use organic paints made from natural materials such as linseed, casein and mineral pigments. These take longer to dry and can be harder to use, but they are safe for allergy- and asthma-sufferers.

If you are picking furniture for a child's room, avoid items made from MDF, laminated wood or chipboard, which contain formaldehyde. Choose furniture made from untreated hardwood from sustainable sources instead. Use natural materials for your child's bedding. For example, get a mattress made from organic latex, wool and cotton, and sheets of unbleached organic cotton.

CUT THE CHEMICALS

Reducing the amount of chemicals you use in the home will lower the risk of your child coming into contact with something harmful.

- If your kitchen cupboard is a jumble of different products, go through it and get rid of any products you don't use. General cleaners may leave a residue on your surfaces, which your child may then touch: so avoid those labelled 'irritant' and choose gentle eco-friendly products or natural cleaning alternatives instead.

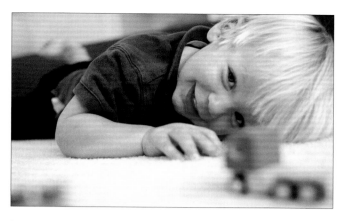

Young children inevitably spend a lot of time on the floor, so it is worth investing in natural coverings that are free from unnecessary chemicals.

- In the same way, go through your bathroom cupboards and throw out any products that you do not need. Avoid wearing perfume, hairspray and a plethora of other products to reduce the amount of chemicals your child breathes in. He or she will prefer your natural smell in any case. Put only natural substances on your baby or toddler – he or she can do without bubble baths, wipes, talc and harsh soaps.
- Get rid of garden pesticides, weed killers and so on. Many common garden products – including creosote – have now been banned, so it is best to dispose of any products you have had for several years. Consider gardening organically to help protect your child from hazardous chemicals. For example, use saucers of beer sunk into the soil to trap slugs rather than poisonous pellets (which a young child could eat).

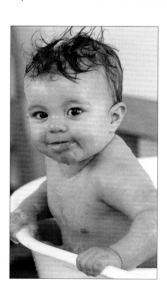

Left: Avoid using unnecessary toiletries. Many bubble baths contain detergent, which irritates the skin, while the ingredients for baby wipes may include propylene glycol – a chemical that is also present in anti-freeze.

Right: Make sure your child spends some time outside every day, whatever the weather.

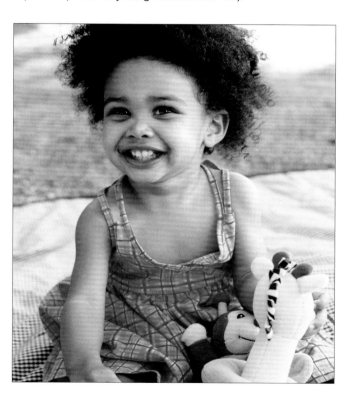

Safety in the home

Young children are naturally curious and have little sense of danger, so it is up to you to make their environment safe. To make your home child-friendly, you need to develop an eye for potential disaster. The best way to do this is to crawl around so that you see each room from a child's perspective. Notice what dangles down, what can be pulled or poked, opened or climbed, and then take steps to make it safe. Be prepared to refine your childproofing at the major stages of your child's development – crawling, walking and so on.

Young children need constant adult supervision: they shouldn't be left in a room alone even for a few minutes. Take extra care when you are under pressure, entertaining guests or trying to get ready to go out: accidents are more likely to happen when you are distracted. It's a good idea to get your child used to a playpen from an early age, so that you have somewhere to put him or her when you need to concentrate on something else.

Babies have a knack of exploring that little bit further when you least expect it, so you need to keep a watchful eye on them at all times.

FIRE!
Smoke inhalation, burns and scalds are all common injuries in childhood. Contact your local fire service for individual advice on protecting your home from fire (fire officers may be willing to fit smoke alarms free of charge).

- Don't overload sockets.
- Don't use an extension lead that isn't powerful enough for the appliance; large appliances should not be plugged into extension leads. Put extension leads away after use.
- Don't leave candles or aromatherapy vaporizers that use a naked flame burning: it's safest not to use them at all. Get in the habit of putting matches and lighters well out of reach.
- Do put smoke alarms on every floor; install a carbon monoxide alarm too.
- Do cover all open fires with a fixed fireguard. Use radiator covers too.
- Do switch off appliances at the socket when they are not in use.

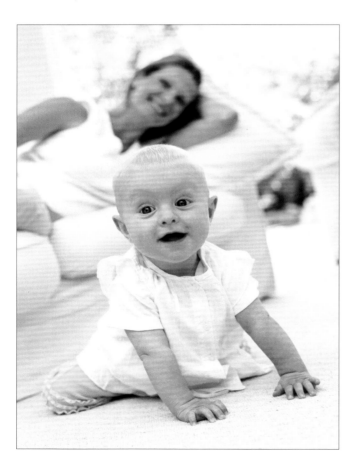

Babies and young children love to rummage through handbags. Be on the safe side and don't ever keep sharp items such as nail clippers or scissors in yours, and make sure any medications you use are in child-safety containers.

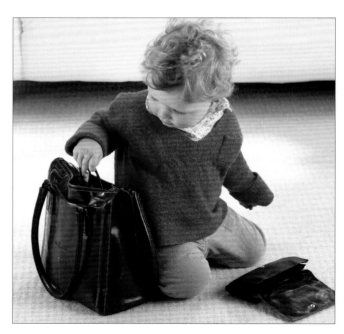

KEEPING ACTIVE CHILDREN SAFE

- Fit stairgates at the top and bottom of stairs once your child is ready to crawl.
- Check your banisters are safe: you need vertical spindles (horizontal ones can serve as a ladder), no more than 10cm/4in apart.
- Put locks on any windows that your child could open.
- Make sure that the locks on the doors to your home are set higher than your child can reach. If not, fit a high bolt and use it.
- Put plug covers on all unused electrical sockets. Turn off the switch at the socket when you are not using it, and replace any worn flexes.
- Cover any child-level glass with safety film.
- Put corner covers on any tables. Consider getting rid of low coffee tables altogether.
- Don't have any flimsy furniture that your child could pull over on top of him or her. Attach freestanding bookshelves to the wall.
- Constantly check floors and other areas for small items that your child could choke on: coins, marbles, pen tops, buttons, rubber tyres from toy cars, small squidgy balls and burst or uninflated balloons are all potential hazards to your child.

IN THE BEDROOM

Children's bedrooms are generally safer than other parts of the home, because they are usually decorated and furnished with the child in mind. But there are some basic things to bear in mind:

The best time to iron is when your child is in bed. If you do need to iron at other times, keep your child well away (in a playpen or behind a safety gate) and put the iron out of reach as soon as you have finished. Put it away when it has cooled down.

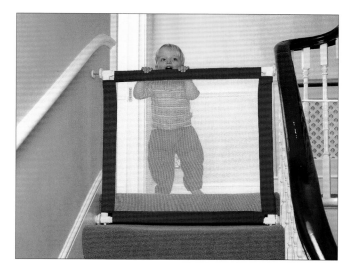

Fit a stairgate at the top and bottom of stairs until your child can safely navigate them independently. Let children practise going up and coming down from time to time: teach your child to come down bottom first.

- Make sure your child's cot is a safe place. The bars should be no more than 7cm/2¾ in apart, and the mattress should fit snugly. Don't give a child under one year a duvet or pillows.
- Position the cot or bed away from windows and radiators.
- Don't put anything under the window (such as low cupboards, bookshelves or toy boxes) that your child could use as a step. Don't forget to fit window locks in your child's room.
- Use a radiator cover to protect your child from burns. Alternatively, turn the thermostat down and cover the radiator with a large towel.

SAFETY WITH TOYS

- Don't let your child play with a toy intended for an older child; age ranges are recommended for safety reasons.
- Don't give toys with long strings to a baby: they are a strangling hazard. Musical cot toys with strings should be removed before the child can get on hands and knees.
- Remove all packaging and labels before giving a toy to your child.
- Check second-hand toys carefully. Old toys may have been made to less stringent safety standards or contain chemicals that are no longer allowed.
- Get rid of broken toys that cannot be repaired.
- If you need to change the batteries in a toy, change all of them: old batteries can get overheated if they are next to new ones.
- Don't get a toy chest that can be locked or one with a hinged lid – it could slam on your child's head.

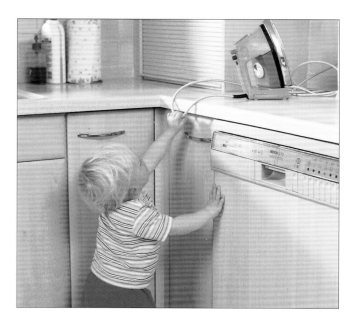

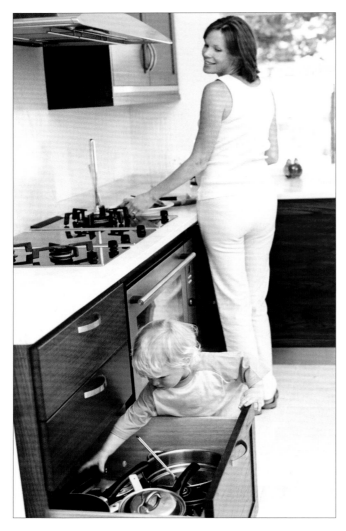

Make sure that your child is sitting in a highchair or booster seat that is appropriate for his or her age, and that they are safely strapped in at mealtimes.

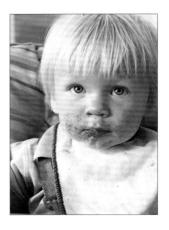

Fit childproof locks to kitchen cupboards and drawers within your child's reach, especially if you store breakable, heavy or harmful items there. But consider letting a child use one cupboard or drawer for play.

IN THE KITCHEN

The kitchen is full of items that are potential hazards for inquisitive children. You need to get into the habit of tidying up after yourself and closing cupboard doors and drawers once you have got what you need. If you can, keep your child out of the kitchen when you are cooking: you may be able to use a stair gate to fence off the cooking area or fit in a playpen to keep your child safe.

Store plastic bags and clingfilm out of reach: young children instinctively want to wear a bag like a hat. Keep knives somewhere safe. Fit locks to low-level cupboards and drawers. Store dishwasher tablets (which are particularly noxious) and other cleaning products in a locked cupboard, and make sure that your child knows this is the "nasty cupboard". If a child does swallow something toxic, get medical advice urgently. If you need to go to hospital, take the packaging with you.

When you are cooking, turn saucepan handles to the back of the hob, and use the rear burners when possible.

Hob guards can make cooking and lifting pans awkward, so are not advisable. Give up deep-fat frying, which is very dangerous, or invest in an electric fryer. Have a small fire extinguisher and a fire blanket to hand.

Put the kitchen bin somewhere your child cannot access. Clean up spills quickly, to avoid slipping, and watch for toys, particularly wheeled ones, left in the kitchen. Ban tablecloths for now, and push chairs in under the table so that your child doesn't use them as a step.

EATING SAFELY

Always get your child to sit down when eating, as he or she is more likely to choke if running around and eating at the same time. Encourage your child to chew well and to eat slowly.

Chop foods that are firm and round. Sausages and hot dogs can block the windpipe, so cut them lengthways and then into small pieces. Cut fruit and raw vegetables into small pieces, not rounds, and quarter grapes before giving them to your toddler. Never give whole nuts to a child under five; popcorn, boiled or sticky sweets and peanut butter eaten from the spoon (rather than spread thinly on toast) are also choking hazards.

Always strap your child into a highchair or booster seat: a five-point harness is safest. Don't use a chair that can be attached directly on to the kitchen table; it may work its way loose unnoticed.

IN THE BATHROOM

Most young children love water, but it is important that you supervise them at all times when they are in the bath and that you don't leave a filled bath unattended: a child can drown in even shallow water and your toddler may be better at climbing than you think. If you need to do something, such as answer the door or attend to another child's needs, get your child out of the bath and take him or her with you.

Keep the toilet seat cover down. A toilet seat lock is useful if your child develops a desire to throw toys and other items down the toilet. Keep mouthwashes, cleaners, razors and medicines in a locked cabinet. Get

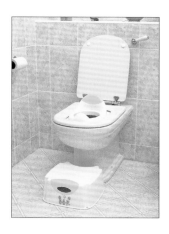

Left: Once your child is toilet trained, you will need to get a step so that he or she can reach the toilet safely and independently.

Right: A garden is a wonderful place for a child to play, so long as it has been made safe.

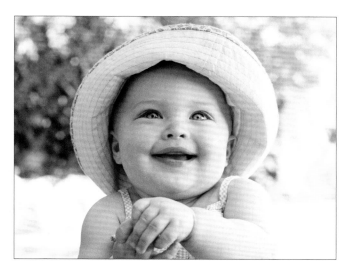

rid of glass thermometers that contain mercury; take them to a pharmacist for safe disposal. Consider turning the hot water temperature down to less than 55°C/130°F.

IN THE GARDEN

A garden allows children to play chasing and ball games much more safely than indoors. And it introduces them to some of the simple wonders of nature: flowers, trees, insects and birds. But you need to plan your garden carefully to ensure that it is safe. Make sure that your child cannot get out of the garden into neighbouring gardens or the street. Maintain fences or walls, make sure there are no gaps that your child can squeeze through, and lock gates after use.

Don't leave your child unattended near any water, even in a bucket. Drain paddling pools and turn them upside-down after use to prevent rainwater from collecting here. Turn any containers kept in the garden, such as dustbins or wheelbarrows, upside-down too.

If you have a slide or climbing frame in the garden, place it on grass rather than a hard surface and check it regularly for safety. Lock away any garden chemicals in a safe place. Always keep garden products in the original bottle so that you know what they are; never decant them

into, say, a lemonade bottle. Better still, get rid of them. Keep garden tools and lawnmowers locked away.

If you have a dog, don't allow it to urinate or defecate in the garden. Teach your child not to eat soil, which may be contaminated by cat faeces. Wash your child's hands after playing in the garden.

Discourage your child from picking flowers or from putting plant material into his or her mouth. Many plants are poisonous and may irritate the skin if they are touched and cause illness or even death if eaten. If you think a child has eaten a poisonous plant, take him or her to hospital (or call an ambulance), and take a sample of the plant with you.

POISONOUS PLANTS
Common garden plants that are toxic include yew, laburnum, lily of the valley, delphinium, deadly nightshade, foxgloves, ivy, hyacinth, mistletoe, daffodil, azalea, privet, rhododendron, toadstools and some mushrooms.

Don't have a pond: it is too easy for a young child to fall in and drown. If you already have one, the safest option is to fill it in; you could turn it into a sandpit.

Don't assume a gate will keep your child in a garden – this one has horizontal bars and an adventurous toddler could easily climb up it.

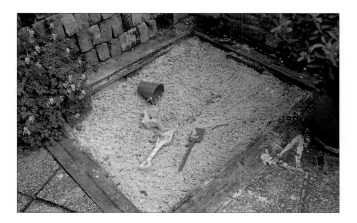

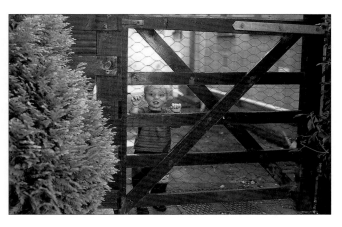

Safety when you are out

However safe you make your own home, you are bound to take your children to other people's homes that are less child-friendly. Get in the habit of scanning any room your child enters for possible hazards. Most people won't mind if you ask them to move something breakable from your child's reach or to move their coffee cup from the corner of a table. Be careful around animals that are unused to children: err on the side of caution and keep your child well away. If you plan to leave your child in another person's care, make sure that you are happy the environment is safe enough – don't leave your child if you are worried.

Be extra vigilant if there is a pond: about 80 per cent of drownings in garden ponds happen when children are visiting friends or relatives. If you go to a park where there is a pond or lake, keep very close to your child.

CAR JOURNEYS

All children should be fastened into properly fitted car seats for car journeys, however short. Never be tempted to take a trip holding your child in your lap; you will not be able to hold on to the child if your car is hit, and you could injure him or her with your body on impact.

Choose a car seat that meets recognized safety standards, and check with the manufacturer that it is suitable for your particular car. Don't buy a second-hand car seat: you won't know if it has been weakened in a previous accident, and it may have been made to less rigorous safety standards than a new seat.

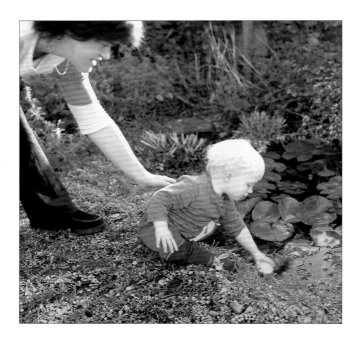

WHICH CAR SEAT?

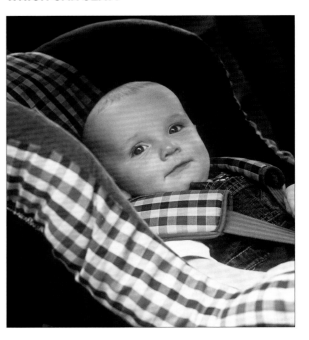

Babies (Group 0): Rear-facing seats are needed for babies from birth to 10–13kg/22–29lb. But it is best to avoid taking a very young baby on a long car journey if you can. Keep your baby in this first car seat until he or she outgrows it.

Older babies and toddlers (Group 1): Forward-facing seats are suitable for children from about nine months (so long as they can sit up well unsupported and weigh at least 9kg/20lb). They last until the child is about four and weighs 18kg/40lb.

Young children (Group 2): Booster seats are suitable for children weighing 15–25kg/33–55lb, usually between the ages of four and six. Like car seats for younger children, they are best fitted in the back of the car rather than the front, and this is essential if there is an airbag in the front of the car. They don't have a separate harness as car seats do; instead the seatbelt goes around both the seat and the child.

Older children (Group 3): Children should use some sort of booster seat until they reach the age of 11. Booster cushions are used for children weighing 22–36kg/48–79lb.

Children are instinctively drawn by water. Never leave your child unattended in a garden with a pond; keep him or her in sight at all times.

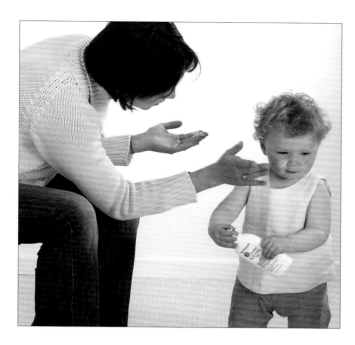

Around 10 minutes of sun early or late in the day helps your child to make essential vitamin D. But he or she needs a high-factor suncream at other times.

Many car seats are fitted incorrectly, so go to a specialist if you need help. If your car is new, go for an ISOFIX car seat, which is much easier to fit.

- Never fit a car seat in the front seat of a car if there is an airbag in front of it – the airbag could seriously harm (and possibly kill) your child if it inflates. It is safer to fit the seat in the back even if there is no airbag.
- Make sure that the seat belt goes through all guides on the seat.
- Check the seat belt is pulled tight before every journey: the seat shouldn't rock sideways or forwards when you try to move it.
- Don't have the buckle of the seatbelt resting on the frame of the car seat; it could snap open in an accident.
- Adjust the harness so it fits snugly. Check it at the start of every journey, as the fit will depend on what your child is wearing. Don't have the buckle resting on your child's tummy.
- If you are using a booster seat, make sure the seatbelt rests against your child's shoulder, not his neck, and from hip bone to hip bone.

OUT IN THE SUN

Children's skin is thinner than adults', so you need to be vigilant about protecting it from sunburn: damage to the skin now could have long-term effects. Babies under six months should be kept out of direct sunlight entirely. If your baby is in a buggy or pram, use a UV sunshade. If you are carrying a baby in a sling, cover his or her arms and legs with a light but closely woven fabric such as cotton and get a wide-brimmed hat.

SUN FOODS
Foods containing the antioxidant beta-carotene may help protect the skin from the harmful effects of the sun. Carrots, melons, mango, apricots and spinach are all good sources that are worth including in your child's summer diet.

Put sunscreen on the baby's hands and feet if they are exposed. Older babies and young children should be kept out of direct sunlight as much as possible during the hottest part of the day (10am–4pm on very hot days). Apply a high-factor sunscreen at least half an hour before you go outside. Use a sunscreen made from natural ingredients with an SPF of at least 20. This will be gentler on your child's skin than very high factor sunscreens that last three or four hours (but which may get rubbed off beforehand in any case). Apply a thick layer and let it sink into the skin rather than rubbing in. Reapply frequently. However, if you know that your child is going to be out in the sun for some time, especially in someone else's care, use a higher factor to be on the safe side. Remember that skin can still burn on warm cloudy days, or in the shade next to water or sand, which reflects sunlight.

Your child will need more fluids when it is hot. If you are breastfeeding, nurse frequently: your milk has a higher water content on hot days so your baby shouldn't need extra drinks.

Some children refuse to hold hands when they are out and about – in which case you will need reins or a wrist strap to keep them safe.

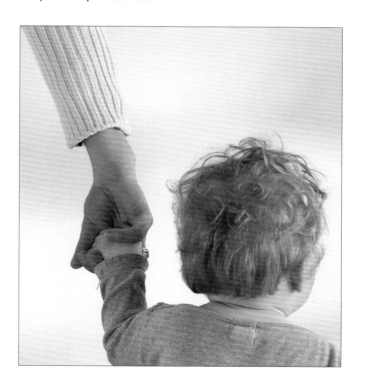

Meal planners and recipes

“ It is always good to include your young child in family meal times and it is easy to adapt your cooking for adults and young children. **”**

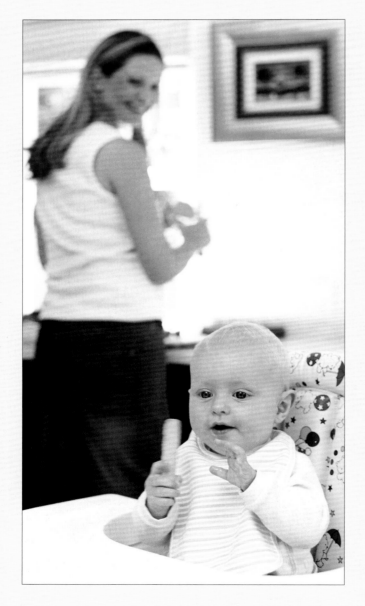

Cooking for children – like most other aspects of childcare – can be very pleasurable but also intensely frustrating. All parents have had the experience of seeing a lovingly prepared meal rejected entirely, flung on the floor or spat out in disgust. Children don't appreciate the effort that you put into making their meals. It's not a criticism of your cooking or your care.

It will take some of the tension out of meal times if you cook batches of food in advance and put them in the freezer. If there is a gap between the time when you cook the food and the time when you serve it, then you will take it less personally if your child merely toys with a couple of spoonfuls. This chapter includes some tried-and-tested recipes that can be spooned into small pots and frozen. Even if you have no home-cooked meals in the freezer, you don't have to resort to processed food. There are plenty of quick meals you can make without much effort: boiled rice with tiny chunks of cheese and peas, pasta with grated fresh tomato, scrambled eggs, and sardines

While your baby still instinctively tests things with his or her mouth, take advantage of this inquisitiveness and offer as many different textures and flavours as you can.

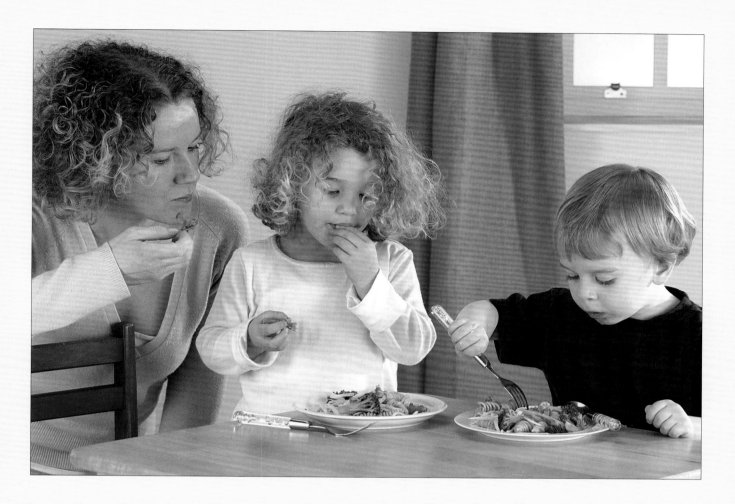

on toast. All these take a few minutes to prepare, and are often a child's favourite meals.

Of course, it is always good to include your young child in family mealtimes and it is easy to adapt your cooking to suit adults and young children. When you make soup or casseroles, for example, get into the habit of using homemade stock or a low-salt bouillon, and then adding salt at the table to your own portion if you need it.

Children are amenable to a little spice in their food, but are unlikely to take to an intensely flavoured, fiery curry. If you are making a curry, stir in the hotter spices once you have taken out your child's portion. Always offer new foods or unusual tastes as something interesting to try rather than something they have to like and eat.

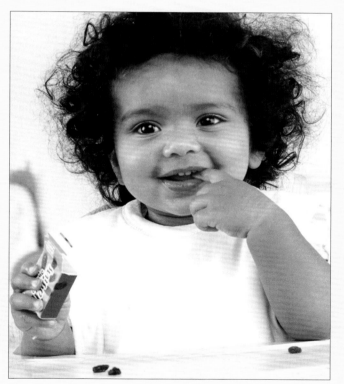

Top: As children get older they enjoy eating in company and start to appreciate the social side of meal times. Encourage this by eating with them whenever you can.

Children love sweet things, but keep their sugary snacks to a minimum and offer dried or fresh fruit rather than biscuits and cakes.

Meal planning for babies

First foods should be easy for babies to eat and digest, so baby rice, puréed root vegetables and pears and apples are ideal, but there is no strict rule about exactly which foods to give first, so it is fine if you want to chop and change. However, do make sure you don't introduce any foods that may cause an allergic reaction until the ages recommended in Chapter 5. The menu planner on the opposite page starts at six months: if you are starting solids earlier, you will have to adapt it slightly so that you don't introduce foods such as chicken, fish or wheat too early.

INTRODUCING SOLIDS

It helps your baby to adjust to new flavours if you mix each food with his or her usual milk or with milky baby rice for the first few times you give it.

FOOD PLANNER

This planner will help you when introducing your baby to solid food. It suggests which foods to introduce when, but remember that each week you will be adding a different food, not feeding your baby only that one, so by week 4, for example, you will be trying baby rice, carrot, squash and pear.

Week	Introduce
1	baby rice
2	carrot
3	squash or swede (rutabaga)
4	pear
5	parsnip, apple
6	banana, potato, rice cakes
7	courgette (zucchini), mango, melon
8	green beans, nectarine/peach
9	natural yoghurt, red lentils
10	leeks, chicken, cauliflower
11	oats, cheese
12	white fish, grain such as quinoa, polenta or millet
13	pasta, onions, grapes
14	bread, lamb
15	beans, spinach
16	apricots, celery, sweet (bell) peppers
17	tomatoes, salmon
18	aubergine (eggplant), mushrooms
19	peas, egg yolk
20	tofu or beef, citrus fruit (such as mandarins)

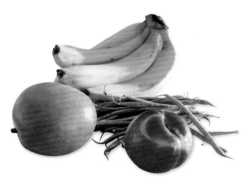

Giving fruits and vegetables of different colours will help your child to get a good range of vitamins.

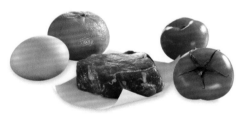

Meat, eggs, tomatoes and citrus fruits can be introduced once the baby is well established on solids.

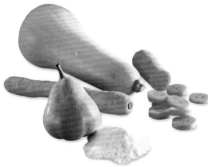

You can gradually introduce a wider variety of fruits and vegetables to your child.

Babies like sweet tastes, so root vegetables, pears and apples mixed with baby rice are good first foods.

Alternate the new food with foods you have already introduced, so that your baby gets used to having different tastes at every meal. You can combine purées, too, mixing squash and carrot, carrot and parsnip, parsnip and apple and so on. Be sure to leave three days before introducing each new food, to allow time for any reaction to show itself. However, once your baby is eating lots of different foods, you can introduce a flavouring such as garlic at the same time as, say, lentils. Remember that you shouldn't cut down on milk feeds until the end of the first year.

PLANNING YOUR MENUS

Once you have a few meals prepared and stored in the freezer, it's easy to give your baby a good and varied diet. Pasta or rice with butter, cheese and a few chopped

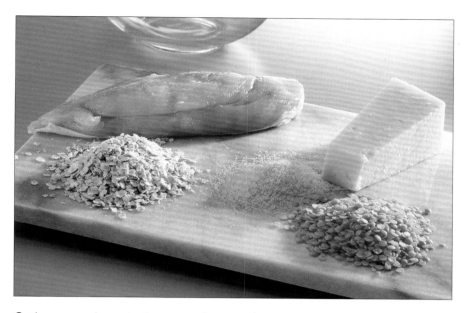

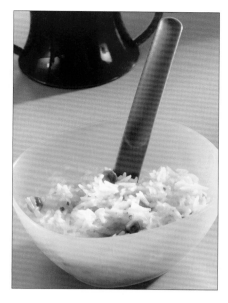

Grains are an important source of energy, while chicken, pulses and dairy foods are good protein foods.

vegetables mixed in, or mashed avocado, make a good quick meal if you run out. Your baby may need a few snacks as well as the usual milk in between meals. Use the menu planner as a guide, and remember that so long as you vary foods throughout a week, your baby will be getting a good mix of nutrients, even if on one day they refuse to eat anything other than grapes.

Breastfed babies will usually have more milk feeds, but a routine might look like this:

A good quick meal is rice with a spoonful of cooked vegetables and some grated cheese.

On waking Milk, then breakfast
11.30 am Lunch with water
2.30 pm Milk and afternoon snack
5.00 pm Supper with water
7.00 pm Milk

MENU PLANNER FOR A BABY FROM NINE TO TWELVE MONTHS

Adapt this to your needs and routine and vary it if you need to.

Day 1
Breakfast Oat porridge with banana
Lunch Tarragon chicken with potatoes
  Plain yoghurt
Snack Pear slices and toast fingers
Supper Vegetable soup with rice

Day 2
Breakfast Oat/millet porridge with pear purée
  Toast fingers
Lunch Lentil dhal with rice or quinoa and spinach
Snack Rice cakes and apple slices
Supper Pasta with peas, olive oil and cheese
  Mango purée

Day 3
Breakfast Wheat biscuit cereal with banana
Lunch Cauliflower and broccoli cheese
  Raspberry and apple purée
Snack Polenta fingers and pear slices
Supper Fish pilau

Day 4
Breakfast Oat porridge with mango and cinnamon
  Toast fingers
Lunch Beany bake
Snack Rice cakes, grapes
Supper Buttery rice with swede (rutabaga) purée and broccoli
  Natural yoghurt with fruit purée

Day 5
Breakfast Millet porridge with pear and banana
Lunch Ratatouille with pitta fingers
  Strawberries or raspberries with

Greek yoghurt
Snack Oatcakes and melon chunks
Supper Lamb casserole with rice

Day 6
Breakfast Wheat biscuit cereal with pear
Lunch Poached salmon with rice, sugar snap peas and cooked tomato
Snack Banana
Supper Vegetable soup and mini cream cheese sandwiches (add pineapple to the cheese and blend to a purée)

Day 7
Breakfast Oat porridge with banana
Lunch Couscous salad
  Apricot compote
Snack Polenta fingers and grapes
Supper Lightly fried chicken fillet, rice and steamed carrot sticks

Recipes for babies: six to nine months

Once your baby is eating a range of foods, you can start combining ingredients to make more interesting meals. Here are some suggestions for easy-to-cook, baby-friendly dishes.

BABY RICE

It's worth making your own baby rice once your baby is eating more than a couple of teaspoonfuls at a time. You won't get it as smooth as the commercial variety, but this is a good way to start introducing texture. Use white rice not brown.

50g/2oz white rice
Breast or formula milk

Bring a small saucepan of water to the boil, add the rice and stir once. Leave to simmer for about 10 minutes, until the rice grains are tender. Drain the rice, then purée with your baby's usual milk.

COURGETTE PURÉE

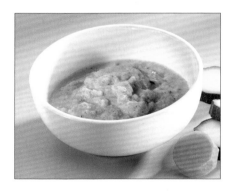

Steamed courgettes (zucchini) go well with sweet carrots. Leave the skin on the carrot if it is organic.

1 courgette
1 carrot

Chop the courgette and peel and chop the carrot. Put the carrot in a steamer and cook for 5 minutes. Add the courgette and steam for another 10 minutes, until both vegetables are very soft. Purée with your baby's usual milk or use a little of the water used to steam the vegetables.

POTATO, SWEDE AND SWEET POTATO MASH

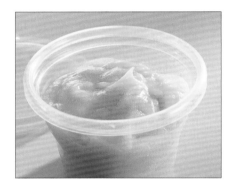

Root vegetables purée well and have a nice sweet taste. You can add a pinch of garam masala to the combination to liven it up once your baby is well established on solid foods and ready for new tastes.

2 large potatoes
Quarter of a small swede (rutabaga)
1 small sweet potato

Peel and dice all the vegetables and steam them for 15–20 minutes, until soft. Blend or mash with your baby's usual milk until smooth.

CHICKEN, PARSNIP AND GREEN BEAN PURÉE

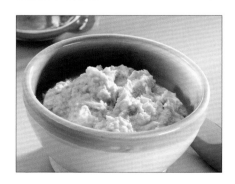

Any vegetable purée goes well with chicken, but parsnip has a wonderfully sweet taste that babies love. Use broccoli or leeks in place of the beans if you like.

1 parsnip
50g/2oz fine green beans
1 small chicken breast
A little olive oil, for frying

Cut the parsnip into quarters lengthways. Cut out the woody core from each piece then chop into small chunks. Top and tail the beans. Steam the parsnip for 5 minutes then add the green beans to the steamer and continue cooking for another 10 minutes, until are soft.

Meanwhile, cut the chicken breast into small pieces. Heat a little olive oil in a frying pan, and fry the chicken for 6–7 minutes until cooked through. Combine the cooked chicken with the vegetables and blend or mash until smooth.

VEGETABLE SOUP

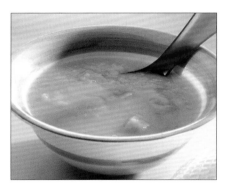

Soup slips down easily, so it is great for times when your baby is tired and doesn't want to eat much. This is a simple recipe that you can also use as a pasta sauce. Substitute celery for the leeks if you like, but in this case add half a chopped onion to the pan and fry for 2–3 minutes before adding the other vegetables.

STOCK

Most commercial stocks are too salty for babies. Good supermarkets and health food stores stock low-salt, good-quality bouillon, but, better still, make your own – it's pretty easy and once you get into the habit of doing it you won't want to go back to cubes. Store stock in the refrigerator for up to 4 days or freeze for up to 3 months.

For vegetable stock

Chop 1 celery stick, 1 large carrot, 1 large leek, 1 onion and 1 garlic clove. Put in a pan with 5 peppercorns, 2 sprigs of parsley (or parsley stalks), 2 sprigs of thyme and a bay leaf. Cover with 1.2 litres/2 pints/5 cups water, and bring to the boil. Skim off any froth, cover the pan, reduce the heat and simmer for 45 minutes. Leave to cool. Pour through a sieve lined with muslin (a baby muslin is ideal).

For chicken stock

Break up the carcass of a cooked chicken. Chop 1 onion, 1 carrot and 1 celery stick and place in a pan with the chicken bones, 5 peppercorns, 2 cloves, a small handful of parsley (or parsley stalks) and a bay leaf. Cover with 1.2 litres/2 pints/5 cups water, and bring to the boil. Skim off any froth, cover the pan, reduce the heat and simmer for 1 hour. Fish out the big bones, then strain through a muslin-lined sieve.

---

2 medium leeks, cleaned
4 large potatoes
2 carrots
A little olive oil, for frying
1.2 litres/2 pints/5 cups vegetable
    stock
Handful of parsley, finely chopped

Slice the leeks. Cut the potatoes into large chunks, and peel (unless organic) and slice the carrots.

Put a little olive oil in a pan over a low heat and add the vegetables. Cook for 5 minutes, stirring all the time. Add the stock, bring to a simmer, cover and cook for 25 minutes. Add the parsley and cook for 5 minutes, then blend.

LENTIL DHAL

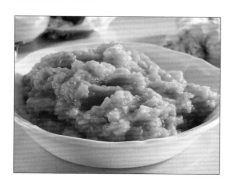

Babies love dhal. You can purée this one with a serving of baby rice and some sliced cooked spinach to make a balanced meal in one – it's good with a spoonful of bio-active yoghurt. You can also add a spoonful of dhal to vegetable soup to make it a more substantial meal.

50g/2oz red lentils, washed
Small slice of ginger
Half a clove of garlic (sliced
    lengthways)
1 bay leaf
1 tomato (optional)

Place the lentils in a small pan. Pour in water up to a level about one and a half times the depth of the lentils. Add the ginger, garlic and bay leaf.

Bring to the boil, skim off any froth, reduce the heat, cover the pan and simmer for about 25 minutes or until the lentils are very tender.

Meanwhile, pour boiling water over the tomato, if using. Leave for a minute or two, remove the skin, cut in half, deseed and chop finely.

When the lentils are soft, discard the ginger and bay leaf, but mash the garlic into the dhal. Add the chopped tomato, if using, and cook for another 5 minutes. Blend if your baby is still eating smooth purées.
Variation: For a spicier dhal, fry half an onion in vegetable oil. Add 1.5ml/ $1/4$ tsp each of ground coriander and ground cumin and fry for a further minute or two. Add this to the dhal.

RASPBERRY AND APPLE PURÉE

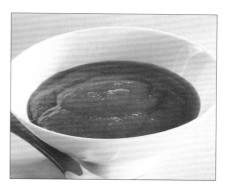

Simple fruit purées are a great way of getting vitamins into your baby.

1 eating apple, peeled and diced
115g/4oz raspberries

Place the fruit in a small pan with a tablespoon of water. Cook over a low heat for 5 minutes, or until soft. Purée the fruit, then pass through a sieve to remove the seeds.

APRICOT COMPOTE

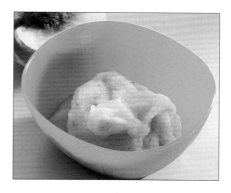

3 ready-to-eat dried apricots
1 eating apple, peeled and diced
1 large nectarine, stoned

Chop the apricots and nectarine. Place all the fruits in a small pan with a little water. Simmer for about 10 minutes, until very soft, then purée.

Recipes for babies: nine to twelve months

Once you have introduced a reasonable number of different foods, cooking for your baby becomes a lot more fun. Here are some baby-friendly meals that older children (and adults) will love too.

CAULIFLOWER AND BROCCOLI CHEESE

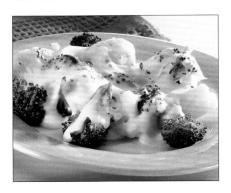

You can add this cheese sauce to any cooked vegetables, or pasta. Use formula or full-fat cow's milk, and choose a cheese with a good flavour – babies like stronger tastes than you might think.

1 small cauliflower, in florets
1 head of broccoli, in florets

For the cheese sauce:
50g/2oz butter
20ml/1 rounded tbsp flour
300ml/½ pint/1¼ cups full-fat milk
115g/4oz Cheddar cheese, grated
Dab of English mustard (enough to cover the tip of a teaspoon)
Pinch of cayenne pepper

Steam the vegetables for about 10–12 minutes until soft.

Meanwhile, to make the sauce, melt the butter in a small pan. Stir in the flour for 1 minute, until the flour is completely cooked. Very slowly pour in the milk, stirring all the time. It will go into a lump at first, but keep stirring and adding the milk slowly. Bring the mixture slowly to the boil, then take the pan off the heat. Add the cheese, mustard and cayenne pepper. Keep stirring.

Add the sauce to the vegetables. Purée in a blender or mash well with a fork, depending on the age of your baby. If you are cooking for an older child, leave the florets whole.

TARRAGON CHICKEN

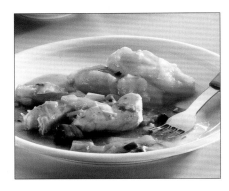

If you are bringing your child up to eat meat, chicken is likely to figure often on the menu. This easy stew contains leeks and mushrooms, but you can add other vegetables as well. Choose organic chicken.

2 large chicken breast fillets
2 medium leeks, washed
A little vegetable oil, for frying
Knob of butter
450ml/¾ pint/2 cups stock, or to cover
Handful of parsley, chopped
1 sprig fresh tarragon (or a large pinch of dried tarragon)
450g/1lb large flat mushrooms
5ml/1 tsp cornflour
Freshly ground black pepper

Cut the chicken into small chunks. Finely chop the leeks.

Heat the vegetable oil in a flameproof casserole or a deep heavy-bottomed frying pan. Fry the chicken in two or three batches over a medium heat for 6–7 minutes, until cooked through. Set aside.

Add the butter to the same pan and cook the leeks for 6–7 minutes until softened but not browned. Return the chicken to the pan. Add the stock and season with a couple of twists of black pepper. Add the herbs and leave to simmer for 10 minutes, uncovered, stirring from time to time, until slightly reduced. Chop the mushrooms very small and add to the pan. Cook for a further 6–7 minutes until cooked down.

When the stew is cooked, put about 50ml/2 fl oz/¼ cup water in a cup. Sprinkle in the cornflour and stir until dissolved. Add the mixture to the stew and cook for a further 2–3 minutes to thicken the sauce.

Variation: You can add 450g/1lb new potatoes, chopped into small dice, to the stew to make a complete meal. If you want to add more vegetables, try half a green (bell) pepper or a large carrot, diced. Cook the potatoes and the extra vegetables with the leeks.

LAMB CASSEROLE

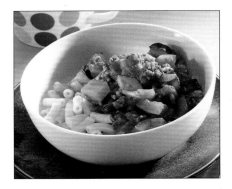

Red meat is the best source of iron, so it is good to include it in your child's diet. Lamb is the first red meat to introduce to your baby: it is very easy to digest and most babies love it. Make sure you choose lean minced (ground) lamb, or trim the meat and mince it yourself, as lamb can be fatty. Choose organic meat if you can.

A little vegetable oil, for frying
450g/1lb minced (ground) lamb
1 large onion, finely chopped
2 large carrots, diced
2 courgettes (zucchini), diced
225g/½lb mushrooms, diced
300ml/½ pints/1¼ cups vegetable stock
400g/14oz can chopped tomatoes
5ml/1 tsp tomato purée
Pinch of mixed herbs
5ml/1 tsp cornflour

Heat a little vegetable oil in a flameproof casserole or a deep, heavy-bottomed frying pan. Brown the meat in two or three batches for about 5 minutes over a high heat. Set aside.

Lower the heat under the pan and add the chopped onion and carrot. Cook for 5–6 minutes, until softened. Add the courgettes and mushrooms and cook until soft.

Return the meat to the pan, then pour over the stock. Stir in the canned tomatoes, the tomato purée and the herbs. Cover and simmer for 40 minutes. Stir from time to time.

Put about 50ml/2 fl oz/¼ cup water in a cup. Sprinkle in the cornflour and stir until dissolved.

Add the mixture to the stew and cook for a further 2–3 minutes to thicken the sauce.

SIMPLE FISH PILAU

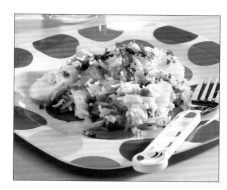

This is a simple fish dish that you can make just as easily with salmon.

200g/7oz cod or haddock fillet
Milk to cover
1 onion, finely chopped
2 garlic cloves, crushed
A little olive oil, for frying
Knob of butter
200g/7oz basmati rice
600ml/1 pint/2½ cups vegetable or fish stock
225g/8oz tomatoes
50g/2oz frozen peas
Small handful of parsley, chopped
Freshly ground black pepper

Place the fish in a small pan and cover with milk. Cook on a low heat until the fish is just opaque – about 5–7 minutes.

Heat a little olive oil in a frying pan. Add the onion and garlic and sweat for 6–7 minutes, until softened but not browned. Add the butter to the pan and let it melt, then add the rice, and stir until coated. Pour in half the stock and stir until it is absorbed into the rice, then add the rest a little at a time until the rice is cooked (about 25 minutes). Skin and deseed the tomatoes and chop, add with the peas to the rice mixture, and cook for a further 5 minutes.

Flake the cooked fish, removing any bones, and add to the rice with the herbs. Season with a twist of black pepper, and cook the pilau for a further 2–3 minutes, stirring.

RATATOUILLE

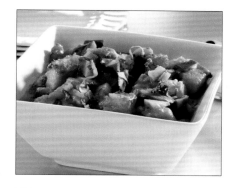

This is great with mashed potato, rice or buttery pasta.

Half a small onion, chopped
A little olive oil, for frying
1 clove garlic, chopped
1 red (bell) pepper, diced
2 courgettes (zucchini), diced
1 aubergine (eggplant), diced
2 large mushrooms, diced
4 tomatoes, peeled and chopped
5ml/1 tsp sun-dried tomato paste
Small handful of basil, chopped

Pour a little olive oil into a frying pan over a low heat and fry the onion for 6–7 minutes, until softened. Add the garlic, pepper, courgette, aubergine and mushrooms and cook for 7–8 minutes. Add the tomatoes, tomato paste and herbs. Cook for a further 15 minutes, uncovered, stirring gently from time to time.

FOOD ON THE GO
Sticks of cheese, mini sandwiches, easy-to-eat fruit or small pots of natural yoghurt are all ideal foods to take out with you. For a more substantial lunch, you could make an easy couscous or pasta salad.

Couscous salad
Pour a serving of couscous into a teacup and cover with boiling water. Add 5ml/1 tsp olive oil, cover and leave for 3–4 minutes for the grains to swell. Cook a few peas, and a chopped tomato in a pan with a tiny amount of water. Add to the couscous with some Cheddar cheese cut into tiny dice.

Pasta salad
Combine some cooked pasta shapes with some finely diced, cooked carrots and peas, flaked canned tuna, chopped parsley and a little olive oil.

Meal planning for toddlers and older children

This two-week plan gives a good, mixed diet with plenty of variety: it uses some simple meals together with recipes from the preceding and following pages. It's a good idea to keep introducing new recipes and ingredients from time to time. But don't worry if your child rejects the unfamiliar at first – children often need to see a new food a few times before they decide to try it.

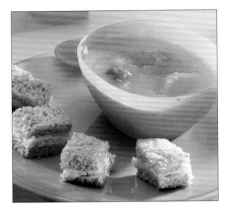

Vegetable soup with sandwiches.

Day 1
Breakfast Oat porridge with pear
  Plain yoghurt
Morning snack Toast with yeast extract, cheese chunks and apple
Lunch Lightly fried chicken, quinoa or rice and peas
Afternoon snack Oatcakes spread with butter and a few raisins
Supper Hummus, vegetable dippers and pitta fingers

Day 2
Breakfast Oat or millet porridge with banana and cinnamon
Morning snack Polenta fingers, cheese slices and apple
Lunch Pasta with pepper sauce
Afternoon snack Pancakes (older children can help to make them)
Supper Fishcakes and green beans
  Mango and yoghurt

Tuna pizza

Day 3
Breakfast Wheat biscuit cereal with apple slices
Morning snack Polenta fingers and grapes
Lunch Sardines on toast
Afternoon snack Rice cakes and grapes
Supper Vegetable soup and mini sandwiches

Day 4
Breakfast Oat porridge and mango
Morning snack Mashed banana on toast
Lunch Fish pilau
  Raspberry and apple purée with yoghurt or fromage frais
Afternoon snack Oatcakes and melon chunks
Supper Pasta with basic tomato sauce

Day 5
Breakfast Millet porridge with raisins and cinnamon
Morning snack Mini nut butter sandwiches
Lunch Homemade pizza with vegetable topping
  Natural yoghurt and/or fruit
Afternoon snack Carrot and cucumber sticks and cheese sticks
Supper Tarragon chicken with steamed potatoes

Day 6
Breakfast Wheat biscuit cereal with pear
Morning snack Toast with yeast extract, grapes
Lunch Spanish omelette with vegetable sticks
Afternoon snack Mini pitta with hummus, grated carrot, shredded lettuce and diced tomatoes
Supper Lamb casserole

Day 7
Breakfast Oat porridge with banana
Morning snack Rice cakes and apple slices
Lunch Borscht served with herby garlic bread or pitta fingers
Afternoon snack Spanish omelette (leftover)

Hummus with vegetables and pitta.

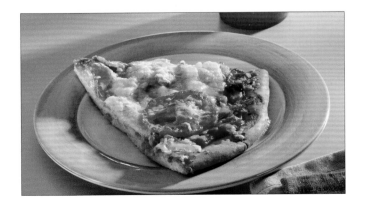

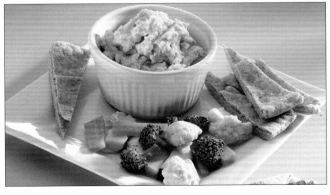

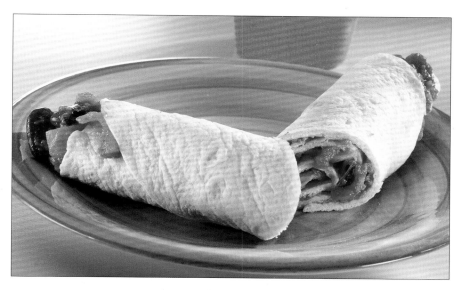

Flatbreads filled with beany bake.

Supper Beany bake in flatbreads with grated cheese

Day 8
Breakfast Wheat biscuit cereal and a plum
Morning snack Polenta fingers with apple slices
Lunch Poached salmon with mashed potatoes, steamed green beans and carrots
Afternoon snack Oatcake and pear
Supper Scrambled eggs on toast

Day 9
Breakfast Yoghurt, pear and toast with yeast extract
Morning snack Rice cakes and apricot or plum
Lunch Butter bean purée on toast
  Grapes and cheese slices

Fish cakes and peas.

Afternoon snack Carrot sticks and hummus
Supper Vegetable soup with a few added haricot (navy) beans

Day 10
Breakfast Millet and oat porridge with apricot compote
Morning snack Oatcakes spread with cream cheese
Lunch Ratatouille with rice or rolled up in flatbreads
Afternoon snack Banana and rice cakes
Supper Dhal with shredded spinach, rice and green beans

Day 11
Breakfast Wheat biscuit cereal with banana
Morning snack Mini sandwiches with peanut butter and grated apple
Lunch Fried chicken fillet, couscous salad and broccoli
  Papaya slices
Afternoon snack Rice cakes and

nectarine slices
Supper Macaroni cheese with peas and carrots

Day 12
Breakfast Oat porridge with apple purée and cinnamon
Morning snack Yoghurt and banana
Lunch Easy fishcakes made with haddock
  Fruit salad of mixed soft fruits sweetened with a little orange juice
Afternoon snack Rice cakes and pear slices
Supper Pasta with pesto

Day 13
Breakfast Scrambled egg on toast, pear slices
Morning snack Rice cakes, raisins and plain yoghurt
Lunch Cauliflower and broccoli cheese
Afternoon snack Polenta slices and an apricot, or apricot purée
Supper Shepherd's pie (Lamb casserole topped with mash)

Day 14
Breakfast Oat porridge with pear and raisins
Morning snack Banana and breadsticks
Lunch Fish pilau made with salmon
  Plain yoghurt
Afternoon snack Apple and cheese sticks
Supper Vegetable soup with pitta fingers

Pasta and pesto with cheese.

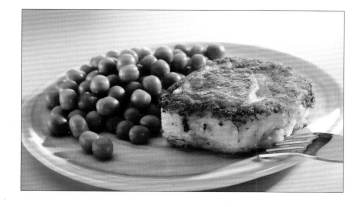

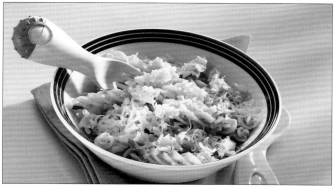

Recipes for toddlers and older children

In theory, older children can eat pretty much what adults do. But you may find that your meals are a bit too spicy or salty for your toddler. These recipes are good for all the family, but they can also be frozen in small portions for the occasions when you want to eat different things or at different times from your child.

BEANY BAKE

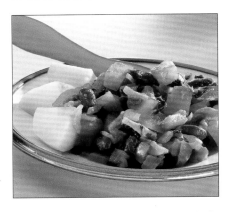

This is a good recipe for the whole family. Older children may like to eat it in flatbreads (Mexican tortillas) with cheese sprinkled on top.

1 onion, chopped
1 green (bell) pepper, chopped
1 garlic clove, crushed
A little vegetable oil, for frying
10ml/2 tsp ground cumin
400g/14oz can chopped tomatoes
5ml/1 tsp tomato paste
Half a small swede (rutabaga), diced
3 carrots, diced
150g/5oz mushrooms, chopped
2 sticks celery, chopped
120ml/4fl oz vegetable stock
400g/14oz can red kidney beans
Handful of coriander (cilantro) or parsley, finely chopped

Preheat the oven to 180°C/350°F/ Gas 4. Heat a little vegetable oil in a flameproof casserole. Add the onion, pepper and garlic and cook for 6–7 minutes, until softened. Add the cumin and cook for another minute.

Add the canned tomatoes, tomato purée, swede, carrots, mushrooms and celery, together with the stock, and season with a couple of twists of black pepper. Cover and cook in the oven for 30 minutes, stirring halfway through the cooking.

Add the kidney beans and cook for another 15 minutes, until the beans are heated through and the vegetables are tender. Stir in the coriander or parsley before serving.

BEETROOT BORSCHT

More of a vegetable stew than a soup, borscht is a great way to get children eating cabbage, which is high in vitamin C and antioxidants. Let your child watch you add the beetroot so he or she can see the soup change colour.

45ml/3 tbsp oil
1 onion, chopped
2 carrots, grated
15ml/1 tsp tomato paste
450g/1lb firm white cabbage, shredded
2 large potatoes, peeled
1.2 litres/2 pints/5 cups hot vegetable or chicken stock
1 cooked beetroot, grated
Sour cream or Greek (US strained plain) yoghurt, to serve
Handful of dill, finely chopped, to serve

Heat 30ml/2 tbsp of the oil in a frying pan and cook the onion and carrot gently for about 10 minutes. Stir in the tomato purée to form a paste.

Chop the shredded cabbage and dice the potatoes. Heat the remaining oil in a large, heavy pan and add the diced potatoes and cabbage. Turn the vegetables for a couple of minutes just to soften slightly, then add the hot stock. Cook for about 15 minutes until the vegetables are soft.

Add the paste from the frying pan and season with a few twists of black pepper. At this stage, you will have an orange-coloured stew.

Add the beetroot to the pan. This will turn the stew a vibrant purple. Bring to the boil and removed from the heat (if it boils too long it loses its colour). Serve the borscht topping with a blob of sour cream and a sprinkling of dill.

HERBY GARLIC BREAD

Any idea that children don't like garlic is quickly dispelled when garlic bread is on offer. If you don't need a whole loaf, cut the prepared bread into portions, wrap each in foil and freeze. This is good with pretty much any soup or vegetable stew.

French loaf
2 cloves garlic, crushed
Handful of parsley and oregano, finely chopped
250g/9oz unsalted butter, softened

Preheat the oven to 180°C/350°F/Gas 4. Cut the bread into 1cm/½in slices, but don't cut right the way through, so that the base of the loaf stays in once piece. Stir the garlic and herbs into the butter, combining well. Spread the garlic butter on both sides of each slice, and spread any leftover butter over the top of the loaf. Wrap the bread tightly in foil and bake for 20 minutes.

SARDINES ON TOAST

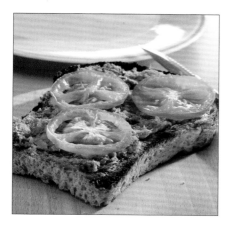

This is a tasty quick meal, and a great way to get your child to eat oily fish. Sardines contain bones that are edible and a good source of calcium, but mash the fish well before using.

Small can of sardines
1 large tomato
2 slices wholemeal (whole-wheat)
bread

Preheat the grill. Halve the fish, remove the backbones if you wish. Mash well. Slice the tomato thinly.

Brown one side of the bread slices under the grill then spread the mashed fish over the uncooked side. Top with slices of tomato.

Grill (broil) until the fish is heated through completely. Any exposed bread will burn in this time, but you can just cut off any charred bits.

BUTTER BEAN PURÉE

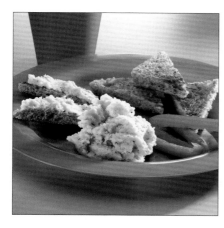

This purée goes wonderfully on toast, or with vegetable dippers such as carrot sticks or slices of red (bell)

pepper. You can add a pinch of paprika or garam masala to spice up the purée if you like.

Small can of butter (lima) beans
50g/2oz Cheddar cheese
30ml/2 tbsp olive oil
½ garlic clove, crushed
10ml/2 tsp very finely chopped
parsley

Mash the butter beans and grate the cheese. Stir the olive oil into the beans with the crushed garlic clove, parsley and cheese. Blend to a thick purée.

SPANISH OMELETTE

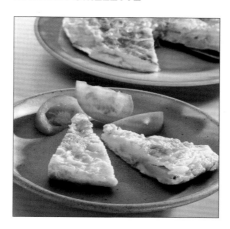

This is an almost universally popular dish. Serve it with sliced tomatoes and carrot sticks. You'll need a small, deep frying pan (about 20cm/8in), and a larger one to fry the onions and potatoes. The omelette is best eaten at room temperature.

1 medium onion
450g/1lb potatoes
30ml2 tbsp olive oil
4 large eggs
Splash of milk
Pinch of sea salt
Good twist of black pepper
Small pinch of cayenne pepper

Halve the onion then slice it thinly into half moons. Peel and slice the potatoes. Heat the oil in a large frying pan and cook the potatoes and onions over a medium heat for 8–10 minutes. Keep stirring so they soften without browning. Turn the

heat as low as possible, cover the pan and leave to cook for 20 minutes, stirring occasionally, until soft. Meanwhile, beat the eggs lightly with the milk and seasoning and set aside.

Transfer the cooked potatoes and onions to a small, deep frying pan and place on the same low heat. Give the pan 1–2 minutes to heat up, then pour in the omelette mixture. It should run into all the gaps between the potatoes and onions. Cook gently, uncovered, for 20 minutes, or until the mixture is cooked through.

When the omelette is done brown the top under the grill for 2–3 minutes. Place a plate over the pan and turn out the omelette. Leave it to cool for 10 minutes or so – it may fall apart if you try to cut it straight away.

BASIC TOMATO SAUCE
This sauce is good for pasta and pizza topping. The sugar balances the acidity of the tomatoes, but you can leave it out. For a more substantial pasta sauce, add flaked canned tuna. Any vegetable can be added to this sauce.

15ml/1 tbsp olive oil
½ onion, chopped
1 clove garlic, finely chopped
400g/14oz can plum tomatoes
5ml/1 tsp tomato paste or sun-
dried tomato paste
Pinch of dried oregano
1 bay leaf
2.5ml/½ tsp sugar

Heat the oil in a saucepan and soften the onion and garlic in it. Cook over a low heat and do not let them brown. Pour in the tomatoes, breaking them up, and add the rest of the ingredients. Cook, covered, over a low heat for 30–40 minutes, until thick, stirring from time to time. Blend or use as it is.

QUICK HUMMUS

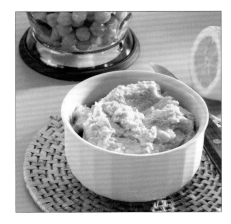

Toddlers love dips, and they are a good way to get them eating raw vegetables. Try thin sticks of carrot, red (bell) pepper, celery or lightly cooked green beans, broccoli and cauliflower florets. Hummus won't freeze but it will keep for a couple of days in the refrigerator.

400g/14oz can chickpeas
½ clove garlic
Squeeze of lemon juice
30–45ml/2–3 tbsp Greek (US strained plain) yoghurt

Blend the chickpeas with the garlic and lemon juice until smooth. Add enough Greek yoghurt to make a good consistency.

EASY FISHCAKES

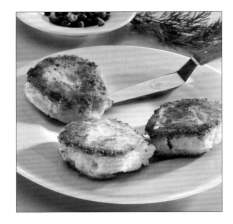

You can make these with any fish – fresh salmon, cod or haddock, or canned salmon or tuna. If you are using canned fish, halve the quantity specified here, as it has a much stronger flavour. The mashed potato should be cold, so this is a good way of using up leftovers.

450g/1lb potatoes
Knob of butter
Milk (see recipe)
200g/7oz salmon fillets, skinned
15ml/1 tbsp capers (optional)
Handful of parsley or dill, finely chopped
Flour
Vegetable oil, for frying

Peel the potatoes and cut into even-sized chunks. Place them in a large pan of water and bring to the boil. Simmer for about 20 minutes or until cooked. Drain, mash with butter and a little milk, then leave to cool.

Place the salmon in a small pan and cover with milk. Bring to a simmer and poach gently for about 6–7 minutes, or until the salmon flesh is opaque all the way through. Drain the fish and flake it very carefully, removing any bones.

Mix the mashed potato and fish together well, adding the capers, if using, and the parsley or dill. Shape the mixture into about six small balls.

Sprinkle the flour on to a plate. Heat some vegetable oil in a large frying pan. Roll each fish ball in flour then place in the hot oil. Cook for about 5 minutes on each side, until golden, pressing the balls down as they cook to make nicely shaped cakes. Drain on kitchen paper, to remove any excess oil.

If you freeze some fishcakes do so before frying, then fry as required when thoroughly defrosted.

Encourage your child to see eating meals as a social activity, something to be enjoyed.

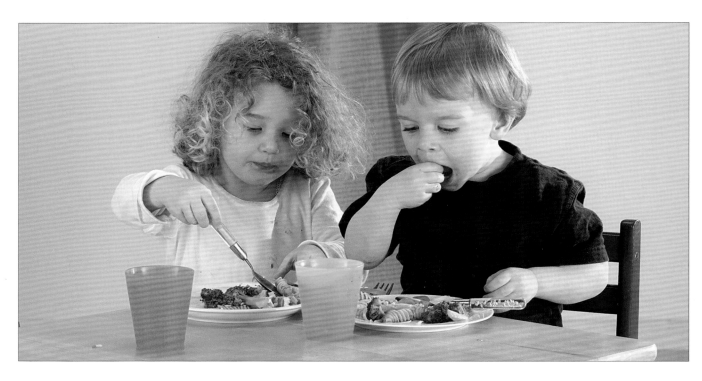

PEPPER PASTA SAUCE

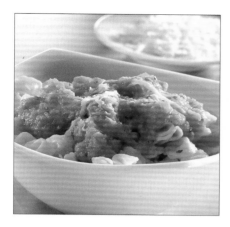

Sweet (bell) peppers are rich in vitamin C, and make a fabulous, quick, healthy sauce for pasta. Grate a little Cheddar cheese over the pasta too, if you like.

1 onion
1 garlic clove
1 red pepper
1 yellow pepper
15ml/1 tbsp olive oil
2 large tomatoes
Small handful fresh basil

Chop the onion and garlic and deseed and slice the peppers. Heat the olive oil in a frying pan and cook the onion, garlic and peppers for 15 minutes over a low heat, until very soft.

Meanwhile, skin, deseed and chop the tomatoes. Add them to the sauce and increase the heat. When it is bubbling, tear the basil leaves and stir them in, and cook for another minute or two, stirring. Add a dash of water if necessary. Blend to a purée.

PIZZA

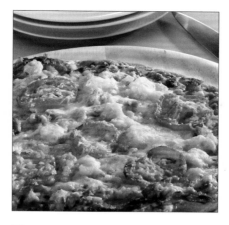

Pizza is popular with all ages, and if you make it yourself rather than rely on storebought or takeaway pizzas, you can make it into a nutritious as well as enjoyable meal. This is a great meal to cook with your children, as they will love flattening out the dough, and adding their choice of topping.

1 quantity of basic pizza dough
1 quantity of basic tomato sauce
Toppings of your choice

Preheat the oven to 230°C/450°F/ Gas 8. Divide the dough into two or four balls and roll each one out to a circle about 1cm/½in thick. Put the pizza on an oiled baking sheet and push the edges up a little to keep the topping in place. Spread a little basic tomato sauce over the base then add the toppings (see below).

Cook for about 12 minutes, until the base is cooked and the topping is bubbling hot.

BASIC PIZZA DOUGH

Making your own pizzas is easy, and older children will enjoy putting on their own toppings. This recipe makes enough dough for two pizzas, or four mini ones. Freeze the spare bases – you can add the toppings and cook them from frozen later on.

350g/12oz strong (hard wheat) plain white flour
1 sachet easy-blend yeast
5ml/1 tsp salt
30ml/2 tbsp olive oil

Place the flour in a bowl and add the yeast and salt. Make a well in the middle and pour in the oil and water. Mix using a wooden spoon, then your hands, to make a smooth ball.

Sprinkle a little flour on the work surface and knead the dough for 5 minutes. Cover with a damp, clean cloth and leave to rest for 5 minutes, then knead for another 5 minutes, until the dough has a slight sheen and is smooth. Place it in an oiled bowl and cover with a warm, damp cloth. Leave in a warm place for an hour or so, until the dough has doubled in size. Knead and shape into the required number of bases.

Pizza toppings: sliced mushrooms, drained, tinned sweetcorn, sliced pitted olives, sliced sweet peppers, sliced tomatoes, cooked peas, steamed, sliced broccoli florets, blobs of pesto, thinly sliced cooked potatoes, flaked canned tuna, small prawns (shrimp), sliced ham, cooked shredded chicken.

When you have finished adding your topping, sprinkle over some sliced mozzarella, or grated Cheddar, parmesan or Gruyère cheese, or a mixture of these, or add blobs of creamy goat's cheese.

POLENTA FINGERS

Made from ground corn or maize, polenta makes a good alternative to toast. Pour polenta in a thin stream into a pan of boiling water (using the quantities recommended on the pack), stirring all the time, then lower the heat and simmer for 5–7 minutes, until it has the consistency of porridge. You can add a little butter or cheese at this point if you like. Then pour it into a flat dish and leave to set for 30 minutes. When the polenta is cool, cut it into fingers, brush with oil and grill. Serve as a snack or serve with a blob of basic tomato sauce and pieces of grilled chicken or fish.

Useful contacts

UK

Allergy UK
3 White Oak Square
London Road
Swanley, Kent
BR8 7AG
01322 619898
www.allergyuk.org

Association of Breastfeeding Mothers
PO Box 207
Bridgewater
TA6 7YT
0870 401 7711

Asthma UK
Providence House
Providence Place
London N1 0NT
08457 01 02 03
www.asthma.org.uk

Bliss
68 South Lambert Road
London SW8 1RL
0500 618140
www.bliss.org.uk
support for parents of premature babies

Breastfeeding Network
PO Box 11126
Paisley PA2 8YB
Tel 0870 900 8787
Information on breastfeeding

Child Accident Prevention Trust
18-20 Farringdon Lane
London EC1R 3HA
Tel 020 7608 3828
www.capt.org.uk

Cry-sis
BM Cry-sis
London WC1N 3XX
Tel: 08451 228 669

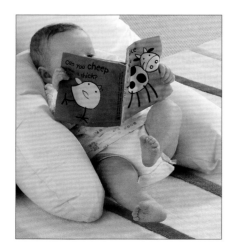

www.cry-sis.com
Helpline for parents with crying child

Eneuresis Resource and Information Centre
Tel 0117 960 3060
www.eric.org.uk
Advice on bedwetting and soiling

Gingerbread
7 Sovereign Close
Sovereign Court
London E1W 3HW
Tel 0800 018 4318
www.gingerbread.org.uk
Local support groups for single-parent families

Institute for Complementary Medicine
PO Box 194
London SE16 7QZ
Tel: 020 7237 5165
www.icmedicine.co.uk

JABS
1 Gawsworth Road
Golborne
Warrington WA3 3RF
Tel: 01942 713565
www.jabs.org.uk
Alternative advice on vaccination

La Leche League
PO Box 29
West Bridgford
Nottingham
NG2 7NP
Tel 0845 120 2918
www.laleche.org.uk

National Association of Toy and Leisure Libraries
68 Churchway
London NW1 1LT
Tel 020 7387 9592

National Childbirth Trust
Alexandra House
Oldham Terrace
Acton
London W3 6NH
Tel 0870 444 8708
Helpline for breastfeeding and postnatal problems

National Childminding Association
8 Masons Hill
Bromley
Kent BR2 9EY
Tel 0800 169 4486
www.ncma.org.uk
Advice on finding a registered childminder

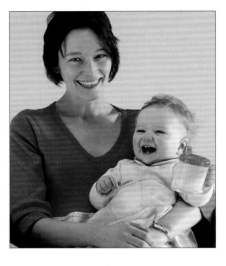

National Eczema Society
Hill House
Highgate Hill
London N19 5NA
Tel: 0870 241 3604
www.eczema.org

St John Ambulance
27 St Johns Lane
London EC1M 4BU
08700 10 49 50
www.sja.org.uk
Information on first aid courses

Single Parents Action Network
Millpond, Baptist Street
Easton
Bristol BS5 0YJ
0117 9514231
www.spanuk.org.uk

Twins and Multiple Birth Association (TAMBA)
2 The Willows
Gardner Road
Guildford
Surrey GU1 4PG
Tel 0870 770 3305
www.tamba.org.uk

Women's Environmental Network
PO Box 30626
London E1 1TZ
Tel: 020 7481 9004
www.wen.org.uk
For information on using real nappies

Other useful websites
www.bygpub.com
www.babyfriendly.org.uk
www.mothering.com
www.raisingkids.co.uk
www.talk-about-twins.com
www.tripletconnection.org

USA
American Holistic Medical Association
12101 Menaul Blvd, NE, Suite C
Alberquerque NM 87112
Tel: 0505 292 7788
www.holisticmedicine.org

American Red Cross
2025 E Street, NW
Washington DC 20006
Tel: 202 303 4498
www.redcross.org

Food Allergy Initiative
41 East 62nd Street, 4th Floor
New York 10021
Tel: 212 572 8428
www.foodallergyinitiative.org

La Leche League
PO Box 4079
Schaumburg
Ilinois 60168-4079
Tel: 0847 519 7730
www.lalecheleague.org

National Organization of Mothers of Twins
PO Box 700860
Plymouth
Michigan 48170-0955
www.nomotc.org

National Safekids Campaign
1301 Pennsylvania Avenue NW
Suite 1000
Washington DC 20004
Tel 0202 662 0600
www.safekids.org

CANADA
Food Allergy and Anaphylaxis Campaign
11781 Lee Jackson Hwy, Suite 160
Fairfax
VA 22033-3309
Tel: 800 929 4040
www.foodallergy.org

La Leche League
12050 Main Street W
PO Box 700
Winchester
Ontario K0C 2KP
Tel: 613 774 1842
www.lalecheleague.org

Multiple Births Canada
PO Box 432
Wasaga Beach
Ontario
L9Z 1Z4
Tel: 705 429 0901
www.multiplebirthscanada.org

Safe Kids Canada
180 Dundas Street W
Toronto

Ontario K1G 5L5
Tel: 416 813 7288
www.safekidscanada.com

St John Ambulance Canada
1900 City Park Drive, Suite 400
Ottawa, Ontario
K1J1A3
Tel: 613 236 7461
www.sja.ca

AUSTRALIA
Anaphylaxis Australia
21 Robinson Close
Hornsby Heights
NSW 2077
Tel: 1300 728 000
www.allergyfacts.org.au

Austprem
www.austprem.org.au
Internet-based support for parents of preterm babies

Australian Breastfeeding Association
1818 Malvern Road
East Malvern
Victoria 3145
www.breastfeeding.asn.au
Telephone numbers of breastfeeding counsellors are posted on the website.

Australian Complementary Health Association
247 Flinders Lane
Melbourne
Victoria 3000
Tel 03 9650 5237
www.diversity.org.au

The Australian Multiple Births Association (AMBA)
Po Box 105
Coogee
NSW 2034
Tel: 1300 88 64 99
www.amba.org.au

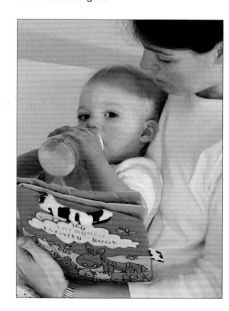

Kidsafe Australia
50 Bramston Terrace
Herston
Queensland 4029
Tel: 07 3854 1829
www.kidsafe.com.au

La Leche League
www.lalecheleague.org/australia
Telephone numbers of breastfeeding counsellors are posted on the website.

St John Ambulance
PO Box 3895
Manuka
ACT 2603
Tel: 02 8788 1388
www.stjohn.org.au

NEW ZEALAND
Allergy New Zealand
PO Box 56 117
Dominion Road
Auckland
Tel: 09 303 2024
www.allergy.org.nz

La Leche League
PO Box 1270
Wellington
New Zealand
Tel: 04 471 0690
www.lalecheleague.org/llnz

St John Ambulance
Level 11, St John House
114 The Terrace
PO Box 10 043
Wellington
Tel: 04 472 3600
www.stjohn.org.nz
First aid courses

New Zealand Multiple Birth Association
PO Box 1258
Wellington
New Zealand
Tel: 0800 489 467
www.nzmba.info

ParentCare
PO Box 8297
Symonds St
Auckland
Tel: 630 9943 ext 3223
www.parentcare.org.nz
Support for parents of premature and poorly babies

Safekids New Zealand
PO Box 26488
Epsom
Auckland
Tel: 09 630 9955
www.safekids.org.nz

Further reading

Penelope Leach, *Your Baby and Child* (Penguin, 1977)

Jan Parker and Jan Stimpson, *Raising Happy Children* (Hodder and Stoughton, 1999)

William Sears, Martha Sears, *The Baby Book* (Little, Brown and Company, 2003)

Dr Benjamen Spock and Dr Robert Needham, *Dr Spock's Baby and Child Care* (Simon and Schuster, 2005)

BREASTFEEDING
La Leche League, *The Womanly Art of Breastfeeding* (Plume Books, 2004)

Norma Jane Bumgarner, *Mothering Your Nursing Toddler* (La Leche League, 1980)

Clare Byam-Cook, *What to Expect if You Are Breastfeeding and What If You Can't* (Vermillion, 2001)

Sandra Lang, *Breastfeeding Special Care Babies* (Bailiere Tindall, 2002)

Penny Stanway, *Breast is Best* (Pan, 2005)

FEEDING YOUR BABY AND TODDLER
Rose Elliot's Mother, Baby and Toddler Book: A Unique Guide to Raising a Baby on a healthy Vegetarian Diet (Hochland Communications, 2003)

Rachael Anne Hill, *Real Food for Kids* (Ryland, Peters and Small, 2005)

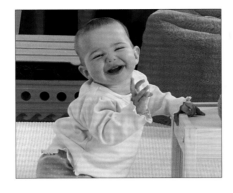

Annabel Karmel, *Feeding your Baby and Toddler* (Dorling Kindersley, 1999)

Sara Lewis, *Veggie Food for Kids* (Hamlyn, 2003)

SLEEP, CRYING AND BEHAVIOUR
Jo Frost, *Supernanny: How to Get the Best from Your Children* (Hodder and Stoughton, 2005)

Penny Hames, *Help Your Baby to Sleep* (Harper Collins, 2002)

Penny Hames, *Toddler Tantrums* (Harper Collins, 2002)

Deborah Jackson, *When Your Baby Cries* (Hodder and Stoughton, 2004)

Elizabeth Pantley *The No-Cry Sleep Solution* (McGraw Hill, 2002)

DEVELOPMENT AND ACTIVITIES
Lynne Murray and Liz Andrews, *The Social Baby: Understanding Babies' Communication from Birth* (CP Publishing, 2005)

Linda Acredolo and Susan Goodwyn, *Baby Signs* (Vermilion, 1996)

Françoise Barbira Freedman, *Water Babies* (Lorenz Books, 2001)

Peter Walker, *Baby Massage* (Carroll and Brown, 2005)

Stella Wellar, *Yoga for Children* (Harper Collins, 1996)

HEALTH CARE
Anne McIntyre, *The Herbal for Mother and Child* (Thorsons, 1992)

Dr John Briffa, *Natural Health for Kids* (Michael Joseph, 2004)

Susan Clark, *What Really Works for Kids: The Insider Guide for Mums and Dads* (Bantam Press, 2002)

Françoise Barbira Freedman, *Postnatal Yoga* (Lorenz Books, 2000)

Joseph Garcia-Prats and Sharon Simmons Hornfischer, *What To Do When Your Baby Is Premature* (Three Rivers Press, 2000)

BEING A PARENT
Naomi Stadlen, *What Mothers Do Especially When it Looks Like Nothing* (Piatkus, 2004)

Kate Figes, *Life After Birth: What Even Your Friends Won't Tell You About Motherhood* (Viking, 1998)

Sean French, *Fatherhood: Men Writing About Fatherhood* (Virago, 1992)

Acknowledgements

With special thanks from the author to Eliza and Jake for the practical experience, and to Jonathan Bastable for the fatherly perspective. Thanks, also to the Brighton Breastfeed Drop-in, and to these parents for their honesty and wisdom: Melanie Davies, Hilary Silverwood, Marta Scott, Juliet Cox and Sally Harper.

Photographs in the book were taken by Scott Morrison, and are the property of Anness Publishing Ltd.
Photographs also taken by: Jo Harrison: 51tl, 65tm, 66b, 69t, 93b, 111t, 113t, 116b, 119tr, 119tl, 133b, 160b, 163b.

Christine Hanscombe: 128 bl, 128 br, 129 both. John Freeman: 192-193 all.

Thank you to the parents and children who took part in the photoshoots: Achael and Amelia Brimson, Alfonso Perez, Andrea and Kiera Thompson, Andrew, Catherine and Scarlett Gordon, Beth and Owen Pierce, Christine and Grace Lewis, Elizabeth and Oliver Allen, Evie and Billie Beswick, Hazel and Isaac Plowman, Heather, Imogen and James Call, Irena and Rose Andrews, Jancien and Arabella Lambeth, Jenny and Lucy Rose, Freddie Lorenz, Kirsty and Olivia Innes, Marion Demoissier and Louisa

Swann, Rose and James Wallis, Sam Beattie and Sienna Brown.

Thanks to the following agencies for supplying additional images:
Alamy: 14rm, 36t & bl, 39tr, 50t, 59tl, 62t, 63t (both), 66t, 67tr, 82b, 102t, 109 both, 112t, 114, 115 both, 118 both, 120, 125 tr, 142b,147b, 149tl, 150b, 151br, 152, 153tl, 159b, 161b, 164, 165 both, 175tr, 181tr, 186b, 191tr &b, 195tr, 209tr, 215tr, 217tl, 220tl, 224b, 234t. Corbis: pp13tr, 23tr, 41tr, 65br, 92bl, 185t, 196, 197 both.
The Science Photo Library: p47bl.

Index

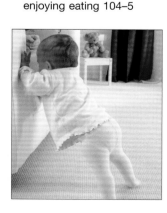
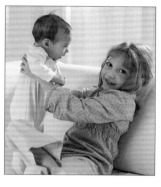

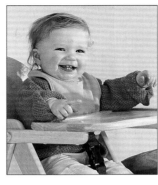

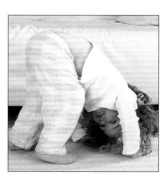

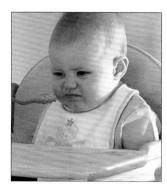
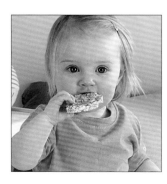

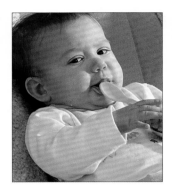

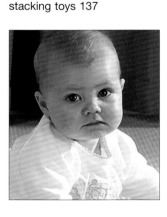

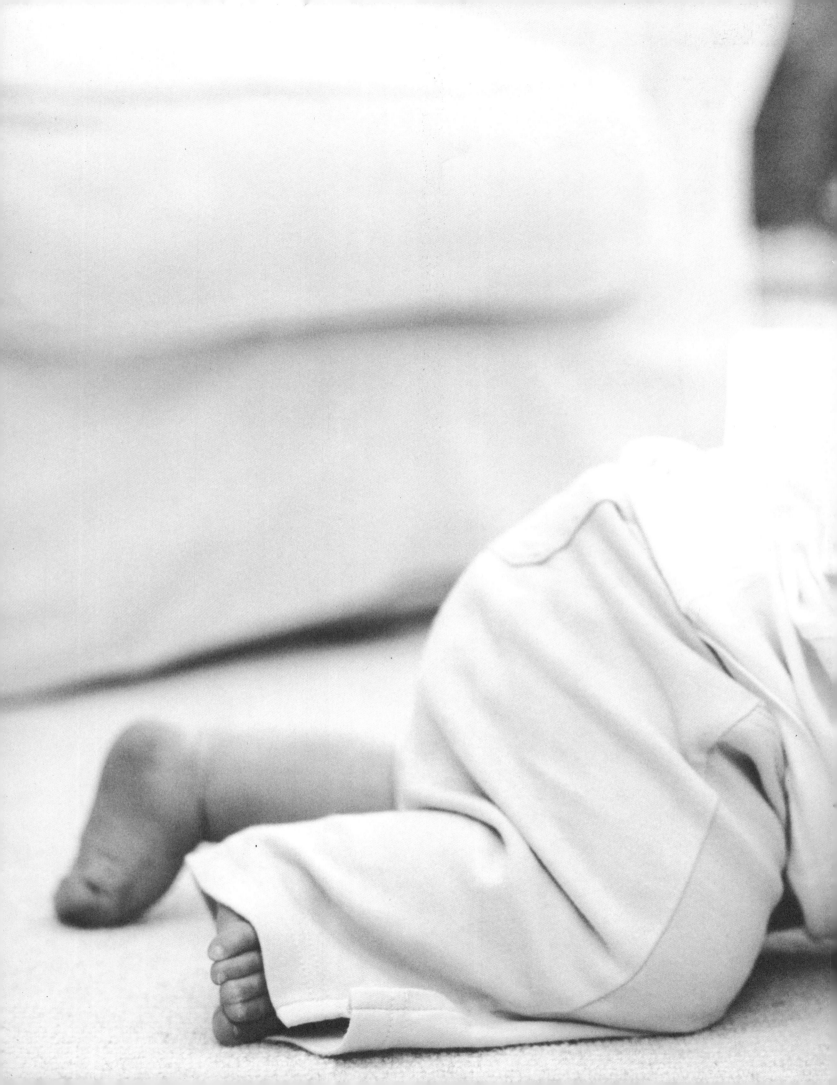